"This collection of essays by a group of distinguished scholars examines the impact of COVID-19 on America's racial and ethnic minorities. I highly encourage anyone interested in this timely and important topic to reflect on these essays from various methodologies on the wide array of lessons learned from the pandemic."

Jason Casellas, *Associate Professor of Political Science,*
University of Houston, USA

"Drawing together cutting-edge scholarship from across multiple disciplines, this collection of essays powerfully details how the COVID-19 pandemic both unveiled and exacerbated systemic and persistent racial inequities for communities of color across the United States. This is a must-read for policymakers and scholars of public health, race, and political science."

Teresa Irene Gonzales, *Assistant Professor of Sociology,*
University of Massachusetts Lowell, USA

"The authors cover disparities in access to healthcare, the effects of a lack of appropriate media coverage, the effects of racism, and almost every institutional aspect that affected the response to COVID-19 to effectively demonstrate the devastating disproportionate effects on the Latinx and African American communities. Indeed, as Navarro and Hernandez claim, it is a 'race war' being waged on communities of color through the failure of the system to respond properly and the inability of these communities to access healthcare generally."

Henry Flores, *Distinguished University Research Professor Emeritus of*
Political Science, St. Mary's University, USA

W0113290

THE COLOR OF COVID-19

The COVID-19 pandemic has disproportionately affected communities of color while highlighting the prevalence of structural racism in the United States. This crucial collection of essays, written by leading scholars from the fields of communications, political science, health, philosophy, and geography, explores the manifold ways in which the COVID-19 pandemic has impacted upon Black, Latinx, and Indigenous communities and the way we see race relations in the United States.

The COVID-19 pandemic has exposed the significance of U.S. health inequalities, which the World Health Organization defines as "avoidable [and] unfair." It has also highlighted structural racism, specifically, institutions, practices, values, customs, and policies that differentially allocate resources and opportunities so as to increase inequity among racial groups. Navarro and Hernandez therefore argue that the COVID-19 pandemic has unleashed a race war in America that has further marginalized communities of color by limiting access to resources by different racial and ethnic minorities, particularly women within these communities. Moreover, the systemic policies of the past that upheld or failed to address the unequal social conditions affecting Blacks, Latinxs, and other minorities have now been magnified with COVID-19. The volume concludes by offering recommendations to prevent future humanitarian crises from exacerbating racial divisions and having a disproportionate impact upon ethnic minorities.

This timely volume will be of great interest to those interested in the study of race and the social impacts of the COVID-19 pandemic in the United States.

Sharon A. Navarro is a professor of Political Science at the University of Texas at San Antonio, United States. Her research interests include women in politics, race and American politics, and Latinx politics. She is author of *Latina Legislator: Leticia Van De Putte and the Road to Leadership* (Texas A&M University Press, 2008) and co-author of *Políticas: Latina Public Officials in Texas* (University of Texas Press, 2008).

She is also co-editor of *Latinas and the Politics of Urban Spaces* (Routledge, 2020), *Race, Gender, Sexuality, and the Politics of the American Judiciary* (Cambridge University Press, 2018), *Latinas in American Politics: Changing and Embracing Political Tradition* (Lexington Books, 2016), and *The Roots of Latino Urban Agency* (University of North Texas Press, 2013).

Samantha L. Hernandez is a visiting scholar at the Institute for Latino Studies at the University of Notre Dame, United States, and Director of Policy and Strategic Affairs at San Antonio City Council. She is co-editor of *Race, Gender, Sexuality, and the Politics of the American Judiciary* (Cambridge University Press, 2018) and *Latinas in American Politics: Changing and Embracing Political Tradition* (Lexington Books, 2016). Her work has also been featured in the *Gender and Politics* journal and various media outlets, including *New York Times*, *NBC Nightly News*, *Marketwatch*, *WIRED*, and *The Wall Street Journal*.

THE COVID-19 PANDEMIC SERIES

This series examines the impact of the COVID-19 pandemic on individuals, communities, countries, and the larger global society from a social scientific perspective. It represents a timely and critical advance in knowledge related to what many believe to be the greatest threat to global ways of being in more than a century. It is imperative that academics take their rightful place alongside medical professionals as the world attempts to figure out how to deal with the current global pandemic, and how society might move forward in the future. This series represents a response to that imperative.

Series Editor: J. Michael Ryan

Titles in this Series:

Creative Resilience and COVID-19
Figuring the Everyday in a Pandemic
Edited by Irene Gammel and Jason Wang

COVID-19 and Childhood Inequality
Edited by Nazneen Khan

The Color of COVID-19
The Racial Inequality of Marginalized Communities
Edited by Sharon A. Navarro and Samantha L. Hernandez

COVID-19, Communication and Culture
Beyond the Global Workplace
Edited by Fiona Rossette-Crake and Elvis Buckwalter

THE COLOR OF COVID-19

The Racial Inequality of Marginalized Communities

Edited by Sharon A. Navarro and Samantha L. Hernandez

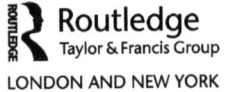

Routledge
Taylor & Francis Group

LONDON AND NEW YORK

Cover image: © zimmytws / iStock images / Getty Images

First published 2022
by Routledge
4 Park Square, Milton Park, Abingdon, Oxon OX14 4RN

and by Routledge
605 Third Avenue, New York, NY 10158

Routledge is an imprint of the Taylor & Francis Group, an Informa business

British Library Cataloguing-in-Publication Data
A catalogue record for this book is available from the British Library

Library of Congress Cataloging-in-Publication Data
A catalog record has been requested for this book

ISBN: 978-1-032-21509-9 (hbk)
ISBN: 978-1-032-21507-5 (pbk)
ISBN: 978-1-003-26871-0 (ebk)

DOI: 10.4324/9781003268710

Typeset in Bembo
by Newgen Publishing UK

CONTENTS

FIGURES

TABLES

CONTRIBUTORS

Elizabeth Alejo is a Ph.D. candidate in Political Science at the University of Illinois at Chicago, United States, and Assistant Professorial Lecturer at Saint Xavier University, United States. Her research focuses on urban development and ethnic communities in Chicago. Her most recent publication (co-authored with Amy Schoenecker) is "Polices of Exclusion: Space, Time, and the Informal Economy in Chicago" in *Space and Culture*.

Nazgol Bagheri is an associate professor of Geography at the University of Texas at San Antonio, United States, where she is also the graduate program coordinator for the Geography and Environmental Sustainability program and the director of the Critical Geographic Information Systems (GIS) Research Laboratory. An award-winning teacher, she teaches a diverse set of courses, including GIS and Feminist Geography. Her current research connects three complementary areas: feminist politics, urban design, and the social production of space. She applies empowering geo-ethnographic approaches to challenge and enrich the Anglo-American hegemonic geographical theories through studying the people whose stories are often unheard, including women and other minorities. Her articles have appeared in *Journal of Cultural Geography, Gender, Place, & Culture, GeoJournal, Papers in Applied Geography, The Geography Teacher, Journal of Social and Cultural Geography*.

Miguel de Oliver is Associate Professor of Geography at the University of Texas at San Antonio, United States. His research explores demographic disparities in the postmodern urban landscape, consumerism and the manifestations of racial/ethnic inequality in the North American built environment, and the increasingly problematic relationship between race, disparity, and alienation.

Leila M. Ensha is Director of Grants, Policy, and Engagement at Planned Parenthood Hudson Peconic (PPHP) in New York, where she oversees the affiliate's grant portfolio, working with State agencies and foundations to support the health services, education programs, and advocacy goals of PPHP. She is a passionate public health advocate with roots in state advocacy, organizing, and campaign work. Her work and research sit at the intersection of health, politics, advocacy, and communications. She completed her Masters in Public Health in Health Policy and Management at the Yale School of Public Health, focusing on the social, political, and legal determinants of health.

Olivia Field recently received her Bachelor of Arts in Politics and International Affairs, with a double minor in French Studies and English, from Wake Forest University, United States. During her time at Wake Forest, Olivia was a Race, Inequality and Policy Initiative (RIPI) Undergraduate Research Fellow and was the Editor-in-Chief of Wake Forest's Student Newspaper, the *Old Gold & Black*.

Tanya E. Gardner is Associate Professor of Communication Studies at Delaware County Community College, United States, and a doctoral student at the Cathy Hughes School of Communication at Howard University, United States. She participated in Howard University's 2019 Research Symposium and the 2015 National Black Families, Black Relationships, Black Sexuality Conference. Her research interests explore health disparities among vulnerable populations.

Sarah V. Gordon-Brilla is the Senior Director of Communications and Brand Experience at Planned Parenthood of Southern New England and Adjunct Professor of Communication at Southern Connecticut State University, United States. She has extensive experience in health communications and has led many health communications campaigns from implementation to evaluation. She was previously the communications lead for the CDC's Racial and Ethnic Approaches to Community Health (REACH) program at the Community Alliance for Research and Engagement, a public health organization co-housed at Yale School of Public Health and Southern Connecticut State University. She is passionate about advocacy work and ensuring that important information about individual's health is accessible to all.

Samantha L. Hernandez is a visiting scholar at the Institute for Latino Studies at the University of Notre Dame, United States, and Director of Policy and Strategic Affairs at San Antonio City Council. She is co-editor of *Race, Gender, Sexuality, and the Politics of the American Judiciary* (Cambridge University Press, 2018) and *Latinas in American Politics: Changing and Embracing Political Tradition* (Lexington Books, 2016). Her work also features in the *Gender and Politics* journal and various media outlets, including *The New York Times*, *NBC Nightly News*, *Marketwatch*, *WIRED*, and *The Wall Street Journal*.

Jackson Higginbottom is the COVID-19 Communications Coordinator for the Centers for Disease Control and Prevention's (CDC) Racial and Ethnic Approaches to Community Health (REACH) program at the Community Alliance for Research and Engagement, a public health organization co-housed at Yale School of Public Health and Southern Connecticut State University, United States. His work focuses on community health and engagement research, community health program evaluation, and stigma and mental health research of sexual and gender minorities. His primary research interests include the social determinants of mental and physical health among sexual, ethnic, and racial minority populations, and developing and evaluating evidence-based interventions to address health needs of under-resourced populations. Prior to his work at Yale, he was heavily involved with free medical clinics that served uninsured and underinsured populations in Oklahoma City.

Jungmi Jun is an associate professor at the School of Journalism and Mass Communications of the University of South Carolina, United States. She is a health and strategic communication scientist. Her research focuses on the intersection of message/media, socio-psychology, and health perceptions/behaviors. Her recent research has focused on health disparities and communicative coping of racism among racial/ethnic minorities, while her research interest in communications surrounding control of emerging tobacco products continues. She is the author of more than 75 peer-reviewed journal and conference papers in the fields of health communication, health disparities, community health, tobacco regulatory science, public health, and public relations.

Tyson D. King-Meadows is Professor of Political Science in the Department of Political Science at the University of Maryland, Baltimore County, United States, where he also holds affiliate appointments in the School of Public Policy, the Department of Africana Studies, and the Language, Literacy & Culture Doctoral Program. His research interests include public opinion, African American Politics, and U.S. election law. He is author of *When the Letter Betrays the Spirit: Voting Rights Enforcement and African American Participation from Lyndon Johnson to Barack Obama* (Lexington Books, 2011) and co-author of *Devolution and Black State Legislators: Challenges and Choices in the Twenty-First Century* (State University of New York Press, 2006). His other recent relevant publications explore residents' attitudes about neighborhood conditions prior to the 2015 protests in Baltimore, the relationship between Black anti-Latino attitudes and support for restrictive immigration policy, and how racial resentment drives White support for Black conservatives.

Jordan Liz is an Assistant Professor of Philosophy at San José State University, United States. His research interests include biomedical ethics, philosophy of medicine, and philosophy of race. His current research focuses on the impact of the COVID-19 pandemic on racial minorities and other marginalized groups.

Mark Martinez is Assistant Professor of Media and Communication studies at Spalding University, United States. His research explores media theory, identity and representation through media, critical race theory, biopolitics, and nonhuman studies. He has recently been working on the application of posthuman and non-human theories to issues of race. He is also currently working on community organizing and antiracism for students of color at Spalding University. His work has been in publications such as MediaCommons, Philosophy of Photography, and Communication +1.

Adam McGlynn is Professor of Political Science at East Stroudsburg University of Pennsylvania, United States. His primary areas of research are Latino/a political behavior and education policy. His research has been published in multiple journals and edited volumes, including the *American Journal of Political Science*, *PS: Political Science and Politics*, and *State and Local Government Review*.

Priscilla Nalubula is currently studying for a Bachelor of Arts in Political Science and a minor in History at the University of Maryland, Baltimore County, United States. She is interested in law, historical research, and public policy, and her expertise includes data analysis of factors associated with Black representation. Her prior professional experiences includes working for King-Meadows as a research assistant and serving as an intern at Capital Christian Fellowship, a nonprofit that addresses community needs, including food insecurity, in Lanham, Maryland. Her extra- and co-curricular activities include membership on the UMBC Mock Trial, in the UMBC Pre-Law Society, and in the UMBC African Student Association. She plans to attend law school after graduation and aspires to utilize her experience in research and in trial advocacy to develop skills in conflict resolution, in public speaking, and in building culturally diverse teams.

Sharon A. Navarro is a professor of Political Science at the University of Texas at San Antonio, United States. Her research interests include women in politics, race and American politics, and Latinx politics. She is author of *Latina Legislator: Leticia Van De Putte and the Road to Leadership* (Texas A&M University Press, 2008) and co-author of *Políticas: Latina Public Officials in Texas* (University of Texas Press, 2008). She is also co-editor of *Latinas and the Politics of Urban Spaces* (Routledge, 2020), *Race, Gender, Sexuality, and the Politics of the American Judiciary* (Cambridge University Press, 2018), *Latinas in American Politics: Changing and Embracing Political Tradition* (Lexington Books, 2016), and *The Roots of Latino Urban Agency* (University of North Texas Press, 2013).

Dani Parker Moore is Assistant Professor of Multicultural Education and Director of the Schools, Education, and Society Minor at Wake Forest University, United States, where she teaches undergraduate and graduate courses on multicultural education, community engagement, and educational psychology. Her research interests include social foundations in education, qualitative research methods, social justice education, and parent-caregiver engagement in schools and community engagement.

Alondra Ramirez is currently an undergraduate student at Wake Forest University, United States, where she is majoring in Mathematical Business with double minors in Politics and International Affairs and Economics.

Dana L. Rogers is an assistant professor in the Department of Communication, Media, and Screen Studies at Southern Connecticut State University, United States. Her research interests are informed by her decade of work in the advertising and public relations industries and focus on the effects of persuasive messaging within such contexts as online communication, health communication campaigns, and cause marketing. She has presented 12 conference papers and co-authored published articles on persuasive communication in *Journal of Broadcasting & Electronic Media* and *Journal of Nonprofit & Public Sector Marketing*.

Amy Schoenecker is an assistant professor in the Politics, Economics, and International Studies Department at the University of Hartford, United States, where she teaches classes on comparative politics with interests in political economy, development, urbanization, the informal economy, and the Global South. She has published articles on the informal economy and has particular interest in the nexus of the state, informality, and gender, ethnic, and racial identities. Her work has been published in *Space & Culture, Spaces and Flows*, and *The Wiley-Blackwell Encyclopedia of Urban and Regional Studies*.

Caitlyn Stout recently completed her Masters in Management and Leadership in Public Administration from East Stroudsburg University, United States. She received her B.A. in Political Science from East Stroudsburg University in May 2020. Her research interests in the field of public policy include education, the environment, and emergency management.

Carolyn A. Stroman is Professor Emeritus in the Department of Communication, Culture and Media Studies at Howard University, United States. As a member of the NOAA Social Science Research Team, she has participated in several research projects and directed three dissertations pertaining to risk and crisis communication. She is a former editor of *The Howard Journal of Communications*.

Wei Sun is Associate Professor and Director of Graduate Studies in the Department of Communication, Culture and Media Studies at Howard University, United States. She is a Fulbright Specialist in Communications/Journalism. Her research interests include intercultural communication, new media studies, and health communication. Her publications have appeared in the *Journal of Faculty Development, The Howard Journal of Communications, Intercultural Communication Studies*, and *World*

Communication and several books. She was recently guest editor for a special issue on COVID-19 for *the Howard Journal of Communications*.

Ryan A. Sutherland is a clinical research coordinator at the Yale School of Medicine, United States, and Partners in Health, which works to coordinate COVID-19 response efforts in Massachusetts. He is also presently serving as a Fellow with the Harvard Public Health Review and is completing an M.Phil. in Development Studies at the University of Cambridge, UK. He is drawn to projects at the intersection of public health, global development, social justice, and health equity. His research focuses on the intersection of international development and public health, centering on homelessness, substance use, refugee rights, and maternal and child health. He was a recipient of the 2020 Dean's Prize for Outstanding MPH Thesis at the Yale School of Public Health for his thesis titled "Tobacco Use, Knowledge of Tobacco Risks, and Perception of Smoking Behaviors Among Urban and Rural Youth in Indonesia" and received the Horstmann Merit Scholarship for academic excellence and potential in public health.

Abigail Timbol is working towards a Bachelor of Arts in Psychology at the University of Maryland, Baltimore County, United States. She previously completed an Associate of Science in Nursing from Montgomery College, Rockville, United States. Her primary research interests include public health, community-oriented care practice, and the provision of frontline healthcare. Her expertise includes quantitative data collection and synthesizing scholarship related to mental health. Her prior professional experiences include working for Dr. King-Meadows as a research assistant and serving as an intern at the Rodham Institute in Washington, DC, a non-profit that provides for community-based health needs aimed at achieving health equity, where she became a trained community outreach intern and planned programs which provided services to underserved populations dealing with inadequate healthcare, food security, and educational attainment. She intends to pursue a graduate degree in clinical psychology, where she can explore psychodiagnostics and intervention procedures that attend to the assessment, diagnosing, and treatment of adverse mental health outcomes.

Betina Cutaia Wilkinson is Associate Professor and Associate Chair of the Politics and International Affairs Department at Wake Forest University, United States. Her research interests are in American politics with a focus on racial and ethnic politics and public opinion. Her book, *Partners or Rivals? Power and Latino, Black and White Relations in the 21st Century* (University of Virginia Press, 2015), won the American Political Science Association REP Section's Best Book Award on Inter-Race Relations in the United States. She is the recipient of the Early Career Award by the Midwest Political Science Association's Latina/o Caucus. She has served as the President of the Midwest Political Science Association's Latina/o Caucus and on the editorial board of *PS: Political Science and Politics*. She currently serves as an executive council member of the Midwest Political Science Association and the director of the Race, Inequality and Policy Initiative (RIPI) at Wake Forest University. Her research has been published in several political science and multidisciplinary journals, including *Political Research Quarterly*, *Social Science Quarterly*, *American Politics Research*, *PS: Political Science and Politics*, and *Race and Social Problems*.

Joshua Yates is a Graduate Student and Teaching and Research Assistant in the Department of Political Science and Geography at The University of Texas at San Antonio, United States. His current research is centered around the dispersion of COVID-19 on diverse populations. His work utilizes community based, theoretically informed research methods along with other socio-spatial visualization tools such as Geographic Information Systems (GIS) that will allow a more in-depth look at how COVID-19 affects people differently

Nanlan Zhang recently completed a doctorate in Mass Communication at the University of South Carolina, United States. Her research interests include gender and racial inequalities, mental health, misinformation, and social and psychological factors associated with health perceptions and behaviors. Her research has been presented at Association for Education in Journalism and Mass Communication and International Communication Association conferences and published in journals, such as *Health Communication* and *Journal of Applied Communication Research*.

FOREWORD

The SARS-CoV-2 virus and the associated COVID-19 pandemic have wrought havoc on the lives of nearly every human being on the planet. They have also magnified existing inequalities, created new inequalities all their own, and placed a megaphone squarely in front of the voices trying to improve our collective social condition. Indeed, the unequal social impact of a virus that is blind to social difference can tell us much about the ways in which our societies are constructed. Diseases do not distinguish their hosts by race, ethnicity, class, gender, sexuality, nationality, religion, or other non-biological social differentiations, but pandemics unearth just how much human beings do.

While the pandemic has impacted all of us, it has not done so in equal ways. Instead, it has highlighted not only biological distinctions as amplifiers of susceptibility to disease, but also, and perhaps more importantly, social distinctions as amplifiers of susceptibility to pandemics. Thus, while some of the unequal impacts of the virus are related to biological factors such as age, sex, and prior medical conditions, the disproportionate impacts of the pandemic are arguably rooted in the seldom acknowledged and often suppressed inequities rooted in structural discrimination and prejudice.

One of the categories of individuals that has been most heavily impacted by both the virus, as well as the associated pandemic, is that of racial and ethnic minorities. As members of these categories are more likely to also be economically disadvantaged, work in jobs that are front-facing and "essential," lack digital access and cultural capital, and live in conditions that allow for physical distancing, they have been disproportionately impacted by COVID-19. As such, the pandemic should, among other things, serve as a wake-up call to structural inequalities and a host of cultural "-isms".

In this insightful volume, Navarro and Hernandez have brought together an impressive range of scholars and scholarship. Collectively, their work goes a long way toward helping us better understand the "color of COVID-19." More than just an intellectual engagement with the topic, the chapters in this volume also represent a moral engagement with injustice and a social engagement with our human collective well-being. The scholarship in this book is sound, and the ethical undertones are loud and clear. That combination is what makes this volume such an invaluable response to the call to not only better understand the impact of the pandemic, but to also move our world toward a more equitable future.

J. Michael Ryan

Series Editor, *The COVID-19 Pandemic Series*

ACKNOWLEDGMENTS

This was truly an exciting project to see from inception to completion. I have many people to thank. First and foremost, my co-author, Samantha, who has one of the sharpest intellectual minds I know. I also thank the contributors for their expertise and belief in this project. I thank Drs. Henry Flores, Jason Casellas, and Teresa Irene Gonzales for taking the time out of their retirement, sabbatical, and teaching to write a review. I thank Routledge's COVID series editor Michael Ryan for his support in our project. I thank my sister, mother, and most of all my father. He passed away a few years ago, but there isn't a day that I do not think of him and thank him for the person I have become.

Sharon A. Navarro

First I would like to thank Sharon for her never-ending belief in me and her continuous friendship and mentorship. I truly have been taught by a pioneer in our field. I'd like to thank my parents and siblings for their love and support. Lastly, I would like to thank my grandmother who passed away before this book was published. She always provided guidance and strength to me in ways I will always cherish.

Samantha L. Hernandez

1

INTRODUCTION

Sharon A. Navarro and Samantha L. Hernandez

On January 20, 2020, the U.S. Centers for Disease Control and Prevention (CDC) diagnosed its first novel coronavirus (COVID-19) infection. Former President Donald Trump's first major remark on January 22, 2020, with regard to the first U.S. case, was this: "We have it totally under control. It's one person coming in from China, and we have it under control. It's going to be just fine" (Keith, 2020). He later promised that the virus would just "magically disappear," and again that "(w) e have it under control" (Boburg et al., 2020), it would not come to the United States, that China was doing a great job controlling it. Over and over in January and February, he assured people in the United States that this was nothing to worry about, that the stock market would recover, and so on. Perhaps most remarkably, at a February press conference at which his own healthcare experts reported that the number of cases would rise, Trump said, "When you have 15 people, and the 15 within a couple of days is going to be down to close to zero, that's a pretty good job we've done" (Keith, 2020).

A few months later, the World Health Organization (WHO) on March 11, 2020 declared the COVID-19 outbreak a global pandemic. Even after then President Trump realized the pandemic was likely to kill thousands of people in the United States and was the greatest crisis of his presidency, Trump had given little thought to his comments, including speculating on unproven remedies (Coronavirus: Outcry after Trump Suggests Injecting Disinfectant as Treatment, 2020). This pattern continued through June 2020, as the Trump administration's one consistency in communication was providing inconsistent, contradictory, confusing, and some-times completely erroneous information (Diamond and Toosi, 2020).

Because past pandemics have led to surges in prejudice, racism, and discrim-ination, the WHO several years ago developed an official policy that no new dis-ease would be given national or geographic names, but simply scientific ones like COVID-19. However, Trump forced his entire administration to use "Chinese

DOI: 10.4324/9781003268710-1

flu," "China virus," or "Wuhan virus," in what can only be seen as an attempt to blame China and the Chinese for the disease (Rogers et al., 2020). Predictably, there was an immediate upsurge in cases of anti-Asian and anti-Chinese assaults and other incidents, as citizens followed the president's lead and blamed China and the Chinese. From March 2020 to August 2021, the StopAAPIHate.org (Asian American Pacific Islander) reported close to 10,000 hate incidents. They point out that this number represents "only a fraction of the number of hate incidents that actually occur" (Stop AAPI Hate Reporting Center, 2021). The violence against Asian Americans was so rampant that in May 2021 Biden signed legislation to curtail the dramatic rise in hate crimes against Asian Americans and Pacific Islanders. The law expedites Justice Department reviews of hate crimes by putting an official in charge of the effort. Federal grants are available to help local law enforcement agencies improve their investigation, identification, and reporting of bias-driven incidents, which go underreported (Behrmann, 2021).

To help us understand how COVID-19 has affected various communities of color and the way we see race relations in the United States, we have brought together some of the best and brightest scholars from communications, political science, health, philosophy, and geography. We define race as a social construct and argue that COVID-19 has unleashed a race war in the United States that has further marginalized the communities of color. We define race wars as the lack of access to resources by different racial and ethnic minorities as well as minority women[1] in varying communities. The systemic policies of the past that either sustained or failed to address the unequal social conditions affecting Blacks, Latinxs,[2] and other racial, ethnic, and gender minorities have now been magnified with COVID-19.

The Intersection of COVID-19 and Systemic Racism

John Hopkins University Center for Global Health has been at the forefront of tracking COVID-19 in the United States. They have reported that "the COVID-19 pandemic has disproportionately affected Blacks, Latinxs and Native Americans in the U.S. at higher rates of infection, more severe disease and higher rates of mortality as compared with Whites" (Golden, 2021). Many scholars of race and ethnicity link these higher rates of infection, disease, and mortality to systemic racism. The question is how the disproportionate effects of COVID-19 on communities of color as compared with Whites must be examined and answered if equity is to be achieved?

In the earliest days of the COVID-19 pandemic in the United States, before the CDC reported demographic data on race and ethnicity, Khanijahani (2021) analyzed county data throughout the United States and found that counties with a high proportion of Whites had lower rates of COVID-19 than counties with higher proportions of Blacks and Latinxs. He found that lack of access to health insurance, employment status, and overcrowded housing were predictors of COVID-19 infections. At the start of the COVID-19 pandemic, Blacks and Latinx living in neighborhoods of Chicago that were redlined in the 1930s (Massey and Denton,

1993), and are still racially segregated, were the first to start dying of COVID-19 in the city, while other races were less affected (Bertocchi and Dimico, 2020). Racial and ethnic minorities are more likely to live in high density, racially segregated and crowded housing as well as multigenerational housing, increasing the risk of COVID-19 infection (Khanijahani, 2021). National estimates show that about 80% of people living in areas of concentrated poverty are either Black or Latinx (Meade, 2014).

Since demographic details are key to understanding how existing social disparities have affected the spread of COVID-19 in the United States, John Hopkins created the Coronavirus Resource Center. As if not to create additional institutional barriers for studying the effects of COVID-19 on minorities, it reported that "no two states report the exact same demographic data," and that "many states do not provide data for several demographic categories, especially for specific ethnicities. Therefore, it is difficult to assess the impact of COVID-19 on certain populations" (https://coronavirus.jhu.edu/data/racial-data-transparency). Those at the Coronavirus Resource Center have worked to "standardize the information with a process that makes it comparable across the U.S" (ibid.). Consequently, we may never know the true impact of COVID-19 on communities of color like lower testing rates, misreported numbers, and so much more.

As of September 2021, CDC data reveal that Latinx persons have a 1.9 and American Indians have a 1.7 higher infection rate with COVID-19, and Blacks a 1.1 times higher rate as compared with Whites. Hospitalizations for COVID-19, a marker of severe illness, show similar disparities, with American Indians being hospitalized at 3.5 times higher rate, Blacks and Latinx are at a 2.8 times higher rate compared with Whites. Mortality rates are 2.0, 2.4, and 2.3 times higher for Blacks, American Indians, and Latinx, than Whites, respectively (CDC, 2021).

One added layer of critical care of Latinx and deaf or hard of hearing individuals is the language barrier. The lack of language access to vaccine information wasn't necessarily the result of poor pandemic planning. In 2020, the Trump administration removed language-access protections that had been written into the Affordable Care Act. Latinxs, at least those who do not speak English, were being left behind by the vaccine rollout (Goodman, 2021). In addition, the U.S. Department of Health and Human Services has acknowledged that the deaf and hard of hearing community has had problems being able to access the vaccine clinics with communication accessibility (Novic, 2021). The institutional marginalization experienced by minority communities is widespread and has no boundaries.

Certain types of employment carry higher risks of COVID-19 infection. Racial and ethnic minorities are more likely to be classified as essential workers and have jobs that cannot be conducted remotely. They are also less likely to have paid sick leave, making them more likely to keep working when sick (CDC, 2021). Overall, people from some racial and ethnic minority groups have less access to high-quality education. Without a high-quality education, people face greater challenges in getting jobs that offer options for minimizing exposure to COVID-19 (The Annie E. Casey Foundation, 2006). The authors culled in this edited volume discuss the systemic challenges marginalized communities faced during COVID-19. However, the inequities borne by minorities stem from historical institutional treatment and memory.

Racism and the Seeds of Distrust

In the past, racist, and at times dangerous, healthcare policies and clinical experiments have targeted particularly Black and Brown communities. Khubchandani and Macias (2021) conducted a review of studies published in the United States from February 2020 to February 2021. Khubchandani and Macias reported that a vaccination hesitancy for adult Americans was 26.3% in contrast to African Americans which stood at 41.6% and for Latinos at 30.2%. Some of the major predictors of vaccine hesitancy in African Americans and Latinos were sociodemographic characteristics (e.g., age, gender, income, education, and so on), medical mistrust and history of racial discrimination, exposure to myths, and misinformation to name a few. The realities of how Black and Brown people have been treated by the U.S. medical establishment are one that views such populations as inferior biologically and intellectually. One of the main examples often pointed to is the Tuskegee experiments, which ran 40 years, from 1932 to 1972 (Reeves, 2021).

The goal of the Tuskegee experiments was to track the natural progression of syphilis. Researchers initially recruited 600 Black men—399 with the disease and 201 without it—and conducted the study without the informed consent of these participants (CDC, 2020). According to the CDC, researchers justified the study by telling these men they were being treated for "bad blood," which referred to conditions like anemia and fatigue as well as syphilis (ibid.).

There was also the long U.S. involvement in the mass sterilization of Puerto Rican women as well as Mexican men and women. Between the 1930s and 1970s, approximately one-third of the female population of Puerto Rico was sterilized, making it the highest rate of sterilization in the world. Countless number of Puerto Rican women were not told they were taking part in a secret trial of the birth control pill (Salvo et al., 1992). Similarly, in California, between 1919 and 1953, Latino men were 23% more likely to be sterilized than non-Latino men. The difference was even greater among women, with Latinas sterilized at 59% higher rates than non-Latinas (Novak et al., 2018). The historic involvement of government in medical abuse, neglect, and exploitation that has jaded generations of minority people into a distrust of public institutions has not aided in the fight against COVID-19. Scholars like Ibram X. Kendi contend that structural racism, systemic racism, and institutional racism are all terms used to describe how societal practices, institutions, and policies maintain White advantage over Blacks, Hispanics, and Asians. Kendi offered a clear definition to explain and incorporate these various terms by stating:

> Racism is a marriage of racist policies and racist ideas that produces and normalize racial inequalities, and that racial inequity is when two or more racial

groups are not standing on approximately equal footing. A racist policy is any measure that produces or sustains racial inequality between racial groups.

Kendi, 2019, p. 17

Racism in healthcare access, employment, education, and discrimination leads to chronic and toxic environments. The chapters in this edited volume provide both a micro and macro view of what communities of color are experiencing as they navigate through COVID-19.

Chapter Outlines

We divided the chapters into five sections. Each section provides a different perspective of how our lives are affected by COVID-19 using systemic racism. Each of our contributors offers his/her own lens for understanding how marginalized communities experience COVID-19. We argue that each perspective offered intersects with structural racism. Let's begin the discussion.

Digital Divide/Education

In Chapter 2, "Placing a Band-Aid on a Bullet Wound? Black and Latinx Educational Experiences During a Pandemic," Dani Parker Moore et al. explore how the COVID-19 pandemic has overwhelmingly impacted Latinxs and Blacks in the United States. In addition to the fact that both groups make up an exorbitant number of COVID-19 cases, evidence suggests that the pandemic negatively influenced the educational attainment of students with limited educational and economic resources. In this study, Parker Moore et al. seek to explore how the pandemic has impacted Latinx and Black educational opportunities and attainment. To address their overarching question, Parker Moore et al. rely upon phone interviews of North Carolina parents, schoolteachers, school administrators, and nonprofit organizations. Their interview conversations center on the connections between Black and Latinx academic achievement and the digital divide, the adverse effects of stay-at-home orders, and racial and ethnic inequities that plague Latinxs and Blacks in the United States. Their results reveal that Black and Latinx students' "education debt" has skyrocketed during the pandemic.

In Chapter 3, "Necessity as the Mother of Invention: Attempting to Overcome the Digital Divide During the COVID-19 Pandemic," Adam McGlynn and Caitlyn Stout contend that digital divide, defined as inequitable access to educational technology and high-speed Internet access, is not a new phenomenon. Practitioners, advocates, and policymakers quickly identified that the COVID-19 pandemic could serve to exacerbate the divide, especially among low-income communities of color. This leads to the question of whether policymakers at the state and local levels rose to the challenge of addressing the digital divide when remote learning became the only safe way to educate our nation's students. This work examines how four school districts predominately serving students of color, Allentown, Pennsylvania; Atlanta,

Georgia; Brownsville, Texas; and Detroit, Michigan, addressed the challenges of remote learning. Applying the literature from the fields of educational inequality and policy change, McGlynn and Stout assess how policymakers, advocacy groups, and business leaders attempted to work collaboratively to overcome the digital divide. They conclude the analysis by discussing the steps stakeholders must take to ensure that students, regardless of race, ethnicity, and income, have the ability to learn remotely in the face of an ongoing pandemic.

Media

In Chapter 4, "COVID-19 Racial Disparities: A Content Analysis of News Media Coverage," Sarah V. Gordon-Brilla et al. argue that with the spread of the COVID-19 pandemic in the spring and summer of 2020, the city of New Haven, Connecticut, saw significant health disparities in rates of infection and death within Black and Latino residents. These health disparities are the result of systemic racial health inequities. Previous research utilizing agenda-setting theory suggests that raising awareness for a public health issue may motivate public support for attention to that issue and thus increase pressure for policy changes. With the need for policy change in mind, this research uses a content analysis approach to examine messaging within New Haven, Connecticut, on the COVID-19 crisis. An analysis of media vehicles used to disseminate information, prominence of coverage related to health disparities by race, and messaging used to share COVID-19 information will enable a better understanding of the public's perception of the salience of this pandemic. Public awareness of health disparities by race and ethnicity is essential to garner support for the development of sustainable public policy changes. This research provides an increased understanding of the messages the public may be receiving to increase awareness of health disparities by race and, thus, impact policy change needed to address such inequities.

In Chapter 5, "Perceptions of COVID-19 and BLM Protesting on Twitter," Tanya E. Gardner et al. point out that since the outbreak of the COVID-19 pandemic, people from various racial backgrounds have been disproportionately impacted by the virus. During the pandemic crisis, the death of George Floyd agitated national protests on racial inequality, and incidences of social unrest and violence were reported all over the country. As the COVID-19 cases kept increasing in many states, and as many businesses reopened, there were fears that the Black Lives Matter (BLM) social movement, inspired by George Floyd's death, contributed to the resurgence of COVID-19 spread. This study investigates how social media users make sense of the relationship between COVID-19 and BLM, and how health disparities of COVID-19 and race have been discussed in Twitter posts. Thematic analysis was used to identify common themes. Ultimately, the findings increase understanding of how social media impacts knowledge regarding public health crises.

Public Health

In Chapter 6, "Same Pandemic, Different Plights: The Conjoined Effects of Socioeconomic Status and Ethnoracial Identity on Psychological Distress at the

Dawn of COVID-19," Tyson D. King-Meadows et al. examine the interaction between ethnoracial identity and socioeconomic status as a shaper of people in the United States' psychological responses to the beginning of the COVID-19 pandemic. King-Meadows et al. use *K*-means cluster analysis and multivariate linear regression to analyze data from a March 2020 Pew Research Center survey of 11,537 U.S. adults and data from an April 2020 Pew Research Center survey of 10,139 U.S. adults. The authors examine whether minorities were more likely than Whites to report high rates of distress and to view the pandemic as a threat to their financial and health well-being. King-Meadows et al. also explore if minorities of high socioeconomic status reported similar levels of distress as equally resourced Whites. These findings will illuminate how minorities' greater propensity to express high psychological distress at the onset of the COVID-19 crisis reflected their structural vulnerability to the economic shocks and social upheaval associated with the pandemic. This chapter concludes by addressing what the findings mean for understanding the effects of racialized economic dislocation on mental health and for understanding how distress and anxiety related to COVID-19 may affect social relations in the future.

In Chapter 7, "The Auto-Immunization of Black Life in Pandemic America," Mark Martinez uses Jacques Derrida's biopolitics to analyze the COVID-19 pandemic and the subsequent resurgent BLM protests as a moment that engages and also exceeds race war in America. Martinez discusses the idea that the pandemic materializes the biopolitical metaphor of auto-immunization of people of color (POC) in America. While touching on the various ways that auto-immunization generally affects non-Whites in America, he focuses on the Black experience from which current protest movements have emerged. American sovereignty, as described by Derrida and other biopolitical theorists, responds to the dangers of POC through an auto-immunization, specifically of Black Americans in urban areas, that is both symbolic and material. An auto-immune response is the attacking of a body by itself, and in America safe spaces for commerce, tourism, and "public" are created through the concerted attack on its own citizenry, arguably one of its most marginalized forms of citizenry, POC. Auto-immunization culminates in spectacle of police violating Black and Brown Americans in public as a sacrifice to the inevitability of safe spaces and a symbol of protecting the American way of life. The chapter also discusses the reframing of biopolitics toward affirmative liberation for POC life in America.

In Chapter 8, "Fight the Virus, Fight the Bias: Asian Americans' COVID-19 Racism Experience, Health Impact, and Activism," Jungmi Jun and Nanlan Zhang contend that stigmatizing and racist terms, such as "Kung flu," "Chinese virus," and "Wuhan virus," have been used to refer to the COVID-19 virus since the first report of COVID-19 outbreak in Wuhan, China. The racist rhetoric has impacted the lives of Asian Americans during the pandemic. This chapter discusses the racist rhetoric of U.S. government officials, the biased COVID-19 news coverage, and their impact on public discourses. Jun and Zhang present the type and prevalence of COVID-19 racist attacks and discrimination experienced by Asian Americans across the nation identified from their recent survey and Asian advocacy groups' incident reports in conjunction with the history of anti-Asian racism in U.S. society. The authors discuss the impact of COVID-19 racism on Asian Americans' mental and physical health and report survey findings regarding Asian Americans' anxiety and behaviors during the pandemic. In addition, Jun and Zhang introduce various activism movements to combat anti-Asian COVID-19 racism. The authors summarize scholars' future directions to assist Asian Americans in coping with the detrimental impact of COVID-19 racism as well as promoting active engagement in racial justice movements.

Working Disparities and Social Distancing

In Chapter 9, "'Balancing It All': The Implications of the COVID-19 Pandemic on Working Mothers in Texas," Nazgol Bagheri and Joshua Yates detail how the COVID-19 pandemic has drastically affected millions of women in Texas who have strived to assert their financial and social independence by working outside the home. In addition to gender-based discriminations—such as gender gaps in housework and childcare, wage gaps, high percentages of women working in an informal, instable labor market—many women are increasingly under pressure to redefine their work–life balance during abrupt school and daycare closures. This chapter is a case study of how COVID-19 has impacted working minority mothers in Texas. Interviewees are either first- or second-generation immigrants to the United States and ethnically belong to a non-White race according to census categorization. They draw on an empirical investigation based on in-depth Zoom and phone interviews of 41 working mothers from diverse family arrangements and professions. Bagheri and Yates tell the socio-spatial stories of women whose contributions to the family and to society have been largely ignored in this crisis. But more importantly, they highlight the disproportional emotional, mental, social, and professional challenges on working mothers. Recognizing the gendered nature of this pandemic, they argue how the lack of gender lens put women, especially vulnerable minority women, at more risk.

In Chapter 10, "Essential, Contingent, Informal, and Infected: Work and Ethnicity During COVID-19," Amy Schoenecker and Elizabeth Alejo suggest that as in other major cities, Chicago's Latinx communities contracted COVID-19 at disproportionate rates. To explain this, reports have emphasized the participation of Latinx communities in "essential" jobs; jobs deemed necessary that cannot be done from home. Schoenecker and Alejo problematize the neutral conceptualization of essential, arguing Latinx workers contracted COVID-19 at disproportionate rates because work is essential to their livelihood. Latinx communities overwhelmingly engage in low-wage contingent and informal work. Since these types of jobs rarely come with a safety net, workers had few options but to work during the pandemic. They use the case of Little Village in Chicago to demonstrate the overlapping elements of job insecurity that contributed to increased exposure to the virus. Little Village, a Mexican American neighborhood, had the highest number of COVID-19 cases early in the pandemic. Using census and original spatial data, they show how staffing agencies recruiting for low-wage contingent, essential jobs, and informal street vending activities are concentrated in Little Village. Schoenecker and Alejo argue that the structure of the U.S. labor market, segmented by race and ethnicity, is key to understanding COVID's disproportionate impact on these communities.

In Chapter 11, "Social Distancing as Lens: Race and Some Instructive Facets of Mass Pathogenic Self-Isolation," Miguel de Oliver examines two racialized aspects of epidemiological social distancing that readily escape the mainstream consciousness. The first section addresses the recommendation to 'shelter-in-place'. The 'place' of the racial other has some features of otherness that have proven therapeutic to the pervasive alienation of contemporary suburban-based consumer capitalism. The intensification of alienation wrought by a 'shelter-in-place' policy contributes to explaining the unusually broad participation of a white mainstream in racial injustice protests in urban centers. The second section of this chapter addresses an unprecedented opportunity for both the mainstream and the minority to perceive each other that is unexpectedly facilitated by the wearing of a respiratory mask. To the racially marginalized of society, the respiratory mask is much more than a deterrent to aerosol contagion; it is a backstage pass to an egalitarian state of individuality that visible minorities regularly see but have scarcely ever experienced.

Vaccine Nationalism

In Chapter 12, "'To Make Live and Let Die': Vaccine Nationalism, Vulnerable Solidarity, and Global Inequalities in the Age of COVID-19," Liz Jordan argues that in September 2020, Oxfam International estimated that wealthy nations representing 13% of the world's population had already purchased 51% of the promised doses of the five leading COVID-19 vaccine candidates. This drastic juxtaposition between the vaccine haves and have-nots is the result of vaccine nationalism. Vaccine nationalism refers to a series of practices, whereby a country attempts to secure vaccines for its own citizens before they are made available to other countries. Such practices have been widely criticized not only for undermining global public health efforts but on moral, political, social, and even economic grounds. Yet, despite these criticisms, many of the world's wealthiest nations continue to engage in vaccine nationalism. This chapter examines how vaccine nationalism operates according to a biopolitical logic aimed at safeguarding the lives of some, while treating the lives of others as expendable. Vaccine nationalism represents a dangerous globalization of biopolitics precisely at a time when the international community should be banding together to combat the COVID-19 pandemic.

In Chapter 13, "Looking Ahead," Sharon A. Navarro and Samantha L. Hernandez contend that COVID-19 has highlighted some ugly realities in American race relations. COVID-19 has wreaked a profound toll on human life with much of its impact being concentrated unequally among marginalized communities and POC, as shown by the collection of research in this edited volume. This chapter reiterates the ways in which systemic racism has intensified how COVID-19 has been experienced by communities of color and minority women. This chapter will suggest some recommendations on how people from the United States can come together to foster a comprehensive and equitable list of solutions.

Notes

1 In the political science field, the normative gender is often overlooked and understudied. For the purpose of this edited volume, we are referring to the politically normative understanding of the concept of gender as being man and woman.
2 Latinxs, Latinos/as, Mexican Americans, and Hispanics will be used interchangeably throughout this edited volume.

References

Behrmann, Savannah. (2021, May 22). COVID-19 Hate Crimes Bill to Fight Asian American Discrimination Passes Senate. *USA Today*. Retrieved from www.usatoday.com/story/news/politics/2021/04/22/covid-19-hate-crime-bill-protect-asian-americans-passes-senate/7290109002/

Bertocchi, Graziella & Arcangelo Dimico. (2020, July). *COVID-19, Race, and Redlining*. CEPR Discussion Paper No. DP15013. Retrieved from https://ssrn.com/abstract=3650128

Boburg, Shawn, Robert O'Harrow Jr., Neena Satija, & Amy Goldstein. (2020, April 3). Inside the Coronavirus Testing Failure: Alarm and Dismay Among the Scientists Who Sought to Help. *The Washington Post*. Retrieved from www.washington post.com/investigations/2020/04/03/coronavirus-cdc-test-kitspublic-health-labs/

Centers for Disease Control and Prevention. (2020). *The Tuskegee Timeline*. Retrieved from www.cdc.gov/tuskegee/timeline.htm

Coronavirus: Outcry After Trump Suggests Injecting Disinfectant as Treatment. (2020, April 24). *BBC News*. Retrieved from www.bbc.com/news/world-us-canada-52407177

Diamond, Dan & Nahal Toosi. (2020, June 10). Trump Team Failed to Follow NSC's Pandemic Playbook. *Politico*. Retrieved from www.polit ico.com/news/2020/03/25/trump -coronavirus-national-security-council-149285

Golden, Sherita Hill. (2021, October 4). Coronavirus in African Americans and Other People of Color. *John Hopkins Medicine*. Retrieved from www.hopkinsmedicine.org/health/conditions-and-diseases/coronavirus/covid19-racial-disparities

Goodman, Brenda. (2021, April 23). Lost in Translation: Language Barriers Hinder Vaccine Access. *WebMD*. Retrieved from www.webmd.com/vaccines/covid-19-vaccine/news/20210426/lost-in-translation-language-barriers-hinder-vaccine-access

Keith, Tamara. (2020, April 21). Timeline: What Trump Has Said and Done About the Coronavirus. *NPR. Org*. Retrieved from www.npr.org/2020/04/21/837348551/timeline

Kendi, Ibram X. (2019). *How to Be an Anti-Racist*. New York, NY: Penguin Random House.

Khanijahani, Ahmad. (2021). Racial, Ethnic and Socioeconomic Disparities in Confirmed COVID-19 Cases and Deaths in the United States: A County-Level Analysis as of November 2020. *Ethnicity & Health, 26*(1), 22–35.

Khubchandani, Jagdish & Yilda Macias. (2021, August 15). COVID-19 Vaccination Hesitancy in Hispanics and African Americans: A Review and Recommendations for Practice. *Brain Behavior Immunity Health*. DOI: 10.1016/j.bbih.2021.100277

Massey, D. and Denton, N. (1993). *American Apartheid: Segregation and the Making of the Underclass*. MA: Harvard University Press.

Meade, E. (2014). Overview of Community Characteristics in Areas with Concentrated Poverty. *ASPE*. Retrieved from https://aspe.hhs.gov/report/overview-community-characteristics-areas-concentrated-poverty

Novak, Nicole L., Natalie Lira, Kate E. O'Conner, Sioban D. Harlow, Sharon L.R. Kardia, & Alexandra Minna Stern. (2018, May). Disproportionate Sterilization of Latinos Under California's Eugenic Sterilization Program, 1920–1945. *American Journal of Public Health, 108*(5), 611–613.

Novic, Sara. (2021, April 13). I was Fortunate to Get My Vaccination, but the Hurdles Are too Great for Many Other Deaf People. *CNN*. Retrieved from www.cnn.com/2021/04/13/opinions/deaf-americans-vaccine-hesitancy-health-care-equity-novic/index.html

Reeves, Jay. (2021, February 2). Infamous Syphilis Study Adds to Town's Vaccine Skepticism. *San Antonio Express News*, A6.

Risk for COVID-19 Infection, Hospitalization, and Death by Race/Ethnicity. (2021). *CDC*, Retrieved from https://www.cdc.gov/coronavirus/2019-ncov/covid-data/investigations-discovery/hospitalization-death-by-race-ethnicity.html

Rogers, Katie, Lara Jakes, & Ana Swanson. (2020, March 18). Trump Defends Using 'Chinese Virus' Label, Ignoring Growing Criticism. *The New York Times*. Retrieved from www.nytimes.com/2020/03/18/us/politics/china -virus.html

Salvo, J.J., M.G. Powers, & R. S. Cooney. (1992). Contraceptive Use and Sterilization Among Puerto Rican Women. *Family Planning Perspective, 24*(5), 219–223.

Stop AAPI Hate Reporting Center. (2021, March 16). *2020–2021: National Report*. Retrieved from https://stopaapihate.org/2020-2021-national-report/

The Annie E. Casey Foundation. (2006). *Unequal Opportunities in Education*. Retrieved from www.aecf.org/m/resourcedoc/aecf-racemattersEDUCATION-2006.pdf

2

PLACING A BAND-AID ON A BULLET WOUND?

Black and Latinx Educational Experiences During a Pandemic

Dani Parker Moore, Betina Cutaia Wilkinson, Olivia Field, and Alondra Ramirez

Introduction

This study relies upon semi-structured interviews in a southern city to obtain a comprehensive understanding of how stay-at-home orders and remote learning affected Black and Latinx students. Building on Ladson-Billings' (2006, 2007) "education debt" argument, we frame this study as a comprehensive examination of the ways in which the education debt that Latinx and Blacks have incurred has skyrocketed since the start of the pandemic. Furthermore, we posit that the education and government institutions attempted to address a monumental problem with limited efforts and resources, much like putting a Band-Aid on a bullet wound. The topics that guide our pandemic study include (1) Latinx and Black children's educational attainment and access to academic resources, (2) parents' assessment of their and their children's struggles, (3) teachers' experiences in and out of the classroom, and (4) potential policy solutions to address the skyrocketing education debt that Latinx and Black students are incurring.

Blacks, Latinxs, and Educational Achievement

What do we know about Blacks, Latinxs, and their academic achievement? The divergence in education attainment between White students and their Black and Latinx counterparts is vast. The national high school dropout rate for Latinxs (12%) and Blacks (7%) is higher than that for Whites (5%), and the percentage of Latinxs who obtain a four-year degree is lower than the percentage of other groups (15%) (Krogstad, 2016). Whites score significantly higher on science knowledge scales than Blacks and Latinxs (Kennedy and Atske, 2019). What is more, Latinx students enter kindergarten with much lower scores in reading and math than their White peers. Interestingly, while the Black-White achievement gap widens throughout

DOI: 10.4324/9781003268710-2

elementary school, the Latinx-White achievement gap narrows between kindergarten and first grade and stays constant throughout children's school attendance, thus revealing some nuances between the experiences of Latinx and Black students (Reardon and Galindo, 2009).

Black and Latinx students face multiple barriers to achieving academic success. One such barrier is attending schools with limited academic resources and educational personnel with Black and Latinx students often attending low-resourced schools in segregated settings. English as a Second Language (ESL) and bilingual staff help non-English speakers' educational attainment and increase their parents' ability to engage in their children's education. Not surprisingly, many immigrant students have limited access to ESL and bilingual staff (Behnke et al., 2010; Olivos and Mendoza, 2010). Another barrier to educational success is not being placed in the gifted or higher track within a school, and we know that Black students are less likely than White students to be placed in higher tracks. The racial makeup of a school's student body also matters. Black students often attend racially homogeneous schools, and thus, they are less likely to achieve academic success relative to students in more diverse academic settings (Mickelson, 2015).

The COVID-19 Pandemic and Its Effects on Mental Health, the Digital Divide, and Education

While physical health has absorbed much of the conversation on the pandemic's health effects, we have some knowledge on the extent that the pandemic affects individuals' mental health. The pandemic has produced a surge in challenges for parents (e.g., financial constraints, working from home while taking care of children, assisting children with remote learning) (Phelps and Sperry, 2020). Children's lives have also changed because of the pandemic, resulting in decreased child health as a function of less physical activity and more sedentary behavior (Moore et al., 2020). A 2020 U.S. study of parents with young children in the midst of the pandemic revealed that 48% do not have regular childcare, 16% have a change in insurance status, and 11% struggle with food security. As to mental health, it is not surprising to find that 27% of parents reported worsening mental health. The researchers also found that struggling with childcare, food insecurity, and healthcare are related to parents' decline in mental health and a rise in children's behavioral problems (Patrick et al., 2020). Thus, in order to address children and parents' needs, schools must increase their efforts to improve food insecurity and provide mental and behavioral health services to children (Drane et al., 2020; Patrick et al., 2020; Phelps and Sperry, 2020). Furthermore, mental healthcare should focus on prevention, promotion, and intervention to meet the community's broad needs during and post the pandemic. Mental health services should be provided face-to-face and digitally using a collaborative network of parents, psychiatrists, psychologists, pediatricians, community volunteers, and nongovernmental organizations (Singh et al., 2020).

The digital divide that existed before the pandemic continued in the spring of 2020. A 2020 Population Reference Bureau analysis of 2018 American Community Survey data revealed that approximately 36% of Blacks and 34% of Latinx residents in the United States do not have access to a computer, internet connection, or both, almost twice as likely as their White counterparts. While some children benefited from the digital transformation in response to the pandemic, others, predominantly those with working-class backgrounds, truly struggled with remote learning (Iivari et al., 2020; also see Drane et al., 2020). Many lacked a reliable computer and/or internet connection along with having a parent or parental figure to guide them. If parents were home (often due to a job loss), they often lacked the computer skills and knowledge to assist their children. Some children were not educated at all (Iivari et al., 2020; see also O'Donnell, 2020). For teachers, the transition to digital instruction provided some advantages but many disadvantages. Some teachers received extensive instruction and numerous resources to develop a strong online curriculum, which they will continue integrating in the future. Other teachers struggled with distance learning and emphasized the numerous challenges that they faced and continue to face, including limited training materials to teach online effectively, laborious lesson planning, lack of ability to address individual student needs and struggles, lack of communication with students, and students' lack of educational resources at home. What concerns many teachers is the fact that once students return to the brick-and-mortar classroom, they will have to address the monumental academic, mental health, and behavioral needs of the students who have been left behind (Iivari et al., 2020).

As to students' actual educational attainment during the pandemic lock-down, all students suffered, but a student's socioeconomic status affected the amount of knowledge they acquired. In a study of students in the Netherlands, Engzell et al. (2020) found that students' learning remotely experienced a learning loss of three percentage points, yet students from less-educated homes experienced a 55% greater learning loss than that of the overall population (Engzell et al., 2020).

Education Debt

Based on the significant academic disparities that exist between White and students of color, we must recognize the "education debt" that exists for Blacks and Latinxs in the United States. Building on critical race theory, Ladson-Billings (2006, 2007) argues that instead of framing the discrepancies in academic achievement between White and students of color as the achievement gap, we must focus on these disparities as the "education debt" that our society has incurred for Blacks, Latinxs, and Native Americans. Our country has a deep history of treating these groups as inferior to Whites and thus developing a racial hierarchy that places these groups at the bottom. Relative to a deficit (the amount that accrues when an entity's spending exceeds its income), debt "is the sum of all previous incurred annual federal deficits" (Ladson-Billings, 2006, p. 4). Approaching the disparities in academic achievement across racial/ethnic groups as "education debt" is the only way to address this perdurable, intrinsic problem.

Thus, in this chapter we recognize the educational struggles that many Blacks and Latinxs experience and argue that the "education debt" (to borrow from Ladson-Billings, 2006) that our society has incurred for these individuals before the COVID-19 pandemic skyrocketed at the onset and throughout the pandemic. Similar to Ladson-Billings (2006, 2007), we do not regard the increasing disparities in educational attainment between Whites and marginalized groups as a burden that many Blacks and Latinxs have to assume but as a failure by the current political, educational systems to respond comprehensively and adequately to the needs of marginalized individuals who were already in vulnerable situations before the pandemic began. In particular, we argue that the mounting "education debt" is a function of the attempt by government and education institutions to address a serious problem in an inadequate way, similar to placing a Band-Aid on a bullet wound.

Data and Methodology

In order to examine how transition to remote learning during the COVID-19 pandemic has affected Blacks and Latinxs in the United States, we conducted semi-structured phone interviews of parents and teachers in Forsyth County, North Carolina. We relied on snowball sampling to produce a robust sample of parents and teachers (Babbie 1998, p. 195). During June to September 2020, we interviewed 52 individuals—18 Latinx parents, 17 Black parents, and 17 teachers. Nineteen of the interviews were conducted in Spanish and translated into English by a bilingual interviewer. The Latinx parent sample consists of 12 individuals who were born in the United States and 25 who were born outside of the United States. The teachers interviewed were predominantly White and taught in elementary, middle, and high schools. The majority taught in public schools with a large percentage of Black and Latinx students. We compensated participants for their participation in the study with a $20 visa gift card sent via mail.

We recorded each of the interviews and transcribed them via a transcription application. To ensure accurate results, one researcher transcribed interviews while the other verified the transcriptions. Each researcher examined the transcriptions and extracted themes individually. The commonality between both researchers was approximately 85%. The appendix contains the interview questions. We conducted interviews until we began to receive little to no new information (e.g., ideas, arguments) (Krueger, 1994, p. 88). We obtained Institutional Review Board (IRB) approval for this study. For more information about our IRB approval, please contact the authors.

The interviewees are residents of Forsyth County, North Carolina, and their experiences and demographic characteristics are fairly representative of larger national trends. Similar to the national average in Forsyth County, Latinxs have one of the highest rates of infection than any other racial/ethnic group. As of November 7, 2020, 35.5% of COVID-19 cases in Winston-Salem are attributed to Latinx individuals (who make up 13% of the population), while White (56% of population) and Black (25% of population) residents accounted for approximately 33.5% and 18% of cases, respectively (COVID-19 Surveillance for Forsyth County, 2020). Comparable to national trends, the share of Black deaths due to COVID-19 (38%) is significantly larger than their share of COVID-19 cases and their share of Forsyth County's population. Furthermore, Forsyth residents are comparable to the U.S. population when it comes to several demographic characteristics such as percentage of those with a college degree, percentage of those in the civilian labor force, percentage of those with a household computer and internet access, and per capita income in the past 12 months (U.S. Census Bureau QuickFacts, n.d.).

Findings

This study seeks to obtain a comprehensive understanding of how stay-at-home orders and remote learning influenced Black and Latinx students' educational attainment with a focus on the extent that the pandemic exacerbated Latinxs' and Blacks'"education debt." In this section, we highlight the themes that emerged from interviewees' answers to the interview questions. The analysis will include actual quotes from participants, though we have changed all of the interviewees' names to protect their identity. A discussion of Latinx and Black parents' perceptions of remote learning is followed by teachers' experiences with online teaching.

Parents' Perceptions of Remote Learning

When speaking with parents about their children's experience with online instruction, the majority of parents reported that learning from home was not effective. When discussing why remote learning did not work, a few mentioned that it was challenging to motivate their children (Iivari et al., 2020).

> LUCIA: *It has affected a lot because the kids, well, virtually they do not receive the same learning as being present in a classroom … online classes are not the same as face-to-face classes.*
>
> KAREN: *It was just horrible … They [teachers] put stuff up, but it was kind like, I don't think my son learned anything because just going online—he was supposed to basically go online and do these assignments, and he's not wired like that … And even though I was on him to do that, he still wasn't doing it.*

Another reason as to why remote learning was not effective is that parents were not able to assist their children with their homework. The two main reasons that they were unable to help were that they were not knowledgeable of the subject matter and that they were not comfortable with the technology (Iivari et al., 2020). As to Latinx parents, many did not feel confident in their English skills to assist with assignments.

ROSA: *I get very frustrated because I can't really help my kids because I do not know how to use technology.*

MARINA: *I don't speak English … in reality, I don't know if he [her son] was doing it right or not … I couldn't help him in anything because I don't understand.*

When asked what parents needed from their children's school, more than half said they wanted teachers to communicate more when using virtual instruction. Several parents provided recommendations.

LESLIE: *Nothing was reiterated for instruction for parents to assist in the virtual learning environment, initially … Some real, live interaction, some facilitation, some question asking, that type of thing.*

TONIA: *For my son, just better communication, and better directions, and more visual aids. And for me, I needed to talk to a live person.*

STACY: *I wish there would have been some way that maybe like at the end of every week there could have been something to kind of summarize like how he's doing and what's the plan for next week.*

However, some parents were satisfied with the amount of communication provided by the teachers and the school system. Parents with children at distinct schools were quite aware of this.

VERONICA: *Their teachers would communicate with me. They would call me, and they would send me messages. The teacher of my other son would also communicate with me, but not as frequently like the other teachers of my other kids.*

Another theme that emerged in conversations with parents is that they were concerned about their children falling behind and not getting the help that they need.

ROSA: *Well, I think [they are learning] half of the percentage of what they were supposed to learn. It was so-so because they do not have a lot of help.*

MARIA: *They did not learn much. I noticed that it was more difficult in subjects that my son already struggled with.*

When discussing how the pandemic has affected children, some parents reported that the lockdown and limited interaction with peers affected their children's mental health, and they were worried about it (Moore et al., 2020; Patrick et al., 2020).

PATTI: *It [the pandemic] also affected her because, you know, being in the middle of a pandemic and being locked up and not being able to do anything, well, it's not easy for you.*

KAREN: *And my son, he's like mom, we can't even play sports. They don't have anything set up for, like, counseling these kids. You gotta think about it, they've been in the house … I'm worried.*

Throughout several interview conversations, it was apparent that some parents struggled with balancing full-time work, taking care of children, and serving as their children's teachers. Some mentioned that their mental health was impacted by the increasing challenges that they faced (Patrick et al., 2020). A few parents felt like they had to choose between quitting their job to help their children with their schoolwork and keep them safe or keeping their job to help pay the bills and thus exposing their kids to the virus.

> LESLIE: *I think I definitely experienced a breaking point … From the mental health perspective, just trying to make sure that they felt safe and secure, even with all of this going on … And yes then also understanding that I would have to stop in the middle of my thought process in the work that I was doing to answer questions from my nine-year old … that was very difficult.*

> ASHLEY: *I knew I was getting snappy and frustrated because I'm trying to separate mom, work, and now teacher at the same time … And then on top of that, I don't want my kid to do bad either. So, now I'm getting mad because I'm like, "You will not be behind." So, I'm trying to make sure they're good to go … it makes me feel like a horrible parent because I have to decide what to do. Do I give up everything so they don't get exposed, but then we have nothing? Or am I selfish because I'm trying to keep what we have? Because there is no other option except for me not to work and I mean that's really not an option because we'd lose the house, we'd lose cars.*

Hence, these results reveal that most parents felt that the pandemic and reliance on remote learning suppressed their children's educational attainment and affected their mental health. While a few parents had strong communication with teachers, several had little interaction with teachers resulting in a limited understanding of how to use the software to access the assignment, limited knowledge of the child's assignments, and heightened frustration that their child was falling behind. Given the heightened stress that remote learning and the lockdown created, some parents' mental health suffered. Most of the findings in this section corroborate the experiences of parents throughout the world.

Teachers' Perception of Remote Learning

Several of the themes that emerged in parents' interviews emerged in the teacher interviews. Of the teachers sampled, most noted that online instruction is not as effective as face-to-face. More specifically, nearly half mentioned that teaching students online was limiting on multiple levels (Engzell et al., 2020). First, many students lacked the necessary resources to learn (Iivari et al., 2020).

> ELAINE: *It [the pandemic] halted all progress. And it forced them to have to make a drastic change that they were ill-equipped to make, dealing with limitations of technology access. I teach a lot of students who are from rural areas who are not that great with computers through no fault of their own, but that just is not widely available where they came from.*

So it's not just that they had the educational barrier that they didn't have a teacher in front of them. They had the access barrier with technology.

JULIA: *I work at a Title 1 school so many of our kids don't have the resources to conduct online learning.*

KAREN: *We had to reach them through like very, very basic platforms like WhatsApp. And that, that was practically the only way to reach them. They of course, most of them didn't have Wi-Fi, reliable Wi-Fi.*

Second, compared to in-person instruction, remote learning prevented students from obtaining additional support from teachers and prevented teachers from gauging what students did not understand and holding students accountable for completing their assignments (Iivari et al., 2020).

GINA: *These kids, they need to be there, so the teacher can actually control the environment, and like call for their attention constantly. When they're at home, it's impossible for us to do any of that. You don't know the environment where they were in, or even if you do know the environment, there's nothing you can do about it. And have to rely on the kids' willingness to do what they're supposed to do, and they are young kids.*

JULIA: *With little kids, I need face-to-face interaction so this can affect them. With limited social interaction, I don't know what they need, what they need to know, what they don't know … Online is not the same as face-to-face.*

Third, the sense of community that teachers and students had in the face-to-face classroom diminished.

IAN: *The brick and mortar system helps a lot, students learn a lot when they are in a classroom. Peer pressure is quite influential. A sense of community is key. I need to build their trust before I teach them, I need to motivate them to value their education. If I can't connect with them, then they won't do well.*

When it comes to teachers' workload, some stated that they are working harder now than they have ever worked in their teaching career (Iivari et al., 2020).

IAN: *I have never worked this hard.*

LISA: *The pandemic has made it much harder to teach … I haven't worked as hard as I have this year.*

As to student performance, some teachers noted that students were distracted from schoolwork. Reasons as to why students were distracted included students not having a quiet place to work, having to work outside the home to contribute financially, being distracted by sick family members, having to help siblings with homework, or having to supervise siblings while parents worked (Iivari et al., 2020).

ANA: *When I tried to get him to pay attention to me and he was focused on the class, his little brother was either watching television or the mother was cooking.*

ELAINE: *… having to go to work instead of being able to attend to their own studies, having to supervise younger siblings, also put a lot of stress and was a hurdle for my students.*

FAITH: *They probably have other stress at home with taking care of siblings … helping the younger siblings with their work. The majority of their parents, as far as I know, were working.*

Some teachers noted that some students were successful with online learning, while some were not (Iivari et al., 2020).

CLAIRE: *It depends on the student-right? Some of my students are very independent and they're very much problem-solvers … They did fine.*

HILLARY: *Well, from those that connected, no, I did not notice any difference. As I said, I had several that did not connect even one day. They practically did nothing. So I imagine that they had more problems. But of those that connected, I never noticed a difference.*

One teacher noted that many of her students accessed food through the nutrition assistance program, but since many do not have access to it, they are concerned since having good nutrition is important for academic success (see Patrick et al., 2020).

JULIA: *Nutrition is also key. For some kids, the only way to get food is to go to the school so now I don't know how they are getting their food.*

When discussing parents, most teachers noted that parents struggled with helping their children because they did not have the knowledge, resources, language, or computer skills required to facilitate online learning (Iivari et al., 2020).

DIANNE: *They don't have that personalized, you know, education that they really need to get … A lot of them … don't even have a computer. Even though their school system provided for them, still some of their parents didn't even know how to use it.*

IAN: *I don't see many language barriers for the kids but I know that there are language barriers with the parents and this is difficult.*

LISA: *The biggest issue that I had was having to teach parents how to use email.*

Some teachers mentioned that parents' financial situations affect their children's learning outcomes (see Engzell et al., 2020; Iivari et al., 2020). A few teachers explicitly noted that parents' financial situations did not impact intellect, but it adds increased stress on the child.

CLAIRE: *I know some people were able to find some babysitters or had, also nannies so that you have to think how much different it was for that student than it was for the one that has to be at home, taking care as well of like the little ones while mom's working. So then at that point, your, your brain is not really considering ... what does the lesson really matter whenever you're more worried about, I mean, your health. Yeah, what you're going to eat the next few days. Oh yeah. I think it absolutely has an effect.*

FAITH: *I do think finances impact students in the fact it is another stressor. I don't think it impacts intellect whatsoever. I think it impacts the ability to procure the resources that other children who have the financial capabilities can. But, I think during the pandemic, it became more evident to the vast public because, it was, everybody was going through the same kind of situation. And so it was easier for all of humanity to see that the kids that don't have a laptop can't do the schoolwork. So therefore, despite IQ, they still can't perform to an ABC, ABCDEF level if they're working at zero.*

When discussing the barriers to students' educational attainment, some teachers mentioned that some parents' financial constraints affected their access to a reliable internet connection.

ANA: *I did have some families that the economic impact was very great. They had no job to keep paying on the internet. They would send me a message related to that ... When the children didn't have the internet, I couldn't contact them.*

When asked about the factors that can be related to students' academic achievement, some teachers recognized that parental support is key. For some, children's academic achievement and parental support are tied to parents' employment situation.

IAN: *Parental support is key, making sure that students complete their homework is essential.*

JULIA: *But we need parental support because parents are working and this has been a problem because they can't help their kids.*

KAREN: *I think that the parental involvement in the academic life of those students, of the children is heavily dependent on the economical situation. So in poor families, you know, parents are working two, three jobs. And not there at night, students are taking care of the little ones. So, of course ... they don't even have physically enough time to learn, to focus on studying*

For others, parental support and not the parents' economic situation is tied to their academic access.

LISA: *Kids who have a lot more parental support through parents making sure that their child has logged on were successful ... Financial resources do not matter as much as parents (or family members) holding kids accountable. There was a student who had a grandmother who was always checking her work and making sure that she completed it. This student did well in my class.*

In line with what parents reported, some teachers noted that the school administration should conduct more parental outreach and supply parents with technology training so that they can assist their children.

> FAITH: *I would say probably the best thing that could happen would be, if each zone would have parent education meetings … to educate the parents on our learning platforms that we're using … I know people would say we did the best we could. I don't believe that. And I think that what we need to do is a better job of community outreach and education of parents in their native language and supply … resources in those communities, meaning like a church or whatever that's available for a hotspot or Wi-Fi … we need better communication between the Hispanic community and our school system to supply those resources.*

It is important to note that in Forsyth County, like in several areas throughout the country, students and teachers were able to obtain hotspots from the school system to partake in/conduct virtual learning. However, some teachers noted that the hotspots were not always effective, thus placing limits on working parents' ability to help their children with school assignments.

> ANA: *We thought that we could have used the hotspots more efficiently, the internet the education department had provided to some children, but they failed the same way. It was not the access but the demand that there was … We had those problems that the network often failed.*
>
> IAN: *They [the school system] provided hotspots to the kids if they needed them but there were problems with them. The hotspots were only good for four hours a day.*

In terms of the teachers' experiences with remote learning, some reported that they struggled with learning the software and how to navigate websites required to teach online (Iivari et al., 2020).

> JULIA: *I had to learn the software to teach online but it was a challenge.*
>
> KAREN: *Making videos through V video … I've never done this, so it was actually a lot of learning how all those platforms are working … like six or nine platforms to learn all of it, all of a sudden we had to create virtual classrooms. So that was just too much to try and figure out all of the websites because they all work differently.*

However, many teachers emphasized that they felt more enthusiastic about their teaching after having time to prepare and learn different web programs over the summer.

> CLAIRE: *We're moving to a new platform now. So that'll be interesting because the one that we were using before, it would crash a lot … I imagine Canvas is going to help us. I hope it does.*
>
> IAN: *I am more enthusiastic about the fall … We will use Zoom … We have had Canvas training and will use Canvas.*

Regardless, some teachers said they still needed access to school resources—paper to print out packets, as well as access to whiteboards or smart boards—in order to teach effectively (Iivari et al., 2020).

ANA: *When we start in August, I have … to see if I can go to school because I have a lot of material in the school, but I do not have it at home.*

DIANNE: *I believe even though we were going to do a virtual class, we need to be in a classroom because in order to us to be able to show them what they need to learn, we need to have, at least the white board or the Blackboard or a smart board to show them.*

MARY: *Paper packets worked well for me and my students since we didn't have to rely on an internet connection to communicate. But, the school only gave us access to the school printer for one month.*

Teachers also requested that the administration pay for their Wi-Fi connection and provide more support and understanding when it comes to the online challenges that they face.

GINA: *Resources. The school, the district is relying on us to pay for Wi-Fi at our houses, so we can do our jobs. To me that doesn't make sense. What else? And it's not resources, but admin to do something about keeping students unchecked about their work, and not just relying on us on calling the parents all the time … it was us calling parents all day every day getting nothing in return, and then … my admin saying like, "Yeah, but your kids have to do the work." And I'm like, "Yeah, but there's nothing else I can do. Like you just told us we cannot go to their house." … a little more admin support would go a long way.*

To shed light on the limited resources that some teachers have, one teacher stated that she knew some teachers who worked from the school parking lot in order to access Wi-Fi.

LISA: *I was fortunate enough to have a computer, laptop and printer at home, but some teachers struggled. They had no Wi-Fi at home so they had to go to the school parking lot to work.*

When asked about how the pandemic has affected their students, some teachers observed that the pandemic affected their students' emotional and mental well-being, as they were unable to interact socially with friends and teachers (Moore et al., 2020; Phelps and Sperry, 2020; Singh et al., 2020).

BETTY: *For them, it's too hard … They want to go outside. They are very afraid. They are very sad. They are confused. They keep their distance, they don't want to be hugged. They feel afraid with people.*

IAN: *The psychological impact on the kids is negative. They hate being away from their friends. Their mental well-being has suffered and they really need to be around their peers.*

JULIA: *Those most affected [by the pandemic] are the kids and their learning was halted … Kids learn from the teacher, each other and this really affects them.*

Furthermore, some teachers reported that the pandemic has affected their own mental and emotional health.

BETTY: *I feel like without hope because I, I cannot give hugs to my students. Yes, because I like that my students feel my love from me, [and I] from them. And that really is impacting too much for me right now.*
MARY: *The pandemic has affected my family and me emotionally.*

In conclusion, some teachers have not noticed a major change in their students' educational attainment, but many have. Teachers have also encountered numerous challenges throughout the pandemic, including having to learn new software, encountering limited access to classroom resources, experiencing difficulty communicating with students and parents, teaching students without reliable technology, and navigating their personal challenges. The themes that emerged from our conversations are comparable to the experiences and struggles that teachers throughout the world are experiencing.

Discussion

This study presents preliminary findings on how the COVID-19 pandemic has affected the educational attainment of Latinxs and Blacks. While some students did not experience academic struggles during the lockdown period, many did. Remote learning was a struggle for most students, parents, and teachers. Students with limited socioeconomic resources are those most susceptible to falling behind during a pandemic. Thus, Black and Latinx students' education debt has skyrocketed during the pandemic.

This study's findings lend credence to some policy recommendations that go beyond placing a Band-Aid on a major dilemma. First, the school district should invest in translators and bilingual staff who can support students and parents who are not English dominant. Teachers should have the educational resources and assistance from staff to communicate with parents regularly. The school system should invest in streamlining the online learning experience and provide teachers and parents adequate equipment, training, and support to navigate these tools (UNESCO, 2020). As students return to in-person classes, the schools must be ready to address the numerous educational, nutritional, mental, and behavioral health needs of the students. School systems should have a group of psychiatrists, psychologists, pediatricians, teachers, parents, and community members ready to assist students to navigate the trauma that they have experienced (Patrick et al., 2020; Phelps and Sperry, 2020). As we look ahead, there are several questions that arise from these findings, including the long-term effects of remote learning on vulnerable populations. A long-term study on this would be extremely useful. Still, this study makes a significant contribution to extant literature by providing an in-depth understanding of how remote learning and stay-at-home orders impacted Latinx and Black students'"educational debt," producing fruitful information about the successes and downfalls of remote learning and shedding light on how to better prepare for the next pandemic.

References

Babbie, Earl R. (1998). *The Practice of Social Research*. 9th ed. Belmont, CA: Wadsworth Thomson.

Behnke, Andrew O., Gonzalez, Laura M., and Cox, Ronald B. (2010). Latino Students in New Arrival States: Factors and Services to Prevent Youth From Dropping Out. *Hispanic Journal of Behavioral Sciences, 32*(3): 385–409. https://doi.org/10.1177/0739986310374025

COVID-19 Surveillance for Forsyth County, NC. (2020, November 7). Retrieved from http://forsyth.cc/publichealth/documents/COVID19Surveillance.pdf

Drane, Catherine, Vernon, Lynette, and O'Shea, Sara. (2020, December 23). The Impact of 'Learning at Home' on the Educational Outcomes of Vulnerable Children in Australia During the COVID-19 Pandemic. *National Centre for Student Equity in Higher Education*. Retrieved from www.ncsehe.edu.au/publications/learning-at-home-educational-outcomes-vulnerable-children-australia-covid-19/

Engzell, Per, Frey, Arun, and Verhagen, Mark. (2020). Learning Inequality During the COVID-19 Pandemic. *SocArXiv*. Retrieved from https://doi.org/10.31235/osf.io/ve4z7

Iivari, Netta, Sharma, Sumita, and Venta-Olkkonen, Leena. (2020). Digital Transformation of Everyday Life – How COVID-19 Pandemic Transformed the Basic Education of the Young Generation and Why Information Management Research Should Care? *International Journal of Information Management,* 55, 1–6. https://doi.org/10.1016/j.ijinfomgt.2020.102183

Kennedy, Brian and Atske, Sara. (2019). Science Knowledge Varies by Race and Ethnicity in U.S. *Pew Research Center*. Accessed on November 16, 2020 from pewresearch.org

Krogstad, Jens Manuel. (2016). 5 Facts about Latinos and Education. *Pew Research Center*. Accessed on November 16, 2020, from www.pewresearch.org

Krueger, Richard A. (1988). Focus groups: A practical guide for applied research. Thousand Oaks, Sage.

Ladson-Billings, Gloria. (2006). From the Achievement Gap to the Education Debt: Understanding Achievement in U.S. Schools. *Educational Researcher, 35*(7), 3–12.

Ladson-Billings, Gloria. (2007). Pushing Past the Achievement Gap: An Essay on the Language of Deficit. *The Journal of Negro Education, 76*(3), 316–323. www.jstor.org/stable/40034574

Mickelson, Roslyn A. (2015). The Cumulative Disadvantages of First- and Second-Generation Segregation for Middle School Achievement. *American Educational Research Journal, 52*(4), 657–692. https://doi.org/10.3102/0002831215587933

Moore, Sarah A., Faulkner, Guy, Rhodes, Ryan E., Brussoni, Mariana, Chulak-Bozzer, Tala Ferguson, Tala J., Mitra, Raktim, O'Reilly, Norm, Spence John C., Vanderloo, Leigh M., and Tremblay, Mark S. (2020). Impact of the COVID-19 Virus Outbreak on Movement and Play Behaviors of Canadian Children and Youth: A National Survey. *International Journal of Behavioral Nutrition and Physical Activity, 17*(85): 1–11. https://doi.org/10.1186/s12966-020-00987-8

O'Donnell, Lisa. (2020, April 29). Thousands of Students Have Not Logged on For E-Learning, Winston-Salem/Forsyth County Schools Say. *Winston-Salem Journal*. Retrieved from https://journalnow.com/news/local/thousands-of-students-have-not-logged-on-for-e-learning-winston-salem-forsyth-county-schools/article_d4877d86-6234-5293-ac62-716018933491.html

Olivos, Edward M. and Mendoza, Marcela. (2010). Immigration and Educational Inequality: Examining Latino Immigrant Parents' Engagement in U.S. Public Schools. *Journal of Immigrant & Refugee Studies, 8*(3), 339–357. https://doi.org/10.1080/15562948.2010.501301

Patrick, Stephen W., Henkhaus, Laura E., Zickafoose, Joseph S., Lovell, Kim, Halvorson, Alese, Loch, Sarah, Letterie, Mia, and Davis, Matthew. (2020). Well-Being of Parents and Children During the COVID-19 Pandemic: A National Survey. *Pediatrics, 146*(4), 1–8. https://doi.org/10.1542/peds.2020-016824

Phelps, Chavez and Sperry, Linda. (2020). Children and the COVID-19 Pandemic. *Psychological Trauma: Theory, Research, Practice, and Policy, 12*(81), S73–S75. https://doi.org/10.1037/tra0000861

Population Reference Bureau. (2020). Children, Coronavirus, and the Digital Divide: Native American, Black, and Hispanic Students at Greater Educational Risk During Pandemic. Accessed on November 16, 2020, from www.prb.org

Reardon, Sean F. and Galindo, Claudia. (2009). The Hispanic-White Achievement Gap in Math and Reading in the Elementary Grades. *American Educational Research Journal, 46*(3), 853–891. https://doi.org/10.3102/0002831209333184

Singh, Shweta, Roy, Deblina, Sinha, Krittika, Parveen, Sheeba, Sharma, Ginni, and Joshi, Gunjan. (2020). Impact of COVID-19 and Lockdown on Mental Health of Children and Adolescents: A Narrative Review with Recommendations. *Psychiatry Research, 293*, 1–10. https://doi.org/10.1016/j.psychres.2020.113429

UNESCO. (2020, June 3). *COVID-19: 10 Recommendations to Plan Distance Learning Solutions*. Retrieved from https://en.unesco.org/news/covid-19-10-recommendations-plan-distance-learning-solutions

U.S. Census Bureau QuickFacts: United States. (n.d.). *U.S. Census.* www.census.gov/quickfacts/fact/table/forsythcountynorthcarolina,US/RHI225219

Appendix

Interview Questions for Black and Latinx Parents:

1. How has the COVID-19 pandemic affected you and your family? Specifically, when it comes to their health? Do you have a family member or someone close to you who was affected by COVID-19? (*Spanish: ¿Cómo ha afectado la pandemia COVID-19 a usted y su familia? Específicamente con respecto a la salud de su familia. ¿Tiene un familiar o alguien cercano a usted que fue afectado por COVID-19?*)

2. How has the COVID-19 pandemic affected your family particularly when it comes to education and remote learning? (*Spanish: ¿Cómo ha afectado la pandemia COVID-19 a su familia específicamente con respecto a su educación y enseñanza virtual?*)

3. How successful has remote learning been for your child(ren)? (*Spanish: ¿Durante el año escolar pasado durante la pandemia, ha sido exitosa la enseñanza de su niño(a)? ¿Como?*)

4. How comfortable did you feel helping your child with his/her/their home-work? (*Spanish: ¿Se siento confortable ayudando a su niño(a) con la tarea? ¿Cuanto?*)

5. Was your child able to complete his/her/their work successfully this past academic year? (*Spanish: Durante la pandemia, su hijo/a pudo completar su tarea escolar con éxito? ¿Como?*)

6. What do you think influenced your child's ability to succeed academically? (*Spanish: ¿Que piensa que afecto el éxito académico a su niño(a) durante la pandemia?*)

7. What do you need as a parent to help your child succeed in school during a pandemic? (*Spanish: ¿Que necesita como padre para que su niño tenga éxito en la escuela durante una pandemia?*)

8. Did you experience any technological issues with remote learning? If so, what can your child's school or local representative do to help you with that issue? (*Spanish: ¿Tuvo unos problemas tecnológicos con respecto a la enseñanza virtual de sus niños? Si respondió si, ¿qué puede hacer la escuela de su niño y su representante político para resolver este problema?*)

9. Is there anything else that you would like to add regarding how the pandemic has affected you or your family? (*Spanish: Hay algo más que quiere decir/agregar con respecto a cómo la pandemia ha afecto a usted o a su familia?*)

Thank you very much for participating in this interview. In order to compensate you for your time, we would like to mail you a $20 gift card. Can you provide me your mailing address so I can mail it to you? (*Spanish: Muchas gracias por participar en esta entrevista. Para compensarla(o) por su tiempo, nos gustaría mandarles por correo una tarjeta de regalo de $20. ¿Me puede dar su domicilio así le mando por correo la tarjeta?*)

Interview Questions for School Teachers:

1. How has the COVID-19 pandemic affected you and your family? (*Spanish: ¿Cómo ha afectado la pandemia COVID-19 a usted y a su familia?*)

2. Now when it comes to your students, how has the pandemic affected your students' ability to learn this past school year? (*Spanish: ¿Cómo ha afectado la pandemia COVID-19 a la enseñanza de los niños de su escuela?*)

3. What resources did you have to assist their learning this past academic year during the pandemic? (*Spanish: ¿Que recursos tuvo este año escolar pasado para ensenar a los niños durante una pandemia?*)

4. What resources do you need to assist their learning this upcoming fall? (*Spanish: ¿Que recursos piensa que necesita para ayudar a la enseñanza de sus estudiantes este otoño?*)

5. How has the pandemic influenced your work? Your ability to carry out your job effectively? (*Spanish: ¿Cómo ha influido la pandemia su trabajo? ¿Su habilidad de hacer su trabajo efectivamente?*)

6. What do you think impacts students' ability to succeed academic-ally? (*Spanish: ¿Que cree que afecta la capacidad de los estudiantes para triunfar académicamente?*)

7. Did you experience any technological issues with remote teaching? If so, what can your school or local representative do to help you with that issue? (*Spanish: ¿Tuvo unos problemas tecnológicos con respecto a la enseñanza virtual de sus niños? Si respondió si, ¿qué puede hacer la escuela de su niño y su representante haga para ayudar a este problema?*)
8. Is there anything else that you would like to discuss regarding how the pandemic has affected you or your students? (*Spanish: ¿Hay algo más que quiere decir con respecto a cómo la pandemia ha afectado a usted o a sus estudiantes?*)

3

NECESSITY AS THE MOTHER OF INVENTION

Attempting to Overcome the Digital Divide During the COVID-19 Pandemic

Adam McGlynn and Caitlyn Stout

Introduction

As COVID-19 began to spread through the United States in March 2020, governors throughout the country closed schools. Classrooms with 20-plus students were viewed as potential breeding grounds for a virus more contagious than influenza by elected officials and health experts. However, the closures came swiftly without time for educators to prepare. In many districts, faculty did not have the time to gather resources to help educate students from home or distribute materials to their students, many of whom would be ill-equipped to learn outside of the classroom.

In this work, we examine how four school districts addressed these challenges; specifically, in ensuring students had access to technology and broadband internet service as teachers implemented remote instruction in the spring of 2020 and for many districts in the 2020–2021 school year. However, for some districts, the absence of access to technology or broadband resulted in having to resort to distributing paper copies of learning materials (Finley, 2020). This creates the question of whether the COVID-19 pandemic propelled upper-income school districts further into the 21st century, while sending low-income school districts serving predominately students of color back to latter half of the 20th century?

An estimated 50 million students began learning from home due to the pandemic with an estimated 15 to 16 million lacking either access to broadband internet service or a device[1] to be able to successfully learn from home, including 26% of Latino/a and 30% of Black students, respectively (Chandra, Chang, et al., 2020). A survey of 501 school superintendents in May 2020 by The School Superintendents Association demonstrated the profound impact the pandemic had on students as 94% of superintendents surveyed stated that their schools had closed for the remainder of the year (AASA, 2020). While 92% of superintendents

DOI: 10.4324/9781003268710-3

reported district supplying laptops, tablets, and/or hotspots to students to provide distance learning, 83% also reported using "work packets," demonstrating that most districts had to diversify their remote instructional practices given likely inequities within their student population. Furthermore, when asked how their district was addressing equity, 92% reported supplying devices to students in need compared to only 38% who stated that home internet access was being provided to students and 71% cited a lack of student access at home would prevent their district from conducting fully online instruction.

The Digital Divide and COVID-19

The concept of the digital divide has evolved over time. While 35 years ago it could be defined as which schools had computers and which did not, today it is a multifaceted concept. As the Organization for Economic Co-operation and Development (2000) explains,

> The digital divide in formal schooling is not simply an equipment differential that can be overcome with further selective investments in hardware, software, and networking. Instead, it derives from both within school and within home differences that extend to learning standards as well as support. Student self-learning ability, and in particular, student ability for independent learning, is an additional factor.

Thus, school districts in the time of COVID-19 must address not only access to tablets, laptops, and broadband internet but also the ability of students and their families to be able to use learning management systems and various software programs to receive instruction. The concept of the digital divide has become more nuanced and is often also discussed as the "homework gap" to highlight those students who may have access to devices and broadband internet at school but not at home. The ACT Center for Equity in Learning found that almost one in five students from underserved backgrounds had access to only one technological device at home from which to do their schoolwork, a rate that was three times higher than those students who were not classified as underserved (Moore et al., 2018).[2] Anderson and Perrin (2018) found that on average 15% of U.S. households with school-aged children lacked broadband internet access with that percentage jumping to 35% in households with annual incomes of less than $30,000. However, the digital divide is not only an economic issue as while 28% of low-income White families lacked broadband access, 41% and 38% of Black and Hispanic households, respectively, in this income category lacked broadband access.[3] Overall, this led to approximately one-quarter of students from low-income households not being able to complete their homework due to not having access to a computer or internet connection (Anderson & Perrin, 2018).

As we examine four school districts with either majority African American or Latino/a populations, we should expect the digital divide to be a significant barrier to instruction during COVID-19. The inequities faced by students of color in urban districts are not new (see Kozol, 1991). However, these inequities persist as those "school districts serving the largest populations of Black, Latino, or American Indian students receive roughly $1,800, or 13 percent less per student in state and local funding than those serving the fewest students of color" (Morgan & Amerikaner, 2018), complicating these districts' ability to overcome the digital divide before and especially during the COVID-19 pandemic. An April 2020 SOMOS Health Care—Latino Decisions poll found that 58% of Latinos were worried about their students falling behind due to COVID-19 school closures. Furthermore, approximately one-third of Latinos stated concern about not having enough computers for learning at home and the increased cost of their cell phone and/or broadband bills created by learning/working at home, with only 11% of respondents saying their schools were providing students with technology. The history of public education is rife with examples of institutional racism from school segregation to racial bias (Perszyk et al., 2019), which creates inequality in academic achievement and attainment and a greater number of dropouts and suspensions for students of color (de Brey et al., 2019). The evidence points to the digital divide as yet another example of institutional racism in American education.

In response, students and families are forced to be creative in getting access to broadband and computers, which often leads to the use of computers at public libraries and free hotspots at fast-food chains. Hampton et al. (2020) found that low-income students in both rural and urban Michigan were more likely to use their cell phones for internet access. The primary vehicle through which the federal government has tried to address access to broadband service is through its Lifeline program, which was originally created in 1985 to provide discounted landline telephone service. Today, it offers a $9.25 subsidy for mobile phone or broadband internet service for families at or below 135% of the federal poverty line. At the school level, the Federal Communications Commission's (FCC) E-rate program allows school districts and libraries to purchase access to telecommunications services, including broadband internet service with discounted rates of up to 90% depending on the area's poverty level (FCC, 2020). Furthermore, Chandra, Chang, et al. (2020) estimated that at the outset of the pandemic as many as 400,000 public school teachers lacked adequate internet connectivity showing the problems faced in educating students remotely is not just limited to student access.

In addition to greater broadband access, one way to address the digital divide is expanding access to devices, with programs that have provided computers to students having been found to improve student interest (Zilka, 2016) while also increasing student achievement and decreasing achievement gaps due to socio-economic status and different learning abilities (Harper & Milman, 2016). In 2013, the Obama administration created the ConnectED program to ensure all public schools had access to high-speed internet and to develop partnerships with corporations and nonprofits to enable schools to purchase technological devices at affordable rates. Thus, school districts were fighting the digital divide on two fronts: first they struggled to ensure students had access to devices and then the broadband access to use them.

COVID-19 as an Impetus for Policy Change

Policy scholars have devoted a great deal of time to understanding the process by which policy change is achieved. Chandra, Chang, et al. (2020) estimated that it would cost anywhere from $6 billion to $11 billion to close the digital divide during the COVID-19 pandemic and another $1 billion to address the divide among teachers lacking access to devices and/or internet connectivity. While this would be a significant investment, Ali et al. (2021) found that the cost of not addressing the digital divide is greater as not educating disconnected students would ultimately yield an annual loss of $22 billion to $33 billion in gross domestic product. In the case of the digital divide and COVID-19, John Kingdon's work on agendas and policy change is especially useful. Kingdon (2003) explains that focusing events are often needed for long-standing problems to be addressed. As discussed in the Introduction, the digital divide is not a new problem, but COVID-19 serves as a focusing event that creates the opportunity for solutions to be brought to bear. Lane McBride, the Managing Director of the Boston Consulting Group, which has authored multiple reports on the digital divide during the COVID-19 pandemic, discusses this possibility stating,

> We are in a unique moment to close the divide—while there is focus and urgency on the issue. To succeed in bridging the digital divide, efforts must take advantage of the momentum on the issue today and maintain the need even beyond the pandemic.
>
> *Lieberman, 2020*

Concurrently, the political environment or what Kingdon identifies as the politics stream must be conducive to achieving policy change and there needs to be available solutions from specialists such as interest groups, bureaucrats, and/or researchers among others which he refers to as the policy stream. When the problem, politics, and policy streams come together, Kingdon explains that a policy window opens that, while fleeting, allows for policy change to occur. In this work, we will assess whether COVID-19 opened a policy window that allowed for these four cities to address the digital divide for the students of color they serve.

The federal government has been providing aid to school districts and states to assist in accessing technology and connectivity. Congress appropriated over $67 billion dollars to K–12 education in the United States, first through the Coronavirus Aid, Relief, and Economic Security (CARES) Act in March 2020 and then the Coronavirus Response and Relief Supplemental Appropriations (CRRSA) Act relief package that was signed in December 2020 (Jordan, 2021). A deeper look at the funding shows why these funds may not fully address the problem. First, the CARES Act funding for K–12 education included $13.5 billion via the Elementary and Secondary School Emergency Relief Fund portion of the bill and was allocated based on the Title I funding formula with school districts having the ability to spend these funds however they wanted (Teich, 2020). With numerous costs associated with COVID-19, including facility improvements, personal protective equipment (PPE) for staff, and custodial needs, not all of this money could go to addressing the digital divide. Chandra, Fazlullah, et al. (2020) found in an October 2020 report that only $1.5 billion of CARES Act funding had been spent on addressing the digital divide in an analysis of 36 states. There was another $3 billion made available to governors to support K–12 education with that money suggested for use to change education models (Teich, 2020), which of course does not come close to the amount required. The CRRSA then provided $54 billion of funding to K–12 education (Jordan, 2021), but much of the motivation for the funding was to reopen schools that remained shuttered since the pandemic and providing remediation for lost learning time. Thus, what we hope to discover in this work is whether four school districts serving majority populations of students of color used the resources available to them to permanently address the digital divide.

Methodology

For this work, we will engage in a qualitative case study of four school districts. Case studies are sometimes criticized for an absence of generalizability to other cases whether those cases be communities, schools, or countries as well as their inability to allow for hypothesis testing (Flyvbjerg, 2016). However, for the purposes of this research, we are not testing existing theory but are exploring how four districts sought to overcome the digital divide when required to transition to remote learning. Furthermore, the absence of quantitative data, as the federal government waived the testing requirements of the Every Student Succeeds Act in response to the pandemic, further reinforces that qualitative research and specifically a case study approach is appropriate. Baškarada (2014) explains the value of case study research as, "case studies provide an opportunity for the researcher to gain a deep holistic view of the research problem" (p. 1).

Our primary sources of data are documents issued by school districts, which detail how they distributed educational resources and provided instruction during the spring and fall of 2020. This includes school district press releases, websites, and instructional and reopening plans. School district websites in some cases lacked consistency in the availability of policy documents online. Therefore, when necessary, we included social media postings and newspaper articles as secondary sources of information for our analysis. Our analysis was guided by assessing how districts provided instruction during the pandemic and worked to provide access to both technology and broadband internet service. Furthermore, we examined, when applicable, the impact of policies and guidelines issued by state governments, which governed district instructional practices during the pandemic. Lastly, we discuss how school districts partnered with community groups and/or corporations to address the digital divide.

TABLE 3.1 School District Demographics 2018–2019

School District	Number of Students Enrolled in District/ Total School Enrollment	Families in Poverty	Percent Hispanic	Percent African American	Broadband Internet Access	IEP Students	English Less Than Well Households
Allentown	16,946/21,930	33.1%	53%	10%	74.9%	3,575	10.9%
Atlanta	52,377/67,775	31.7%	4%	52%	78.1%	5,819	1.2%
Brownsville	44,402/47,885	40.5%	94%	0%	46.5%	5,383	12.5%
Detroit	49,931/127,340	45.5%	8%	78%	59.3%	7,738	3.5%

Source: U.S. Department of Education, National Center for Education Statistics, Common Core of Data, and Education Demographic and Geographic Estimates.

Note: The table provides data on enrollments, poverty, racial and ethnic makeup, Individualized Education Plans (IEP), broadband access and English language usage for students and families in the Allentown, Atlanta, Brownsville, and Detroit school districts.

In the field of education policy, scholars have focused on the inequities present in both large urban centers and even to some extent rural areas. However, smaller cities along with suburban and exurban communities are seeing increased populations of people of color. As such, we wanted to diversify the communities assessed with a balance of traditional urban school districts (Atlanta and Detroit) with growing communities of color (Allentown and Brownsville). From 2010 to 2019 for instance, Pennsylvania saw a 38% increase in its Latino population (Krogstad, 2020). This growth was driven in large part by Latinos settling in smaller cities such as Allentown where Latinos now comprise 52.2% of the city's population (U.S. Census Bureau, 2019). Brownsville, while being 94% Latino, grew from a city of 85,000 residents in 1980 to having an estimated 182,781 residents in 2019 (U.S. Census Bureau, 2019). Table 3.1 presents the demographic data of each of the four districts studied along with data on internet accessibility, the special education population, and the percentage of households in each district that speak English "less than well" according to data from the U.S. Department of Education.

A Tale of Four Districts

Allentown School District

On Wednesday, March 11, 2020, a single Allentown School District (ASD) employee became symptomatic, prompting a two-day school closure that would continue for more than a year. An online technology needs survey distributed to parents and students showed approximately 60% of students did not have access to a device at home, which led to 4,000 Chromebooks being loaned to students. As well, 20% of students did not have broadband access. This led to the district waiting until April 27, 2020, more than six weeks after they initially closed, to begin required remote instruction. The district established an At-Home Learning webpage where they posted optional enrichment and review materials for students to complete before mandated learning began. Paper copies of the materials for all grades could be picked up from elementary school buildings in conjunction with the distribution of grab-and-go lunches (ASD, 2020b). Thus, while many other districts in the Lehigh Valley re-started instruction within two weeks of the state shutdown (Palochko & Merlin, 2020), the digital divide prevented the ASD from engaging in required instruction.

The district used part of its $9.8 million from the CARES Act to purchase another 5,000 Chromebooks (Palochko, 2020a). The UNIDOS Foundation, a local nonprofit, raised $13,000 to provide over 100 Chromebooks to students in need. The district's website stated broadband access was available to students through two local cable companies, which offered free service to new customers for a limited time and that eligible families could use the Lifeline program to receive assistance for broadband service (ASD, 2020b). The district also purchased 3,500 more hotspots over the summer of 2020 for students to use in preparation for remote learning, which was funded by a grant from the Pennsylvania Department of Community and Economic Development. Thus, the district was relying on myriad sources for student connectivity and did not procure full access to broadband for their students. In January 2021, a partnership with T-Mobile through their Project 10Million program was announced, which would provide broadband access to 2,000 district families using wireless hotspots. The partnership will last for five years and was paid for with grant money (Peterson, 2021).

In July 2020, the district announced that they would not be reopening schools in the fall, "Due to the uncertainty surrounding the COVID-19 pandemic and gaps in the national supply chain of personal protective equipment (PPE)" (ASD, 2020a). They would reimagine their existing Virtual Academy as the ASD Virtual Campus for all students and highlighted three tenets—(1) expanding the use of technology, (2) implementing a 1:1 device model, and (3) developing community partnerships to ensure student accessibility. A Parent University website was set up with videos to show parents how to do everything from using Zoom and Google Classroom to how to create an email account (ASD, 2020c). The videos were presented in English, Spanish, and Arabic. Furthermore, the late-fall spike in COVID-19 cases and guidance from the Pennsylvania Department of Education that districts should consider remote instruction in such instances also accounted for why the district did not reopen their schools. Parents were once again surveyed on their instructional preference for the fourth quarter of the academic year with the district announcing a plan for elementary students to return to in-person learning on April 19, 2021, with secondary students to follow a week later in a hybrid instructional model. As these plans were being developed, the superintendent of the district, Thomas Parker, announced his resignation effective May 1, 2021.

Allentown struggled to overcome the digital divide during the pandemic. Despite beginning remote learning in the spring of 2020, access and technology issues persisted as the district remained closed to in-person learning to start the 2020–2021 school year. The district did seek out community partnerships to address these challenges, but there is evidence that the Commonwealth of Pennsylvania could have done more to help the district. When schools were closed for the remainder of the 2019–2020 school year, the Pennsylvania Department of Education announced a $5 million grant program for low-income districts to purchase technology, but Allentown received no funds from the program, possibly due to previously receiving state funding unrelated to the pandemic (Palochko, 2020b). Additionally, a study published by the PA Budget and Policy Center found that Pennsylvania not using the Basic Education Funding formula to distribute state-allocated CARES Act funding cost the ASD over $4 million, with similar shortfalls for districts across the Commonwealth with majority African American and/or Latino/a populations (Polson & Henninger-Voss, 2020).

Atlanta Public Schools

On March 12, 2020, ten days after the first confirmed COVID-19 case in Georgia, the Atlanta Public Schools (APS) released a memo stating that all school buildings will be closed until at least March 31, 2020. APS would not reopen as Governor Brian Kemp ordered all schools in the state of Georgia to remain closed for the rest of the academic year on April 1, 2020 (Carstarphen, 2020b). The district responded quickly to this impending crisis for their students. On March 14, 2020, they announced that Xfinity Wi-Fi hotspots would be available to those who need them, for free. The district also notified families that Comcast would be offering free internet for 60 days to families who receive public assistance. Teachers were instructed to prepare six weeks' worth of instructional packets for their students to utilize while they were learning from home (Carstarphen, 2020a).

On March 23, 2020, APS began distributing 7,500 iPads to first- and second-grade students as part of a Tablet2Read program. The district also distributed 8,000 laptops to sixth- to eighth-grade students. Nine thousand hotspots were available for students in seventh to eleventh grades, with many families taking advantage of Xfinity's free Wi-Fi program. Families had until March 31, 2020, to pick up their child's school-issued device for online learning (Carstarphen, 2020a).

The district released a "Sustained Distance Learning" schedule at the end of March in response to public outcry from parents. Parents claimed their children were overwhelmed with the transition to online learning and the amount of work they were given to complete while at home. The district set virtual instruction time limits for each grade, with Kindergarten through fifth grade receiving three hours maximum of virtual instruction a day and ninth- to twelfth-grade students receiving five hours maximum of virtual instruction a day. Toward the middle of April, the district transitioned to a four-day instructional week to allow one day for teachers to have remediation time with students who were struggling (Carstarphen, 2020c).

The state of Georgia received $450 million in funding provided by the CARES Act. APS received $22 million; however, that number dwindled to $17 million once indirect costs, administrative overhead, and shares to private schools were covered. The CARES Act money went toward school lunches, the cleaning of facilities along with hazard pay for maintenance workers, mental health initiatives, professional development for teachers and staff, and supplemental learning materials (Bracken, 2020).

APS also received financial help from many community partners. The Get Our Kids Connected Campaign was formed by Comcast and APS to help bridge the digital divide, and Intercontinental Exchange, a technology firm based in Atlanta, donated $1.3 million to the campaign to help the district purchase computers for students. Trinity HealthShare, a nonprofit healthcare ministry, also donated $50,000 to the campaign. The United Way, Atlanta Tech Village, Caring for Others, and Rainbow Village were among other companies and nonprofits to donate and provide financial aid to the digital divide crisis among students in the district (APS, 2020).

APS decided on fully virtual instruction for at least the first nine weeks of the 2020–2021 school year, which was extended to the end of 2020 to ensure administration and staff could formulate a reopening plan that was safe for educators and students. Pre-Kindergarten through second-grade students along with Special Education students returned to in-person learning on January 25, 2021. Grades 3 through 5 returned to in-person learning on February 8, 2021, and Grades 6–12 returned to in-person learning on February 16, 2021. All students adhered to a four-day school schedule with one day for asynchronous learning, and parents and guardians did have the option to keep their children fully remote if they preferred (APS, 2021).

Brownsville Independent School District

The Brownsville Independent School District (BISD) closed on March 13, 2020, for spring break and students never returned as schools throughout Texas were closed by order of Governor Greg Abbott. The district was unable to implement a fully online learning model as it would not have been able to provide devices to more than half of its students. The district was able to instruct approximately 60% of the student population online, while the remaining 40% of students who lacked access to devices or broadband were given printed instructional packets to continue their learning (Long, 2020a).

At the conclusion of the academic year, BISD distributed over 22,000 learning packs to elementary school students, which included books and other instructional materials in math, science, and social studies to mitigate the regression in learning that took place due to the pandemic (Long, 2020c). Approximately one-third of the materials were distributed in Spanish. BISD maintained virtual instruction to begin the 2020–2021 school year as the Rio Grande Valley faced its largest COVID-19 surge in the summer of 2020. The district participated in the state of Texas' Operation Connectivity initiative. Under the initiative, Governor Greg Abbott allocated $200 million of state CARES Act funding to match CARES Act funding used by Texas school districts to purchase over one million devices and Wi-Fi hotspots. The program allowed the state to make bulk purchases on behalf of the participating school districts that not only helped with supply chain problems but created costs savings of 20%–40% (Abbott, 2020). The district was also able to procure some additional technology via donations and contributions from local retailers, such as Boost Mobile, Walmart, and Sam's Club (Long, 2020b).

The district purchased 10,000 iPads, 21,000 Chromebooks, and 19,000 hotspots (some of which were provided via Sprint's 1Million Project); however, thousands of devices and hotspots did not arrive prior to the start of the school year. In response, the district enabled 20 school buses to serve as Wi-Fi hotspots, most of which parked at district schools from 7:30 a.m. to 4:30 p.m. each day. Additionally, for those without devices, which was estimated to be less than 15% of students at the start of the school year,

> The district is providing non-digital, paper-based versions of instructional content, including the consumable Elementary, Middle and High School textbooks in the core content area(s), or instructional packets will be available for content areas to access exercises and supports. Students and parents are encouraged to submit student work information via text messages, remind app, and Class Dojo or other means. The district will implement traditional grading and phone check-ins to measure academic progress in these situations.
>
> *BISD, 2020b*

In October 2020, after operating remotely to start the year, the district put into place a staggered reopening plan starting with those students who did not have access to technology. Also coinciding with the beginning of the school year, the district announced a partnership with local stakeholders, including the Brownsville Public Utilities Board, Port of Brownsville, Texas Southmost College, The University of Texas Rio Grande Valley, the Greater Brownsville Incentives Corporation, and the City of Brownsville to create a plan that will improve broadband access and speed to the residents of Brownsville. Following the staggered soft reopening, BISD reopened to students at every grade level on November 30, 2020, but gave students the option to continue distance learning for the remainder of the school year if they desired (BISD, 2020c). As of March 2021, 14% of students were attending in-person instruction (Long, 2021).

Detroit Public Schools Community District

On March 16, 2020, the Detroit Public Schools Community District (DPSCD) closed all Kindergarten through 12th-grade schools for three weeks in response to COVID-19. Governor Gretchen Whitmer signed Executive Order 2020-35 on April 4, 2020, which ordered all schools to close their doors for the remainder of the school year. Kindergarten through eighth-grade teachers at the DPSCD were instructed to create learning packets that would be available for students to pick up by March 18. The high school students were provided with PSAT/SAT workbooks until students were able to obtain school-issued laptops. Students and families also received regular check-ins and phone calls from school staff to ensure students had the materials necessary for them to continue learning from home. Work packets were used late into April for students who did not have access to technology (DPSCD, 2020a).

The district estimated that over 90% of their students needed the devices and technology required to succeed in online learning (DPSCD, 2020b). Although the district had been working on bridging the digital divide for the past three years, the COVID-19 pandemic ultimately uncovered that the vast majority of Detroit's public school students were falling victim to the digital divide. A community partnership between Quicken Loans, DTE Energy, the City of Detroit, and Skillman Foundation pledged to donate over $23 million in tablets and high-speed internet connections to students in the DPSCD. The Rocket Mortgage Classic golf tournament raised approximately $1.4 million to help end the digital divide in Detroit as well (DPSCD, 2020c). DPSCD was given $85,120,566 from the CARES Act, with the money being used for PPE and technology. Approximately $25 million was spent on PPE including face masks, hand sanitizing stations, plexiglass barriers, and improvements in the heating, ventilation, and air conditioning systems. The district also announced that first-year teacher salaries would be increasing from $38,000 to $51,071 to help retain teachers (DPSCD, 2020d).

DPSCD schools reopened on September 8, 2020, with reduced class sizes and social distancing practices; however, that did not stop COVID-19 cases from rising within the district. On November 16, Detroit public schools transitioned to fully remote learning citing an uptick in cases throughout the city. The school district did not return to in-person instruction until March 8, 2021. Families still have the option to have their children learn remotely from home. Teachers were also given the option to teach from home or return for in-person instruction. The district released new COVID-19 guidelines that include a limit of no more than 20 students per classroom (DPSCD, 2021).

Discussion

All four of the districts studied struggled both to provide fully online instruction during the pandemic and to return to in-person instruction in the fall of 2020. The African American and Latino/a students from these communities likely fell further behind their fellow students in wealthier districts because of the pandemic given the experiences we have described. While the federal government and, to a lesser extent, states and community partners contributed to overcoming the problem, the digital divide cannot be solved solely by money. Chandra, Fazlullah, et al. (2020)

discusses a multistep process for addressing the divide, including an analysis of curriculum and device compatibility as well as broadband infrastructure. Furthermore, the Council of Chief State School Officers (2020) designed an assessment blueprint for school districts to explain the data collection needed to make these decisions. This explains why the pandemic on its own did not bring about the elimination of the digital divide.

In looking at these four districts, we see that the size of the municipality and the presence of potential corporate benefactors can be impactful. Allentown and Brownsville as smaller cities had fewer corporate and community partners to work with and were more dependent on their state governments. In this case, Allentown struggled to get adequate support from the Commonwealth of Pennsylvania given the questionable model they employed in distributing CARES Act funding. While Brownsville had some success in acquiring devices and hotspots through Operation Connectivity, they struggled to get local governments in the Rio Grande Valley to contribute their funds to creating broadband infrastructure (Reyba, 2020). Atlanta and Detroit had their own challenges in overcoming the digital divide, but the pool of corporate resources they could draw from was much larger, which enabled them to secure millions of dollars in outside donations.

Despite the less-than-rosy findings presented here, it is possible that the pandemic has provided the funding and motivation to address the problem. If local education agencies were able to obtain data during the pandemic to help them understand how to best eliminate the divide in their communities, the streams of problems, policy, and politics may have finally aligned. Ali et al. (2021) find that federal aid "closed 20% to 40% of the K–12 connectivity divide and 40% to 60% of the device divide as of December 2020" (p. 5), but their report notes that these efforts have been more successful in shrinking the divide among Black students compared to Latino/a students.

The American Rescue Plan (ARP) brings another approximately $130 billion to K–12 education. While the Biden administration has been focused on reopening schools, there is funding in the ARP to help overcome the digital divide. School districts are required to spend 20% of their funds on addressing learning loss through evidence-based programs, but educational technology is listed as one of the areas that qualifies (Alliance for Excellent Education, 2021). Additionally, the law includes $7.171 billion to create the Emergency Connectivity Fund, which will address "the Homework Gap" for students who do not have access to devices or broadband at home through the E-rate program. This will enable school districts to be reimbursed for 100% of the purchase costs of "eligible equipment and/or advanced telecommunications and information services" (FCC, 2021), including connected devices, modems, routers, and Wi-Fi hotspots.

Future research should examine how districts are developing plans to address the divide if those assessments did not take place during the pandemic. Our work found that districts were examining which devices would best serve their students but were often dependent on multiple means of providing broadband access. Partnerships between local governments and school districts to provide broadband should be looked at for cost savings and providing what has become a vital utility for people of all ages in the 21st century. School districts cannot produce this infrastructure on their own, and this type of intergovernmental partnership would be invaluable in ensuring racial and ethnic equity for broadband access. Under the ARP, the funding to address the digital divide exists, and how these funds are spent will provide a fruitful pathway for future research. The concern for many districts serving majority African American and Latino/a populations is that as vaccination rates climb and more schools are able to reopen, these school districts could decide to focus more on in-person remediation, facility concerns, or any of the other countless inequities that exist for their students, which could divert funding from technological investments that address the digital divide.

Notes

1 A device for this work is defined as a laptop, tablet, or desktop computer regardless of brand or operating system. It does not however include cell phones.
2 Underserved students were defined by a student being classified in any of these three categories: (a) a family income of less than $36,000, (b) parents' highest education level being a high school diploma or less, or (c) the student's race or ethnicity is African American, Hispanic/Latino, Native American/Alaska Native, or Native Hawaiian/Other Pacific Islander.
3 It should be noted that while this work focuses on the experience of urban districts educating students of color, the digital divide is also an issue in rural areas. In low-income urban communities, access to devices and broadband is often an economic issue in terms of having access to but not being able to afford technology and internet service. Whereas in low-income rural communities, financial and infrastructure issues exist in that the FCC estimates that most of the 21 million people in the United States who cannot access broadband internet service live in rural areas (Reston, 2020).

References

AASA—The School Superintendents Association. (2020, June 12). Report of Initial Findings: COVID Survey 2 Impact on Public Schools. Retrieved from https://aasa.org/uploadedFiles/AASA_Blog(1)/COVID-19%20and%20Schools%20Detailing%20the%20Continued%20Impact_Intial%20Findings_6_16_2020_FN.pdf

Abbott, G. (2020, August 20). Governor Abbott Announces Procurement of over 1 Million Services, Wi-Fi Hotspots Through Operation Connectivity. Office of the Governor. Retrieved from https://tea.texas.gov/sites/default/files/covid/Governor-Abbott-Announces-Procurement-Of-Over-1-Million-Devices-WiFi-Hotspots-Through-Operation-Connectivity.pdf

The Administration of President Barack H. Obama. (2013). ConnectED Initiative. Retrieved from https://obamawhitehouse.archives.gov/issues/education/k-12/connected

Ali, T., Chandra, S., Cherukumilli, S., Fazlullah, A., Hill, H., McAlpine, N., McBride, L., Vaduganathan, N., Weiss, D., & Wu, M. (2021). *Looking Back, Looking Forward: What It Will Take to Permanently Close the K–12 Digital Divide*. San Francisco, CA: Common Sense Media. Retrieved from www.commonsensemedia.org/sites/default/files/uploads/kids_action/final_-_what_it_will_take_to_permanently_close_the_k-12_digital_divide_vjan26_1.pdf

Allentown School District. (2020a, July 22). ASD Announces Plans to Open Schools Virtually. Retrieved from www.allentownsd.org/cms/One.aspx?portalId=521953&pageId= 12149919

Allentown School District. (2020b). Corona Virus (COVID-19) Updates. Retrieved from www.allentownsd.org/departments/community_and_student_services/health_services/ COVID19

Allentown School District. (2020c). Virtual Campus Parent University. Retrieved from www.allentownsd.org/cms/One.aspx?portalId=521953&pageId=12242843

Alliance for Excellent Education. (2021). American Rescue Plan Act summary of K-12 Education Provisions. Retrieved from https://all4ed.org/wp-content/uploads/2021/ 03/American-Rescue-Plan-Act-Summary.pdf

Anderson, M., & Perrin, A. (2018, October 26). Nearly One-in-Five Teens Can't Always Finish Their Homework Because of the Digital Divide. *Pew Research*. Retrieved from www.pewresearch.org/fact-tank/2018/10/26/nearly-one-in-five-teens-cant-always- finish-their-homework-because-of-the-digital-divide/

Atlanta Public Schools. (2020). Get Our Kids Connected. Thank You to Our Donors. *Atlanta Public Schools*. Retrieved from www.atlantapublicschools.us/Page/62089

Atlanta Public Schools. (2021). Return + Learn Phase II. Retrieved from www.atlanta publicschools.us/reopen

Baškarada, S. (2014). Qualitative case studies guidelines. The Qualitative Report, 19(40), 1–25.

Bracken, L. (2020, May 21). Budget Commission Meeting. Finance Division. *Atlanta Public Schools*. Retrieved from www.atlantapublicschools.us/site/handlers/filedownload. ashx?moduleinstanceid=62170&dataid=82555&FileName=May%2021%20Budget%20 Commission%20Final.pdf

Brownsville Independent School District. (2020a, October 8). Update: Soft Reopening Plan by Grade Level and Programs – Faculty and Staff. Retrieved from www.bisd.us/ news-and-events

Brownsville Independent School District. (2020b). BISD Asynchronous Plan. Retrieved from https://resources.finalsite.net/images/v1616784951/bisdus/esqbx20n3vglcbk9v1lg/00- BISDAsynchronousPlanningFinal9-17-2020.pdf

Brownsville Independent School District. (2020c). BISD Reopening Plan. Starting Strong. Retrieved from https://resources.finalsite.net/images/v1605020319/bisdus/ zrqumgbkxyofylkveo8c/01_ReopeningPlan.pdf

Carstarphen, M. J. (2020a, March 23). *Important COVID-19 Updates for APS Families and Stakeholders*. [Memorandum]. Superintendent. Retrieved from www.atlantapublicschools. us/cms/lib/GA01000924/Centricity/Domain/25/MJC%20COVID-19%20Parent%20 Memo%203.23.2020%20Final.pdf

Carstarphen, M. J. (2020b, March 26). *Important School Closure Update*. [Memorandum]. Superintendent. Retrieved from www.atlantapublicschools.us/cms/lib/GA01000924/ Centricity/Domain/25/MJC%20COVID-19%20Parent%20Memo%203.26.2020%20 Final.pdf

Carstarphen, M. J. (2020c, March 31). *Important COVID-19 Updates for APS Families*. [Memorandum]. Superintendent. Retrieved from www.atlantapublicschools.us/cms/lib/ GA01000924/Centricity/Domain/25/MJC%20COVID-19%20Parent%20Memo%20 3.30.2020%20FINAL.pdf

Chandra, S., Chang, A., Day, L., Fazlullah, A., Liu, J., McBride, L., Mudalige, T., & Weiss, D. (2020). *Closing the K–12 Digital Divide in the Age of Distance Learning*. San Francisco, CA: Common Sense Media; Boston, MA: Boston Consulting Group.

Chandra, S., Fazlullah, A., Hill, H., Lynch, J., McBride, L., Weiss, D., & Wu, M. (2020). *Connect All Students: How States and School Districts Can Close the Digital Divide*. San Francisco, CA: Common Sense Media.

Council of Chief State School Officers (2020). Restart & Recovery: Home Digital Access Data Collection: Blueprint for State Education Leaders. July. Retrieved from: https://ccsso.org/sites/default/files/2020-07/7.22.20_CCSSO%20Home%20Digital%20Access%20Data%20Collection%20Blueprint%20for%20State%20Leaders.pdf

de Brey, C., Musu, L., McFarland, J., Wilkinson-Flicker, S., Diliberti, M., Zhang, A., Branstetter, C., & Wang, X. (2019). *Status and Trends in the Education of Racial and Ethnic Groups 2018*. National Center for Education Statistics. U.S. Department of Education. Retrieved from https://nces.ed.gov/pubsearch/pubsinfo.asp?pubid=2019038

Detroit Public Schools Community District. (2020a, March 13). DPSCD Rolls Out Action Plan to Families During COVID-19 Three-Week Closure. Retrieved from www.detroitk12.org/cms/lib/MI50000060/Centricity/Domain/5833/R%2020.03.13%20COVID%2019%20FINAL.pdf

Detroit Public Schools Community District. (2020b, April 23). Connected Futures Frequently Asked Questions. Retrieved from www.detroitk12.org/cms/lib/MI50000060/Centricity/Domain/84/Connected-Futures-FAQ_FINAL-4.23.20-.pdf

Detroit Public Schools Community District. (2020c). Connected Futures and Technology and Family Resource Hubs. Retrieved from www.detroitk12.org/Domain/37

Detroit Public Schools Community District. (2020d). FY 2020–2021 Budget Detail. Retrieved from www.detroitk12.org/cms/lib/MI50000060/Centricity/Domain/4019/FY%2021%20Budget%20Detail%20Final.pdf

Detroit Public Schools Community District. (2021, February 25). *2/25 Return to In-Person Update*. Detroit Public Schools Community District. Retrieved from www.detroitk12.org/site/default.aspx?PageType=3&DomainID=4&ModuleInstanceID=7278&ViewID=6446EE88-D30C-497E-9316-3F8874B3E108&RenderLoc=0&FlexDataID=50449&PageID=1

Federal Communications Commission. (2020). E-Rate: Universal Service Program for Schools and Libraries. Retrieved from www.fcc.gov/consumers/guides/universal-service-program-schools-and-libraries-e-rate

Federal Communications Commission. (2021). Wireline Competition Bureau Seeks Comment on Emergency Connectivity Fund for Educational Connections and Devices to Address the Homework Gap During the Pandemic. Public Comment. WC Docket No. 21-93. Retrieved from https://docs.fcc.gov/public/attachments/DA-21-317A1.pdf

Finley, K. (2020, April 9). When School Is Online, the Digital Divide Grows Greater. *WIRED*. Retrieved from www.wired.com/story/school-online-digital-divide-grows-greater/

Flyvbjerg, B. (2016). Five Misunderstandings About Case-Study Research. *Qualitative Inquiry*, *12*(2), 219. Retrieved from https://doi.org/10.1177/1077800405284363

Hampton, K. N., Fernandez, L., Robinson, C. T., & Bauer, J. M. (2020). Broadband and Student Performance Gaps. James H. and Mary B. Quello Center, Michigan State University. Retrieved from https://doi.org/10.25335/BZGY-3V91

Harper, B., & Milman, N. B. (2016). One-to-One Technology in K–12 Classrooms: A Review of the Literature from 2004 Through 2014. *Journal of Research on Technology in Education, 48*(2), 129–142.

Jordan, Phyllis W. 2021. What Congressional Covid Funding Means for K-12 Schools. FutureEd. December 20. Retrieved from https://www.future-ed.org/what-congressional-covid-funding-means-for-k-12-schools/

Kingdon, J.W. (2003). *Agendas, Alternatives, and Public Policy* (2nd ed.). New York: Addison-Wesley.

Kozol, J. (1991). *Savage Inequalities: Children in America's Schools*. New York: Harper Perennial.

Krogstad, J. M. (2020, July 10). Hispanics Have Accounted for More Than Half of Total U.S. Population Growth Since 2010. *Pew Research Center*. Accessed December 15, 2020, from www.pewresearch.org/fact-tank/2020/07/10/hispanics-have-accounted-for-more-than-half-of-total-u-s-population-growth-since-2010/

Lieberman, Mark. 2020. 5 Insights for How to Tackle the Digital Divide During the Coronavirus and Beyond. Education Week. April 21. Retrieved from: https://www.edweek.org/technology/5-insights-for-how-to-tackle-the-digital-divide-during-the-coronavirus-and-beyond/2020/04

Long, G. (2020a, May 20). BISD: Summer School Online Only; In-Person Instruction Ruled Out. *The Brownsville Herald*. Retrieved from https://myrgv.com/local-news/2020/05/20/bisd-summer-school-online-only-in-person-instruction-ruled-out/

Long, G. (2020b, June 10). Getting Connected: CIS, BISD Distribute Free Tablets. *The Brownsville Herald*. Retrieved from https://myrgv.com/local-news/2020/06/10/getting-connected-cis-bisd-distribute-free-tablets/

Long, G. (2020c, June 17). Summer Learning: BISD Hands Out Books Ahead of Next School Year. *The Brownsville Herald*. Retrieved from https://myrgv.com/local-news/2020/06/17/summer-learning-bisd-hands-out-books-ahead-of-next-school-year/

Long, G. (2021, March 15). Adapting to Challenges; Schools Mark Year of Pandemic. *The Brownsville Herald*. Retrieved from https://myrgv.com/local-news/education/2021/03/15/adapting-to-challenges-schools-mark-year-of-pandemic/

Moore, R., Vitale, D., & Stawinoga, N. (2018, August). The Digital Divide and Educational Equity: A Look at Students with Very Limited Access to Electronic Devices at Home. *ACT* (Iowa City, IA). Retrieved from www.act.org/content/dam/act/unsecured/documents/R1698-digital-divide-2018-08.pdf

Morgan, I., & Amerikaner, A. (2018). Funding Gaps 2018. The Education Trust. Retrieve from https://edtrust.org/resource/funding-gaps-2018/

Organization for Economic Co-operation and Development. (2000). The Digital Divide Within Formal School Education: Causes and Consequences. Retrieved from www.oecd.org/site/schoolingfortomorrowknowledgebase/themes/ict/thedigitaldividewithinformalschooleducationcausesandconsequences.htm

Palochko, J. (2020a, April 17). Allentown School District Buying 5,000 Chromebooks for Students During Coronavirus Closure. *The Morning Call*. Retrieved from www.mcall.com/news/education/mc-nws-allentown-school-board-20200417-dlt4qy4h4rc6njv3vdy3uhbo4q-story.html

Palochko, J. (2020b, April 25). Allentown School District Shut Out of State Money to Buy Computers for Students During Coronavirus. *The Morning Call*. Retrieved from www.mcall.com/coronavirus/mc-nws-coronavirus-allentown-schools-state-money-computers-20200428-dgny4udtmfaklmfnen5tm4atny-story.html

Palochko, J., & Merlin, M. (2020, March 25). Coronavirus Highlights Inequity Among Lehigh Valley Schools, as Students with Least Stand to Lose Most During Closure, Advocates Say. *The Morning Call*. Retrieved from www.mcall.com/coronavirus/mc-nws-coronavirus-school-districts-closures-online-learning-20200325-vkkkehs2wngurnugbhga5wqety-story.html

Perszyk, D. R., Lei, R. F., Bodenhausen, G. V., Richeson, J. A., & Waxman, S. R. (2019). Bias at the Intersection of Race and Gender: Evidence from Preschool-Aged Children. *Developmental Science*, *22*(3). https://doi.org/10.1111/desc.12788

Peterson, M. (2021, January 19). Over 2,000 Allentown School District Homes to Get Free Internet in Partnership with T-Mobile. *The Morning Call*. Retrieved from www.mcall.com/news/local/allentown/mc-nws-allentown-schools-hot-spots-20210118-22lcoduk4bbonlssqxcboncvr4-story.html

Polson, D., & Henninger-Voss, E. (2020, December). Pennsylvania Distributes Emergency K–12 School Funding Backwards: The Fewest Dollars Go to School Districts with the Greatest Need. *PA Budget and Policy Center*. Retrieved from https://krc-pbpc.org/wp-content/uploads/PBPC-CARES-Act-Dist.-FINAL.pdf

Reston, M. (2020, April 9). Pandemic Underscores Digital Divide Facing Students and Educators. *CNN*. Retrieved from www.cnn.com/2020/04/09/politics/digital-divide-education-coronavirus/index.html

Reyba, N. (2020, September 30). Brownsville Tables Item to Enter Into CARES Relief Funding Agreement with BISD. *The Brownsville Herald*. Retrieved from https://myrgv.com/featured/2020/09/30/brownsville-tables-item-to-enter-into-cares-relief-funding-agreement-with-bisd/

Somos Health Care and Latino Decisions. (2020, April). SOMOS: COVID-19 Crisis National Latino Survey. Retrieved from https://latinodecisions.com/wp-content/uploads/2020/04/SOMOS-COVID19-Svy-Exec-Summary.pdf

The State of Michigan. (2020, March 10). Michigan Announces First Presumptive Positive Cases of COVID-19. *Michigan.gov*. Retrieved from www.michigan.gov/coronavirus/0,9753,7-406-98158-521365--,00.html

Teich, A. G. (2020, July 15). CARES Act Funding: A Stimulus Primer for Districts. Tech and Learning. Retrieved from www.techlearning.com/how-to/cares-act-funding-a-stimulus-primer-for-districts

U.S. Census Bureau. (2019). Quick Facts. Accessed May 24, 2021. Retrieved from www.census.gov/quickfacts/fact/table/brownsvillecitytexas/PST045219 www.census.gov/quickfacts/allentowncitypennsylvania

Zilka, G. C. (2016). Reducing the Digital Divide Among Children Who Received Desktop or Hybrid Computers for the Home. *Journal of Information Technology Education: Research, 15*, 233–251. Retrieved from www.informingscience.org/Publications/3519

4

COVID-19 RACIAL DISPARITIES

A Content Analysis of News Media Coverage

Sarah V. Gordon-Brilla, Dana L. Rogers, Jackson Higginbottom, Leila M. Ensha, and Ryan A. Sutherland

Introduction

In 2020, the COVID-19 pandemic created an urgent need for effective communication in shaping the public's understanding of the contagious viral disease, its impact on populations, and its spread. The news media played a vital role in providing the public with important information about the health threat. As a communication vehicle, it has the power to inform and educate as well as shape public perceptions and attitudes (Bullock et al., 2001). Research suggests this effect is even more pronounced during catastrophic events (Ball-Rokeach & DeFleur, 1976; Shih et al., 2008). As COVID-19 spread across the United States, it became clear that certain populations were disproportionately impacted by its effects.

COVID-19 and Racial Health Disparities

Information from the Centers for Disease Control and Prevention (CDC) shows significant racial disparities in COVID-19 rates and prevalence (CDC, 2020). Black and Indigenous people contracted the disease at five times the rate of White people, and Hispanic/Latino communities experienced COVID at a rate four times higher than that of White people (CDC, 2020a, 2020b). While noteworthy, such racial health disparities are not specific to COVID-19 and have been a major focus of public health research for years (CDC, 2020b). The National Institutes of Health (n.d.) defines health disparities as when members of certain populations do not experience the same health status as other groups.

Research suggests there is a positive association between discrimination or racism and chronic health conditions or other self-reported indicators of ill-health (Williams & Mohammed, 2008). Racism is defined as a system that uses race to preferentially allocate resources and goods to groups regarded as superior

DOI: 10.4324/9781003268710-4

and/or dominant (Bonilla-Silva, 1996; Williams & Mohammed, 2008). Racism is deeply embedded in the systems, culture, and institutions of American society, allowing discrimination to persist in institutional structures and policies (Williams & Mohammed, 2008). Calling attention to societal racism and racial inequities is required for significant change. The extent to which this issue is reported and how it is framed by the media can impact the public's understanding and assessment of its importance (Niederdeppe et al., 2013). With this in mind, we examined the news coverage of the COVID-19 pandemic in New Haven, Connecticut, a nationally representative city, to help provide a better understanding of the public's perception of the salience of the racial disparities that the crisis highlighted.

Theoretical Framework

Research on agenda setting and framing suggests the reporting of news significantly influences perceptions and attitudes (Bullock et al., 2001; McCombs & Shaw, 1972). Given the public's reliance on the media during times of crisis, this influence may be significantly enhanced. Raising awareness about a public health issue and influencing public understanding may motivate public support and increase pressure for policy changes (Barnes et al., 2008; Pacheco & Boushey, 2014; Walsh-Childers, 1994; Winsten, 1985). With this in mind, we used the theoretical frameworks of agenda setting and framing to examine local media coverage of racial inequities within COVID-19 media stories to provide a better understanding of the messages being conveyed to the public.

Agenda Setting Theory

Agenda setting theory asserts that the media effectively tells people what they should be thinking about and the issues they should focus on (McCombs & Shaw, 1972; McCombs, 2004). On a macro level, it posits a link between the issues that are being emphasized in the media and the importance the public assigns those issues (Dearing & Rogers, 1996). The more extensive the media coverage of an issue, the more cues media consumers receive regarding the relative significance of that issue. The media make certain issues more salient to the audience through coverage and positioning and, conversely, depress the importance of other information via a lack of coverage. Especially pertinent to the subject of this study, research examining agenda setting effects suggests the media agenda displays the perspectives of a ruling class (Rogers & Dearing, 1988). Specifically, a study by Chow and Knowles (2016), conceptualizing agenda setting as a process bolstering in-group dominance by barring issues related to social inequities, found evidence that some members of the dominant racial group set the racial agenda by removing the issue of racial inequity from public discourse. An absence of information about race and racial disparities in the media may inhibit public perception of the salience of the issue, diminishing awareness of the topic among policymakers leading to a lack of effort from a systems level to reduce such disparities.

Framing Theory

Framing theory may be used to examine how an issue is portrayed by the media. According to Cappella and Jamieson (1997), the process of framing in mass communication is when the media is able to focus the viewer's attention on a particular issue or subject. What is salient and what is unimportant is determined by the inclusion or exclusion of selected words, angles, themes, and concepts. Thus, framing draws attention to certain aspects of an issue while minimizing attention to others (Cappella & Jamieson, 1997). Framing theory rests on the assumption that the way an issue is portrayed in the news can impact the way audiences understand it (Scheufele & Tewksbury, 2007). Notably, journalistic framing has been shown to influence public opinion of particular issues and, in turn, policy formation (Gans, 1983; Pan & Kosicki, 1993). Research has examined different framing devices, such as emotional appeals, tone, and source, that influence people's perceptions, attitudes, and behavior. Framing studies examining emotional appeals, such as fear and anger, suggest fear can help facilitate persuasion, indicating that the expectancy of a negative outcome may reduce the likelihood of a specific behavior (Rogers, 1985; Rosenstock, 1990). Similarly, the tone of a news story has been found to significantly affect audiences' perception of and support for an issue. For example, Wanta et al. (2004) found that the more negative the tone of news coverage a nation received in the media, the more likely respondents were to think negatively about that nation. Another dimension of framing in the news media is the choice of information source. In using officials representing both government and professional entities as information sources, journalists present a particular picture of the issue they are covering (Steele, 1995). Officials are often used as sources for news stories by journalists, and research in this area indicates that official sources are deemed more credible than unofficial sources (Armstrong & Nelson, 2005). As people tend to believe official figures, citing expert sources in news stories can have a significant impact on public opinion (Page et al., 1987). The way in which the media frames coverage of health issues and diseases impacts audiences' understanding of those issues as well as their attitudinal and behavioral reactions (Freimuth et al., 1984; Jordan, 1993; Snyder & Rouse, 1995; Tian & Stewart, 2005). Research suggests the framing of health-related news stories may affect an individual's search for care, create alarm, motivate support for a resolution, impact regulation, or even direct research and development (Gorman, 1993; Nelkin, 1989; Winsten, 1985). It is important to examine the extent of issue coverage in the media and how the issues are framed, as coverage may significantly impact public health and public health policy.

In this study, we examine issue coverage and issue framing within the New Haven news media during the first six months of the COVID-19 pandemic. This research helps to broaden the understanding of agenda setting and framing during a crisis. It also provides an increased understanding of the messages the public may have received within the pandemic news stories concerning racism and racial disparities and, thus, potentially impact policy change needed to address such inequities.

Research Objectives

Based on research indicating that news message exposure may play a role in the public's awareness of an issue and their perception of the salience of that issue, we ask: *To what extent are racial disparities and racism addressed in news coverage of the COVID-19 pandemic, distributed within the New Haven area between March 1, 2020, and August 31, 2020?*

Journalists often frame their stories through the sources they use, and these sources can be influential in how people view issues (Cohen, 1963; Kim & Weaver, 2003). One factor that may influence how the public thinks around an issue is whether the sources in news stories are considered credible. Research in this area suggests that expert sources, such as scientists, research reports, and health professionals, lend greater credibility to news stories (Ramsey, 1999). As a result, we posit the following research question: *How many of the news stories feature experts as sources of information?*

Additional framing mechanisms that could affect public perception and understanding of issues include the tone of the story and the extent emotional appeals are used (Rogers, 1985; Rosenstock, 1990; Wanta et al., 2004). With this in mind, we posit the following research questions: *How often are emotional appeals used in the news media reporting? Is the overall tone of the news coverage positive, neutral, or negative?*

Method

We conducted a content analysis of news coverage of the COVID-19 pandemic for the New Haven area from March 1, 2020, through August 31, 2020. The population of New Haven, Connecticut, is 130,331 as of 2019 and consists of 32% of residents who identify as Black or African American, 30% Latino, and a staggering 48% of the city's residents are considered low income. The racial makeup of New Haven's population mirrors the same proportions of the population of the United States, making it a nationally representative state (U.S. Census Bureau, 2020). Additionally, 87.5% of households in New Haven have a computer, and 81.6% of households have a broadband internet subscription (U.S. Census Bureau, 2019).

Sampling

Media news outlets were selected based on their exposure and readership in the New Haven area. Sources include WFSB Channel 3, NBC Connecticut, WTNH Channel 8, *New Haven Register*, *New Haven Independent*, *CT Mirror*, *Hartford Courant*, and *Connecticut Post*. To find distribution data, we consulted with:

- Library of Congress,
- Hearst News Media,
- Media Intelligence Center at Cornell University,
- Electronic Resources Librarian at Southern Connecticut State University

News reports from these outlets were collected using each organization's Twitter account (see Figure 4.1). This method was chosen because most news outlets utilize Twitter to promote their organizations' work and report by linking stories and sending users back to their websites (Stocking et al., 2018). In fact, 93% of major news outlets' Twitter accounts share a link to a story on the organization's own website (Holcomb et al., 2011).

Tweet Retrieval and Preprocessing

Tweets were collected from the news media organizations' Twitter timelines using Twython. Twython is a Python library that provides an easy way to access and store Twitter data (Twython 3.8.0 Documentation, 2013; Pilgrim & Willison, 2009). After the tweets were collected using Twython, a list of a priori keywords that were generated prior to analysis were applied to articles. A total of 2,431 tweets contained a URL to an article and featured at least one keyword from all three thematic categories (race, health disparities, and COVID-19 pandemic) (see Table 4.1).

TABLE 4.1 Keywords Used for Articles Coded

Race	Health	Pandemic
Race	Inequality	COVID-19
Racial	Inequality	Covid/COVID
Black	Inequity	Coronavirus
African American	Unequal	Coronavirus
African	Disparity	Pandemic
Latino	Disparities	
Latina	Health	
Latinx	Outcomes	
Hispanic		
People of color		
POC		
African American		
Racism		
Racist		
Immigrant		
Migrant		
Communities/community of color		
Indigenous		
Asian		
China		
Chinese		

Note: The table contains the keywords used in the search for tweets. The first column contains words related to race (e.g., Black, people of color, racism). The second column contains words related to health (e.g., inequality, disparities, health). The third column contains words related to the pandemic (e.g., COVID-19, pandemic, coronavirus).

SUPPLEMENTARY TABLE 4.1 Intercoder Reliability Analysis

	kappa*	z	p value
Focus			
Health	0.665	8.95	0
Healthcare	0.757	9.95	0
Personal Finances	0.646	8.4	0
Economy	0.538	7.46	<0.001
Education	0.838	10.9	0
Average	0.6888		
Race			
Racism + Implied Racism	0.879	11.5	0
Health Disparities	0.436	6.72	<0.001
Frames			
Quoted Experts	0.452	6.9	<0.001
Emotional Appeal	0.629	8.18	<0.001
Tone¥	0.634	10.6	0

Note: This table contains the results of our intercoder reliability analysis. The first column contains the issues discussed, race, and frames codes. The second column contains the kappa values. The third column contains the z score. The final column contains the p value of the intercoder reliability analysis.

* Cohen's kappa for 2 Raters (Weights: unweighted).
¥ Cohen's kappa for 2 Raters (Weights: equal).

Article Screening

Coders screened all articles collected from Twython according to this inclusion criterion: (1) article tweeted by the selected news organizations; (2) news report must be directly about or related to the COVID-19 pandemic; (3) news report must have occurred during the study timeframe (March 1, 2020, through August 31, 2020); (4) must mention race, racial disparity, or racism.

Coding Framework and Procedure

The content of each article was coded according to the presence or absence of the following categories: (1) discussion on racism/implied racism, (2) use of words "racial disparities," (3) issues discussed (personal health, healthcare system, personal finances, economy, education), (4) framing through sources cited (expert source, data, testimonials), (5) emotional appeal, and (6) framing through tones (positive, neutral, and negative).

Racial Disparities and Racism

Racial Disparities

Articles were coded with "racial disparities" if the story either specifically mentioned "racial disparity" or "racial inequity" or demonstrated disparities between groups of people.

Racism/Implied Racism

Articles had to either explicitly mention racism or imply racism. Examples of keywords indicating implied racism: Black Lives Matter, BLM, police accountability, redlining, George Floyd (any victim of state violence), Jim Crow laws, Tuskegee Experiment, segregation (see Table 4.2).

TABLE 4.2 Excerpts from Articles and Issues Discussed

Story ID	Issues Discussed in Article	Quote
1151	Health Racial Disparities Racism	A protestor held a sign that read, "We are suffering from two pandemics: COVID-19 and racism."
1153	Health Healthcare System Socioeconomic Implications Racial Disparities Racism	"As we've been watching the protests that have erupted across our country in response to the killing of George Floyd and others, we know now that even in the midst of the pandemic, structural racism and the racism that shows up as people navigate social space are still alive and well," said Wizdom Powell, director of the Health Disparities Institute at UConn Health. "We've long been arguing for a systems change around health care access and insurance." People of color here are also more likely to work in high-risk, "essential" jobs, such as those in nursing homes, grocery stores and retail, and to live in densely populated communities and have higher rates of pre-existing conditions like diabetes and asthma that are caused or worsened by systemic racism; "We don't do a good job in the state of reporting actively and fully on racial, ethnic, and language data," Everette said. "So we can't solve a problem—even though we know it exists—if we don't have the tools to monitor our progress in that way."
1163	Health Socioeconomic Implications Educational Racial Disparities Racism	COVID-19-related deaths and infection rates are disproportionately higher among minorities, as is unemployment.; Minorities comprise a significant share of Connecticut's nursing home workers, who insist they risked infection daily caring for vulnerable seniors—while lacking adequate protective gear.; But inequalities in "health care, housing, and economic opportunities—these are all interlinked," he added.
1191	Health Healthcare System Racial Disparities	Black and Latino residents in major cities are particularly vulnerable to COVID-19 for several reasons: They are more likely to live in densely populated areas, where spread occurs more easily; they are more likely to work front-line jobs that require in-person contact with co-workers or customers; and they disproportionately face pre-existing health conditions that increase their likelihood of serious symptoms.

TABLE 4.2 Cont.

Story ID	Issues Discussed in Article	Quote
1227	Health Healthcare System Personal Finances Socioeconomic Implications Racial Disparities	For months now as the coronavirus pandemic upended everyday life, people in Connecticut's Latino and Black communities have done more than their share—and suffered more than their share—to keep hospitals operating, grocery stores open, buses running and nursing homes staffed.; "Long-standing systemic health and social inequities have put some members of racial and ethnic minority groups at increased risk of getting COVID-19 or experiencing severe illness, regardless of age," the Centers for Disease Control and Prevention determined, based on nationwide data of hospitalizations and coronavirus-linked deaths.
1565	Personal Finances Socioeconomic Implications Racial Disparities	Black and Hispanic people, and those living in the state's largest cities are disproportionately affected by this economic downturn and the resulting housing crisis.
2344	Health Personal Finances Socioeconomic Implications Racial Disparities Racism (Implied)	Black and Latino people in the state have not only borne disproportionate loss of life due to COVID-19, but have also been hardest hit financially, according to data released Thursday. The multi-faceted analysis tells a tale of two pandemics as COVID-19 exacerbates existing health and economic inequities. Among the most striking findings is that Black people are nearly twice as likely to have lost a loved one or friend to the coronavirus as White people. They are also much less likely to feel that their employers are keeping them safe at work. From an economic standpoint, Latinos experienced higher rates of job layoffs and greater housing insecurity.
2519	Health Healthcare System Racial Disparities	"My concern is communities of color won't participate in these trials at high enough rates and so we won't know if there are differences in certain communities or certain groups," said Summer Johnson McGee, Ph.D. and dean of the University of New Haven School of Health Sciences. The history of syphilis trials among Tuskegee Airmen and Guatemalan women nearly 90 years ago still casts a shadow over medicine. But she says the process of clinical trials has come a long way. "So, we have to start now building that groundwork in the community with trusted leaders, to get folks to understand we're not experimenting on you, we're not asking you to do something risky, we're trying to help everyone protect the public health," said McGee.

Note: The table contains excerpts from articles and issues discussed. The first column contains the unique story ID assigned during coding. The second column contains the issues discussed in the article. The third column contains an excerpt from the article.

Issues Discussed

To indicate the context in which the COVID-19 information was presented, the primary topic of each article was noted. This was determined by coding the main subject identified in the lead paragraphs of the article or introduction in the news broadcast. The categories were not mutually exclusive, and each news story was coded for one or more of the following primary topics.

Health

If the story specifically mentioned the impact of COVID-19 on the health of individuals or populations.

Healthcare System

If the article focused on the delivery of healthcare or healthcare systems and infrastructure, including keywords such as pharmaceutical, vaccine, testing, health insurance, hospitals and hospitalizations, nursing homes, assisted living, community health workers, contact tracing, or mention of the impact on another healthcare system, like dentistry.

Personal Financial Implication

If the article specifically mentioned the impact of COVID-19 on the personal finances of individuals such as losing income, employment, housing/homes.

Societal Economic Implication

If the story mentioned specific socioeconomic impacts of COVID-19 on restaurants, bars, travel, hospitality, housing, among other industries, and/or the impact on the stock market, unemployment rates, and/or community food banks.

Educational

If the article mentioned the impact of COVID-19 on the educational system, specific schools, and/or specific students. Keywords include digital divide, school reopenings, and school attendance.

Expert Sources of Information

For each article, it was noted whether or not the journalist included an expert in the report. An expert source was defined as someone with stated credentials, high status within an organization or field, or considerable tenure within the field. Examples include physicians, healthcare providers, Public Health Commissioners, subject matter experts, leaders of relevant organizations, heads of hospital departments, and/or academic centers. References and links to academic studies were also coded as expert opinion.

Emotional Appeals

If the story appealed to the reader on an emotional level either through descriptive language, images, or video. Examples include phrases such as "tragic loss" or images of people in distress. Emotional appeals of resilience were also included, such as "beating the odds" or images of people overcoming something (i.e., being released from the hospital).

Tone

Coded as either positive, neutral, or negative, the tone was determined by weighing the presence of positive images, words, or phrases (e.g., "On the rebound," 1922) to negative words and phrases (e.g., "all of us are struggling," 2528). If the presence of positive and negative phrases were equal within the article, coders determined the

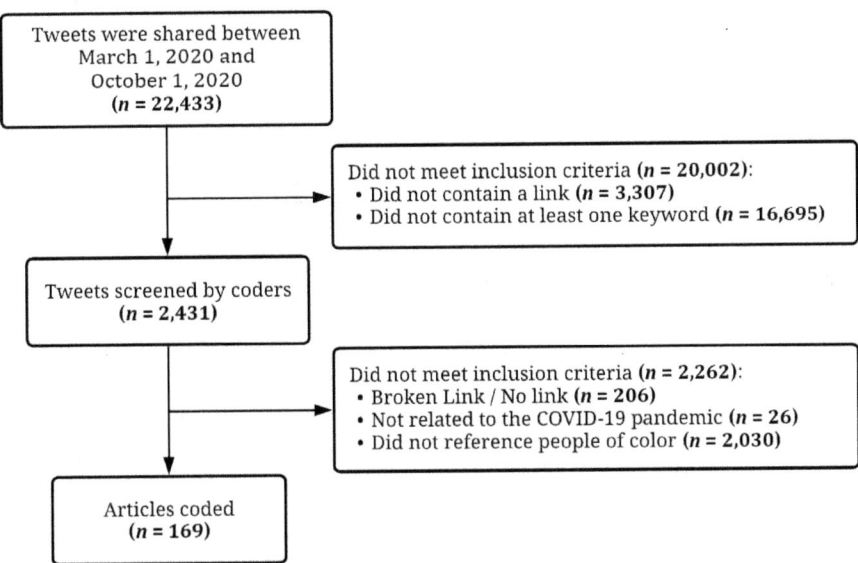

FIGURE 4.1 PRISMA Diagram of Analysis Process

The figure describes the diagram of our tweet search, screening, and coding process. A total of 22,433 tweets were authored by local news organizations between March 1 and October 1, 2020. Of these, 20,002 tweets did not contain at least one of the inclusion criteria keywords or a working URL; 2,431 articles were screened by coders; 2,262 did not meet the inclusion criteria due to broken links, not related to COVID-19 pandemic, or did not reference people of color; and 169 articles were coded.

article was neutral. The title of the article was often very instructive—setting the tone for the whole article (see Table 4.2).

Coding Procedure

Coding was conducted by two authors, who independently reviewed all transcripts. Coders were trained on the codebook that explicitly defined each category and variables within each category. Pilot coding was conducted to ensure comparability within the coding scheme. The intercoder reliability (Cohen's kappa, unweighted unless otherwise noted) before consensus was estimated as 0.879 for racism/implied racism, 0.436 for racial disparities, 0.689 on average for issues discussed (range 0.538–0.838), 0.452 for expert sources, 0.629 for emotional appeals, and 0.634 (weighted) for tone (see Table 4.3).

Statistical Analysis

The coded news stories included breaking news; the reporting of timely events within 24 hours; news bulletins, brief and timely news stories; and features that are not time-sensitive. Each news story is considered a single unit of analysis. All statistical analytical procedures were conducted in R Studio.

TABLE 4.3 Intercoder Reliability Analysis

	kappa*	z	p value
Focus			
Health	0.665	8.95	0
Healthcare	0.757	9.95	0
Personal Finances	0.646	8.4	0
Economy	0.538	7.46	<0.001
Education	0.838	10.9	0
Average	0.6888		
Race			
Racism + Implied Racism	0.879	11.5	0
Health Disparities	0.436	6.72	<0.001
Frames			
Quoted Experts	0.452	6.9	<0.001
Emotional Appeal	0.629	8.18	<0.001
Tone¥	0.634	10.6	0

Note: The table contains the results of our intercoder reliability analysis. The first column contains the issues discussed, race, and frames codes. The second column contains the kappa values. The third column contains the z score. The final column contains the p value of the intercoder reliability analysis.

* Cohen's kappa for 2 Raters (Weights: unweighted).
¥ Cohen's kappa for 2 Raters (Weights: equal).

Results

Local Media Coverage of Racial Disparities in COVID-19

Out of the 169 articles that met the inclusion criteria, the articles coded as having a focus on personal health (84.0%) were the most common, followed by articles focusing on the economy (53.8%). In all, 79.3% ($n = 134$) of articles discussed two or more issues. Racial disparities were discussed in 87.9% of economy-focused stories ($n = 80$), 87.8% of personal finance-focused stories ($n = 36$), and 84.9% of healthcare-focused stories ($n = 62$) (see Table 4.4).

News Stories Featuring Experts

In the articles examined, 81.6% quoted experts directly or cited research studies ($n = 139$). In our sample, the articles discussing personal finances had the highest proportion of stories that quoted experts (92.7%), followed by articles covering the healthcare system (91.8%). Articles discussing personal health were the least likely to quote experts (85.2%). When discussing race-related issues, 86.8% of articles that discussed racial disparities quoted expert sources compared to 80.1% of articles that discussed racism.

Use of Emotional Appeals in News Media Reporting

Many articles included statistics (81.1%), testimonials (69.8%), and emotional appeals (63.3%). Of the articles that included an emotional appeal, we found that the issues discussed tended to be education focused (80.0%) followed by personal finance stories (75.6%) (see Table 4.5).

Overall Tone of News Coverage

To examine tone in news coverage, articles were coded as having a positive, neutral, or negative tone. In all, 37.2% of the articles were coded with negative tone, 46.7% of the articles were coded as having a neutral tone ($n = 79$), and 9.4% of articles with a positive tone ($n = 16$). Additionally, we examined how tone was used in articles discussing racism and racial disparities. When discussing racism, a higher proportion of articles were coded as having either negative (42.5%, $n = 31$) or neutral tones (46.6%, $n = 34$) compared to having a positive tone (11.0%, $n = 8$). Similarly, when discussing racial disparities, a higher proportion of articles contained either a negative (41.9%, $n = 57$) or neutral tone (50.1%, $n = 69$), compared to positive tone (7.4%, $n = 10$) (see Table 4.4).

Limitations

While this study provides important information about how the media in New Haven reported on racial disparities within their COVID-19 coverage, there were some

TABLE 4.4 Frequency of Issues in Articles Tweeted by Local News Organizations

Organization Type	Twitter Account of News Organization	Issues Discussed					Race-related Issues	
		Health n (%)	Healthcare n (%)	Finances n (%)	Economy n (%)	Education n (%)	Racism¥ n (%)	Racial Disparities n (%)
Local Newspapers and Online Journalism	Conpost (n = 5)	3 (60.0)	2 (40.0)	0 (0)	1 (20.0)	1 (20)	0 (0)	2 (40.0)
	CTMirror (n = 81)	67 (82.7)	42 (51.9)	19 (23.5)	49 (60.5)	13 (16.0)	35 (43.2)	72 (88.9)
	Hartfordcourant (n = 36)	30 (83.3)	15 (41.7)	10 (27.8)	21 (58.3)	9 (25.0)	17 (47.2)	28 (77.8)
	Nhregister (n = 10)	10 (83.3)	4 (33.3)	3 (25.0)	3 (25.0)	2 (16.7)	3 (25.0)	10 (83.3)
	Newhavenindy (n = 7)	7 (100)	4 (57.1)	2 (28.6)	2 (28.6)	3 (42.9)	2 (28.6)	3 (42.9)
Local TV News	NBCConnecticut (n = 13)	10 (76.9)	4 (30.8)	2 (15.4)	6 (46.2)	1 (7.7)	5 (38.5)	8 (61.5)
	WFSBnews (n = 2)	2 (100)	0 (0)	0 (0)	1 (50.0)	0 (0)	1 (50.0)	1 (50.0)
	WTNH (n = 11)	11 (100)	1 (9.1)	5 (45.5)	7 (63.6)	1 (9.1)	8 (72.7)	10 (90.9)

Note: The table describes the frequency of issues in articles tweeted by local news organizations. The first column identifies the type of media organization (e.g., local newspapers and online journalism, local TV news). The second column contains the Twitter account of the news organization. Columns 3 through 7 contain the counts of the issues discussed by news organization (e.g., health, healthcare, personal finances, economy, education). Columns 8 and 9 contain the counts of race-related issues by news organization (e.g., racism, racial disparities).

N = 169.

¥ Racism includes articles covering racism and implied racism.

TABLE 4.5 Frequency of Race–Related Content, Tone, and Frames by Issues Discussed in Article

Issues Discussed	Total Count	Race-related Issues		Tone			Frames	
		Racial Disparities	Racism	Positive	Neutral	Negative	Quotes Experts	Emotional Appeal
	n	n (%)	n (%)	n (%)	n (%)	n (%)	n (%)	n (%)
Health	142	119 (83.8)	66 (46.5)	14 (9.9)	69 (48.6)	59 (41.5)	121 (85.2)	89 (62.7)
Healthcare	73	62 (84.9)	30 (41.1)	7 (9.6)	36 (49.3)	30 (41.1)	67 (91.8)	45 (61.6)
Personal Finances	41	36 (87.8)	14 (34.1)	1 (2.4)	18 (43.9)	22 (53.7)	38 (92.7)	31 (75.6)
Economy	91	80 (87.9)	41 (45.1)	6 (6.6)	45 (49.5)	40 (44.0)	79 (86.8)	61 (88.4)
Education	31	24 (77.4)	9 (29.0)	1 (3.2)	14 (45.2)	16 (51.6)	27 (87.1)	22 (71.0)

Note: The first column has the issues discussed in the article (e.g., health, healthcare, personal finances, economy, and education), followed by the total count of articles that contain that issue. Other columns show the counts and percentages of race-related issues (e.g., racial disparities and racism), tone of the article (e.g., positive, neutral, negative), and frames used in the article (quotes experts, emotional appeal).

limitations. Twitter was a convenient way to collect and analyze articles published by local news media; however, we were unable to confirm if every article was printed or broadcasted, and the quantity of articles shared on Twitter varied significantly by news organizations. Additionally, some tweets collected by Twython were truncated at 140 characters, which may have interfered with our keyword screening process.

A limitation in the codebook was the requirement of the word "disparities" or "inequities" for that article to be coded for racial disparities. One coder was more liberal in their understanding of the code and included examples of racial disparities, which may have impacted the analysis of this variable.

Additionally, the agenda setting effects we propose may be impacted by paywalls limiting public access to news. The extent to which this news is reaching New Haven residents may be somewhat limited, as out of the eight news organizations, one had a paywall (New Haven Register).

Discussion

News media play a vital role in communicating important information to the public during crisis. Our pilot study examining news coverage of the COVID-19 crisis provides an understanding of the media's agenda setting practices and framing tools, bringing awareness to communication that influences public perception and systemic change.

Agenda setting theory suggests that the media can influence the public and policy through issue awareness and salience (McCombs & Shaw, 1972; [McCombs, 2004;] Scheufele & Tewksbury, 2007). This is especially vital during times of crisis. Our analysis of news coverage during the start of the COVID-19 pandemic showed little acknowledgment of the racial disparities in virus contraction and death. This is evidenced by the omission of the word "disparities" in the news media. This omission supports previous research, suggesting that members of the one racial group can set public agenda by not including terms identifying inequities in media coverage (Chow & Knowles, 2016).

However, a different crisis changed the media's intended agenda and brought racial injustice and its language to the forefront of the world's stage. In June 2020, the Black Lives Matter movement surged after the killing of George Floyd, a Black man killed by a White police officer in Minneapolis, Minnesota. People worldwide demanded police accountability for Floyd, and all Black lives harmed by state violence. Nationally and in New Haven, media covered the protests, actions, and conversations about racial equity and police brutality. Increased attention to racial injustice was reflected in the news coverage on COVID-19 racial disparities, especially following the death of Floyd (see Figure 4.2). The convergence of crises—the killings of Floyd, Breonna Taylor, and the many Black victims of state violence combined with the disproportionate number of cases and deaths from COVID-19 in communities of color—increased coverage in news media about the policies driving inequity and equity in healthcare, education, labor, environmentalism, and housing (see Figure 4.2).

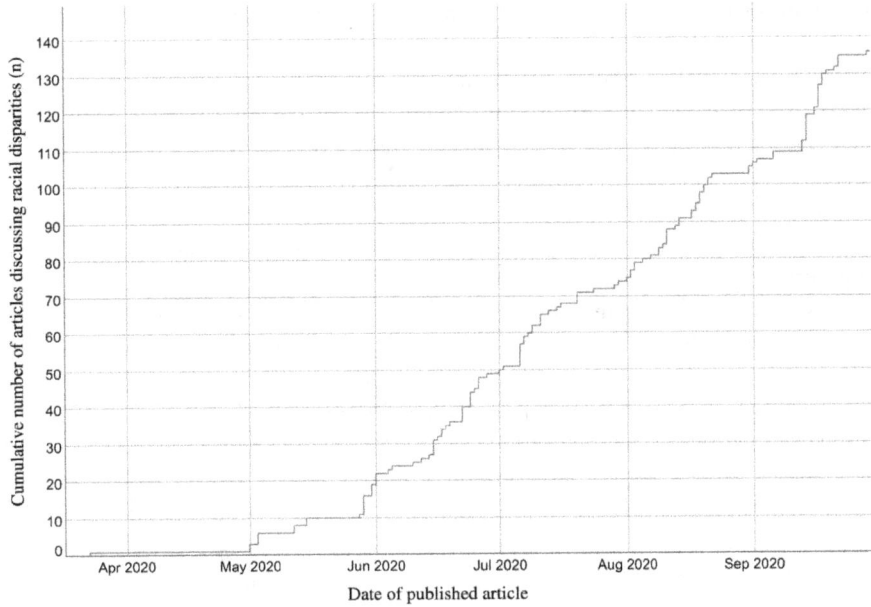

FIGURE 4.2 Number of Articles Discussing Racial Disparities by Date

The figure depicts the cumulative number of articles discussing racial disparities by publication date.

While we are not able to make a causal connection between the news coverage of racial disparities and policy changes related to this issue, it is important to note that New Haven, like many U.S. cities, issued an ordinance declaring racism a public health crisis. Such declarations represent a policy shift and are the first step in advancing racial equity. For policymakers to understand and frame racism as a public emergency, it should be ensured it receives the same or similar time, allocation of resources, commitment, and urgency as COVID-19. Future researchers should examine the impact of such legislation on communities.

In addition to considering issue salience under agenda setting theory, we examined how the media framed news stories. Research suggests that experts are considered important sources of information to the public (Page et al., 1987) and journalists utilize this as many news stories we reviewed incorporated experts in the reporting. Framing information in this way not only lends credibility to the topic but also provides a sense of issue importance to the public. Interestingly, the highest percentage of news stories that used experts as sources focused on racial inequities in terms of the personal financial implications of the pandemic (nearly 93%) and stories reporting on healthcare (nearly 92%). This may be because expert sources were needed to help explain the disproportionately negative impact communities of color were experiencing as a result of the COVID-19 pandemic. The inequities in these areas and others were not simply a result of the pandemic but were illuminated by COVID-19 in ways that could not be ignored. Advocates for racial equity should continually encourage journalists to utilize expert sources on racial equity, to increase the issue salience for the public, and to encourage policy change. However, it is important to note here that the perception of an "expert" in medicine or healthcare may widely vary to Black, African American, Hispanic, or Latino/a individuals due to historical and ongoing medical racism.

Another framing technique used in the media is emotional appeal. Our analysis showed most of the news stories incorporated an emotional appeal with a personal testimonial to humanize news stories. However, some research indicates that when coverage is highly personalized with individual characteristics, the audience is more likely to assume there is individual responsibility to the circumstance, opposed to a societal/systemic responsibility (Shah & Nah, 2004).

The use of tone was also examined as a framing technique in the news stories: we found the majority of articles used a neutral tone (46.7%) and those using a negative tone close behind (37.2%). While it is understandable that few stories used a positive tone during the first six months of the pandemic coverage, it is important to note the possible impact of more frequent negatively toned stories. Research in this area indicates that negatively toned news stories show an agenda setting effect on the public's perception of the subject, while neutral and positively toned stories have no significant effect (Wanta et al., 2004). Consequently, the number of negatively toned news stories covering the pandemic and touching on racism or racial inequalities may have a more significant effect on the public's perception and understanding.

While we measured frequency of keywords and framing techniques within the media, the next potential steps include examining levels of cultural competency. In other words, to what extent does the audience and readership come to understand the implications of racial disparities?

An additional consideration in terms of the coverage of racism and racial disparities in COVID-19 news stories is the news outlet's commitment to diversity and inclusion. Of the eight news media organizations we collected articles from, approximately 48% of the total articles that met our inclusion criteria were from the *CT Mirror*, with 65 of the 81 articles from *CT Mirror* coded for racism and racial disparities (see Table 4.4). This reflects *CT Mirror*'s strategic plan prioritizing diversity in journalists, viewpoints, and stories (CT Mirror, 2019). Also important to note, the *CT Mirror* has a dedicated health reporter focusing on "health access, affordability, quality, equity and disparities, social determinants of health, health system planning, infrastructure … and other health policy" (CT Mirror, n.d.). Such an organizational structure in a news organization appears to increase coverage, and thus public awareness, of equity and disparities.

Conclusion

This content analysis reveals a lack of coverage of racial disparities and racism within COVID-19 news reporting. The pandemic impacted Black and Latino populations in New Haven at a rate of five and four times higher than White populations, highlighting the racial inequities within the city, and yet there were only 169 news articles in New Haven covering racism and racial disparities during the first six months of the pandemic (see Table 4.4).

To understand racial disparities, it is pivotal to understand how racism continually operates in our society. Many of the articles we analyzed reported on disparities without acknowledging racism as a root cause. Racial disparities are the outcomes of hundreds of years of systemic racism, set within a context of racial inequities of larger societal institutions (Williams & Rucker, 2000). These disparities are not incidental or naturally occurring due to differences between races, rather they are outcomes borne of deep institutionalized racism. Particularly in medicine and health, there is a deeply entrenched history of racism and bias that persists today.

The impact of the Black Lives Matter movement is evident in our analysis with increased coverage of racism and racial inequities in the COVID-19 reporting. The increased awareness and understanding of the issue led to the declaration of racism as a public health crisis in New Haven. Across the country, 14 cities, 73 counties, and 8 states have taken similar measures (American Public Health Association, n.d.). While these are important first steps, they must be backed by continued communication with the public to increase attention and help motivate support for additional policy changes and actions.

References

American Public Health Association. (n.d.). *Racism Is a Public Health Crisis.* Retrieved from www.apha.org/Topics-and-Issues/Health-Equity/Racism-and-health/Racism-Declarations

Armstrong, C. L., & Nelson, M. R. (2005). How Newspaper Sources Trigger Gender Stereotypes. *Journalism and Mass Communication Quarterly, 82*(4), 820–837. https://doi.org/10.1177/107769900508200405

Ball-Rokeach, S. J., & DeFleur, M. L. (1976). A Dependency Model of Mass-Media Effects. *Communication Research, 3*(1), 3–21. https://doi.org/10.1177/009365027600300101

Barnes, M. D., Hanson, C. L., Novilla, L. M., Meacham, A. T., McIntyre, E., & Erickson, B. C. (2008). Analysis of Media Agenda Setting During and After Hurricane Katrina: Implications for Emergency Preparedness, Disaster Response, and Disaster Policy. *American Journal of Public Health, 98*(4), 604–610. https://doi.org/10.2105/ajph.2007.112235

Bonilla-Silva, E. (1996). Rethinking Racism: Toward a Structural Interpretation. *American Sociological Review, 62,* 465–480. https://doi.org/10.2307/2657316

Bullock, H. E., Wyche, K. F., & Williams, W. R. (2001). Media Images of the Poor. *Journal of Social Issues, 57*(2), 229–246. https://doi.org/10.1111/0022-4537.00210

Cappella, J. N., & Jamieson, K. H. (1997). *The Cognitive Bases for Framing Effects.* New York, NY: Oxford University Press, 58–86.

Centers for Disease Control and Prevention. (2020). *COVID Data Tracker.* Retrieved from https://covid.cdc.gov/covid-data-tracker/#cases

Centers for Disease Control and Prevention. (2020a, February 11). *COVID-19.* Retrieved from www.cdc.gov/coronavirus/2019-nCoV/index.html

Centers for Disease Control and Prevention. (2020b, December 10). *Health Equity: Promoting Fair Access to Health*. Retrieved from www.cdc.gov/coronavirus/2019-ncov/community/health-equity/index.html

Chow, R., & Knowles, E. (2016). Taking Race Off of the Table: Agenda Setting and Support for Color-Blind Public Policy. *Personality and Social Psychology Bulletin, 42*(1), 1–15. https://doi.org/10.1177/0146167215611637

Cohen, B. (1963). *The Press and Foreign Policy*. Princeton, NJ: Princeton University Press.

CT Mirror. (n.d.). *Staff*. Retrieved from https://ctmirror.org/about-us/staff/

CT Mirror. (2019, July 24). *The CT Mirror 2019 to 2022 Strategic Plan*. Retrieved from www.documentcloud.org/documents/6222548-Strategic-Plan-July-2019-to-June-2022.html

Dearing, J., & Rogers, E. (1996). *Agenda-Setting*. Thousand Oaks, CA: Sage. www.doi.org/10.4135/9781452243283

Freimuth, V. S., Greenberg, R. H., DeWitt, J., & Romano, R. M. (1984). Covering Cancer: Newspapers and the Public Interest. *Journal of Communication, 34*, 62–73.

Gans, H. (1983). News Media, News Policy, and Democracy: Research for the Future. *Journal of Communication, 33*, 174–184.

Gorman, J. (1993). Postmodernism and the Conduct of Inquiry in Social Work. *Affilia, 8*(3), 247–264. https://doi.org/10.1177/088610999300800302

Holcomb, J., Gross, K., & Mitchell, A. (2011, November 14). *How Mainstream Media Outlets Use Twitter*. Pew Research Center's Journalism Project. Retrieved from www.journalism.org/2011/11/14/how-mainstream-media-outlets-use-twitter/

Jordan, D. (1993). Newspaper Effects on Policy Preferences. *Public Opinion Quarterly, 57*(2), 191–204.

Kim, S. T., & Weaver, D. H. (2003). Reporting on Globalization: A Comparative Analysis of 535 Sourcing Patterns in Five Countries' Newspapers. *The International Journal for Communication Studies, 65*, 121–144.

McCombs, M. (2004). *Setting the Agenda: The Mass Media and Public Opinion*. Malden, MA: Polity Press.

McCombs, M. E., & Shaw, D. L. (1972). The Agenda-Setting Function of Mass Media. *Public Opinion Quarterly, 36*(2), 176–187.

National Institutes of Health. (n.d.). *Minority Health and Health Disparities: Definitions and Parameters*. Retrieved from www.nimhd.nih.gov/about/strategic-plan/nih-strategic-plan-definitions-and-parameters.html

Nelkin, D. (1989). Journalism and Science: The Creative Tension. In M. Moore (Ed.), *Health Risks and the Press* (pp. 53–71). Washington D.C.: Media Institute.

Niederdeppe, J., Bigman, C., Gonzales, A., & Gollust, S. (2013). Communication about Health Disparities in the Mass Media. *Journal of Communication, 63*, 8–30.

Pacheco, J., & Boushey, G. (2014). Public Health and Agenda Setting: Determinants of State Attention to Tobacco and Vaccines. *Journal of Health Politics, Policy and Law, 39*(3), 565–589.

Page, B., Shapiro, R., & Dempsey, G. (1987). What Moves Public Opinion. *American Political Science Review, 81*(1), 23–43.

Pan, Z., & Kosicki, G. M. (1993). Framing Analysis: An Approach to News Discourse. *Political Communication, 10*, 55–76.

Pilgrim, M., & Willison, S. (2009). *Dive into Python 3* (Vol. 2). Amsterdam, Netherlands: Springer.

Ramsey, S. (1999). A Benchmark Study of Elaboration and Sourcing in Science Stories for Eight American Newspapers. *Journalism & Mass Communication Quarterly, 76*(1), 87–98.

Rogers, E. M., & Dearing, J. W. (1988). Agenda-Setting Research: Where Has It Been, Where Is It Going? *Communication Yearbook, 11*, 555–594.

Rogers, R. W. (1985). Attitude Change and Information Integration in Fear Appeals. *Psychological Reports, 56*(1), 179–182. https://doi.org/10.2466/pr0.1985.56.1.179

Rosenstock, I. M. (1990). The Health Belief Model: Explaining Health Behavior Through Expectancies. In K. Glanz, F. M. Lewis, & B. K. Rimer (Eds.), *Health Behavior and Health Education: Theory, Research, and Practice* (pp. 39–62). New York, NY: Jossey-Bass/Wiley.

Scheufele, D. A., & Tewksbury, D. (2007). Framing, Agenda Setting, and Priming: The Evolution of Three Media Effects Models. *Journal of Communication, 57*, 9–20.

Shah, H., & Nah, S. (2004). Long Ago and Far Away: How US Newspapers Construct Racial Oppression. *Journalism, 5*(3), 259–278. https://doi.org/10.1177/1464884904041659]

Shih, J., Wijaya, R., & Brossard, D. (2008). Media Coverage of Public Health Epidemics: Linking Framing and Issue Attention Cycle Toward an Integrated Theory of Print News Coverage of Epidemics. *Mass Communications and Society, 11*(2), 141–160. https://doi.org/10.1080/15205430701668121

Snyder, L. B., & Rouse, R. A. (1995). The Media Can Have More Than an Impersonal Impact: The Case of AIDS Risk Perceptions and Behavior. *Health Communication, 7*, 125–145.

Steele, J. E. (1995). Experts and the Operational Bias of Television News: The Case of the Persian Gulf War. *Journalism & Mass Communication Quarterly, 72*(4), 799–812. https://doi.org/10.1177/107769909507200404

Stocking, G., Barthel, M., & Grieco, E. (2018, January 29). *Sources Shared on Twitter: A Case Study on Immigration.* Pew Research Center Journalism & Media. Retrieved from www.journalism.org/2018/01/29/sources-shared-on-twitter-a-case-study-on-immigration/

Tian, Y., & Stewart, C. M. (2005). Framing the SARS crisis: A computer-assisted text analysis of CNN and BBC online news reports of SARS. *Asian Journal of Communication, 15*(3), 289–301. https://doi.org/10.1080/01292980500261605

Twython—Twython 3.8.0 Documentation. (2013). Twython 3.8.0 Documentation. Retrieved from https://twython.readthedocs.io/en/latest/

U.S. Census Bureau. (2019). *U.S. Census Bureau QuickFacts: New Haven City, Connecticut.* Census Bureau QuickFacts. Retrieved from www.census.gov/quickfacts/newhaven cityconnecticut

U.S. Census Bureau. (2020). *American Community Survey 5-Year Data (2009–2019).* Retrieved from www.census.gov/data/developers/data-sets/acs-5year.html

Walsh-Childers, K. (1994). Newspaper Influence on Health Policy Development. *Newspaper Research Journal, 15*, 89–104.

Wanta, W., Golan, G., & Lee, C. (2004). Agenda Setting and International News: Media Influence on Public Perceptions of Foreign Nations. *Journalism & Mass Communication Quarterly, 81*(2), 364–377.

Williams, D. R., & Mohammed, S. A. (2008). Discrimination and Racial Disparities in Health: Evidence and Needed Research. *Journal of Behavioral Medicine, 32*(1), 20–47. https://doi.org/10.1007/s10865-008-9185-0

Williams, D. R., & Rucker, T. D. (2000). Understanding and Addressing Racial Disparities in Health Care. *Health Care Financing Review, 21*(4), 75–90.

Winsten, J. A. (1985). Science and the Media: The Boundaries of Truth. *Health Affairs, 4*, 5–23.

5

PERCEPTIONS OF COVID-19 AND BLM PROTESTING ON TWITTER

Tanya E. Gardner, Wei Sun, and Carolyn A. Stroman

Introduction

Since the outbreak of the COVID-19 pandemic, people from various racial backgrounds have been disproportionately impacted by the virus. By December 2020, more than 280,000 Americans had died of COVID-19, with African Americans representing 18.5% of all deaths of a known race, despite representing only 12.4% of the population (APM Research Lab, 2020). "Black, Latino and Native American communities, in particular, have suggested higher rates of infection and deaths, laying bare deep inequities in the American healthcare system and social factors underlying health" (University of Southern California, 2020). Undoubtedly, COVID-19 has hit minority communities harder in the United States, and minority members are more susceptible to contracting the virus and more likely to die of it (Nania, 2020). The Centers for Disease Control and Prevention's (CDC) National Center for Health Statistics reported the distribution of pandemic-related death according to race and ethnicity (CDC, 2020a). Nationally, the total COVID-19 death rates were 52.1% White, 21.2% Black, 6.1% Asian, and 16.1% Latino. In many states, a staggering number of African Americans died from the disease. By May 2020, the death distribution percentages of African Americans in the following states were as follows: Mississippi 61%, Louisiana 51.7%, South Carolina 51.2%, Georgia 46.5%, Alabama 44.5%, Maryland 42.1%, Missouri 38.7%, Michigan 33.4%, and Illinois 31.7%. By October 2020, the CDC vital report showed the trend that 51% of COVID-19-related deaths were of Whites, followed by 20% and 19% of Blacks and Latinos, respectively (CDC, 2020c).

On May 25, 2020, in the midst of the pandemic crisis, an innocent Black man, George Floyd, died as a result of police brutality. This event sparked nationwide protests against racial inequality, led by the Black Lives Matter (BLM) movement. While the number of COVID-19 cases continued to increase in many states, and

DOI: 10.4324/9781003268710-5

as businesses began to reopen, there were fears that the BLM movement protests contributed to the resurgence of COVID-19 spread (Meyer, 2020). In a time of political and racial division, people expressed their support for, or opposition to, the claim that there was a connection between the protests and the rising number of cases.

This study aims to investigate how social media users make sense of the relationship between COVID-19 and BLM, and how health disparities of COVID-19 and race have been discussed in Twitter posts. The findings of the research will increase our understanding of how social media impacts knowledge regarding public health crises.

Literature Review

This section reviews the literature pertaining to BLM and online social movements, media framing of the COVID-19 pandemic, and racial and health disparities during the pandemic.

Black Lives Matter and Online Social Movement

Researchers have debated the roles and efficacy of social media usage in recent social movements. Some believe that digital media technologies help activists achieve and promote citizens' participation in democracy, such as in the cases of Tunisia, Egypt, the Occupy movement, and Hong Kong protests (Castells, 2015; Kidd & McIntosh, 2016; Lee et al., 2015). Other scholars believe that slacktivism and clicktivism are not real social movements, and they create an illusion that people are interested in supporting a cause or an organization (Fuchs, 2015; Glenn, 2015). However, a recent Pew Research study reported that 23% of respondents indicate that they have changed their views because of social media (Perrin, 2020). People report having changed their views due to some issues discussed on social media, including the BLM movement, police brutality, political parties, ideologies, and political figures. In 2018, only 13% of people believed that social media made them change their viewpoints (Perrin, 2020). Mundt et al. (2018) assert that social media have played salient roles in building connections, forming coalitions, and mobilizing resources to scale up social movements.

Blevins et al. (2019) presented a big data analysis of #BlackLivesMatter tweets and related hashtags used on Twitter during two specific targeted time periods. The hashtag #MikeBrown was created after Michael Brown was shot to death in 2014 in Ferguson, Missouri. Another hashtag, #Ferguson, was created after a grand jury chose not to indict Darren Wilson, the police officer who shot Brown. Blevins et al. (2019) identified three hashtag schemas. The first was places and proper names; this type of hashtag identified specific names and locations involved in incidents (i.e., #MikeBrown or #Ferguson). The second was ideological hashtags, which identify a belief or position on the political nature of the incident (i.e., #BlackLivesMatter). The third was conceptual hashtags, such as #Icantbreathe. Network analysis of data found that Twitter provided a public sphere for previously unheard voices to be expressed and an opportunity for users to frame the meaning of Brown's murder as relatable to their personal lives and experiences. This was reflected in the posters' use of first-person personalization of the issue (i.e., #IfTheyGunnedMeDown).

In another study on the social media response to BLM that analyzed 66,159 tweets over three targeted timeframes (before Michael Brown shooting, after Michael Brown shooting, and after release of the grand jury report acquitting the officer involved in the shooting), researchers explored how social media users attach meaning to the BLM hashtag movement and reframe the movement through co-occurring hashtag use (Ince et al., 2017). They concluded that co-occurring hashtags show how users associate with words that describe the social movement, and how these additional words reflect the movements' intended meaning. Twitter provides social media users space to engage in mobilization strategies, form collective identities, and create and sustain social movement narratives (Ince et al., 2017; Ray et al., 2017). Wilkens et al. (2019) examined the rhetorical functions of social media used by the BLM social movement, which include defining the nature of the problem and targeting injustice. Activists used race and racism to help justify who and what was included in the movement. Social movement advocates were characterized as those who perform movement-endorsing acts of discourse, rather than undermining acts of discourse. The analysis shows how activists used Twitter to balance different and competing priorities of expanding the BLM movement while defining and preserving the movement's focus.

Media Framing of the COVID-19 Pandemic

Scholars have studied global media framing on COVID-19 since the outbreak of the pandemic. Ogbodo et al. (2020) studied the global media framing of COVID-19 in terms of media reports' word choices; the researchers asserted that

> when a message is released through the media, what matters most is not what is said but how it is said. As such, the media could either mitigate or accentuate the crisis depending on the major frames adopted for the coverage.
>
> *Ogbodo et al., 2020, p. 257*

Jo and Chang (2020) believed there were political consequences of COVID-19 media framing in South Korea. South Korea's ruling party received a higher approval rating during the pandemic, and the ruling party won reelection. When the government's capacity is visible to its people, their attitudes toward government could change. Poirier et al. (2020) analyzed 12 major media resources in Canada and identified "health crisis," "social impact," and "Chinese outbreak" as Canadian media frames on COVID-19.

Wicke and Bolognesi (2020) examined two metaphors Twitter users applied to frame the COVID-19 discourses in the United States. In war metaphors, Twitter users employed "fight," "combat," "threat," and "battle" to reflect the severe situations the country was facing. Words such as "storm," "monster," and "tsunami" were comparable to war metaphors. In family metaphors, "house," "parents," and "kids" indicated the control of the spread of the virus in terms of healthcare and treatment. Bolsen et al. (2020) also studied the two theories on the origins of COVID-19. One claim was that the virus is zoonotic, transmitted at a Chinese seafood market from bats to human beings. Another claim was a conspiracy theory: the virus was human-made and leaked from a Chinese laboratory. They found that framed messages about COVID-19 origins have a powerful impact on people's beliefs; people who tend to believe in the conspiracy theory cause of COVID-19 are reluctant to take preventive measures, such as wearing facial masks and keeping socially distanced. The authors believed the misinformation and conspiracy theory could pose a public health threat (Bolsen et al., 2020).

Grinberg et al. (2019) studied fake news on Twitter during the 2016 presidential election. They concluded that misinformation spread during the election indicated that about 1% of users created 80% of fake news. This study also concluded that 80% of all tweets were associated with the top 10% of frequent Twitter users (Grinberg et al., 2019). A group of Kuwaiti researchers explored the top concerns of Twitter users on COVID-19 during the initial days of the pandemic spread. They analyzed a total of 167,073 tweets posted from February 2, 2020 to March 15, 2020 and observed that fear of the pandemic spread in nations that were ill-equipped with basic personal protective equipment supplies. Moreover, at the beginning of the pandemic, there was a shortage of facial masks reported all over the world.

Public health agencies were challenged to correct misinformation and conspiracy theories in fast-moving information channels like Twitter (Abd-Alrazaq et al., 2020). Racist attacks against Chinese people centered around misinformation suggesting that the novel coronavirus was created in a Chinese biolab. Chen et al. (2020) tracked the social media discourse on the COVID-19 pandemic. Their analysis of English-language tweets collected from January 21, 2020 to March 31, 2020 showed a shift in the discourse and public mood in initial tweets from understanding the pandemic (naming and identifying the pandemic origin) to the need for preparedness and expressions of panic over lack of personal protective equipment. Meanwhile, researchers urged public officials to provide accurate public information through online engagement.

Das and Dutta (2020) explored an understanding of public emotions and sentiments during the pandemic in India. The researchers performed a corpus-level emotion mining analysis on tweets using the National Research Council (NRC) Emotion Lexicon. Eight emotions were identified: anticipation, anger, surprise, joy, fear, trust, sadness, and disgust. Three sentiments (positive, negative, and neutral) were also identified (Das & Dutta, 2020). This study extracted emotions and sentiments over time, providing insight into public expressions during the COVID-19 pandemic.

Researchers have previously studied public health crises during the pandemics of H1N1 flu and Ebola (Ahmed et al., 2019; Lazard et al., 2015; Miller et al., 2017). Researchers in the United Kingdom explored the public perception of the H1N1 swine flu at its peak in April 2009. Through coding and analysis of 7,679 swine flu-related tweets, researchers found that fear, information seeking, and misinformation were salient themes (Ahmed et al., 2019). The pandemic's name was also cited as a cause of confusion in understanding the virus's source, as users commented that abstaining from pork would prevent one from contracting the virus (Ahmed et al., 2019). The outbreak of the Ebola virus in 2014 primarily affected Western Africa and is cited as the largest epidemic of this pathogen's history (CDC, 2019). Public concern over an Ebola diagnosis in the United States prompted the CDC to conduct a live Twitter chat. Through an analysis of 2,155 Ebola-related public tweets, Lazard et al. (2015) determined the public concerns that needed addressing through public health communication included information about the virus's life span, symptoms, and transmission.

Racial and Health Disparities During the Pandemic

The CDC confirmed that during the COVID-19 pandemic, certain racial minority groups were affected disproportionately (CDC, 2020b). Barriers such as discrimination, inadequate housing, lack of access to and utilization of healthcare services, and socioeconomic status have been associated with COVID-19 morbidity and mortality. Some preventive strategies, such as closing businesses, may have created unintentional harms (e.g., job loss, stress, and reduced access to services, especially for some racial and ethnic minority groups). Wen and Sadeghi (2020) observed two kinds of inequity during COVID-19. First, minority members living in urban areas and working in higher-risk jobs were unlikely to have the flexibility to work from home, due to the nature of their work. In California, Latinos accounted for 95% of positive COVID-19 cases, and 90% of that positive test population could not work from home (Wen & Sadeghi, 2020). These authors also cite data from the Bureau of Labor Statistics which reported that compared to White workers, more African American workers were unable to work from home (Wen & Sadeghi, 2020). Workers from minority-member overrepresented industries experienced higher COVID-19 infection rates. Second, minority groups with higher rates of preexisting medical conditions had risk factors of severe COVID-19 symptoms (Wen & Sadeghi, 2020). Van Beusekom (2020) reviewed several studies related to race and COVID-19. In a Milwaukee hospital study, among 2,595 patients positive for COVID-19, 59.1% were Black, which was 5.4 times higher than other races. More Black patients were hospitalized, especially those who were poor (Van Beusekom, 2020). Furthermore, poor Black patients were 3.6 times more likely to require intensive care. Scientists claimed that structural racism, not race, created the COVID-19 inequality (Egede & Walker, 2020; Khazanchi et al., 2020). As stated by Egede and Walker (2020):

> These systems affect health through a variety of pathways, including social deprivation from reduced access to employment, housing, and education; increased environmental exposures and targeted marketing of unhealthy

substances; inadequate access to health care; physical injury and psychological trauma resulting from state-sanctioned violence such as police brutality and chronic exposure to discrimination; and diminished participation in healthy behaviors or increased participation in unhealthy behaviors as coping mechanisms.

e77

George Floyd's death during the pandemic angered the public, which led to protests during a health crisis. While there exists an emerging body of literature on COVID-19, research exploring the connection between COVID-19 and the BLM movement is lacking. This current study will add to our understanding of the topic.

This study asks the following research questions (RQs):

RQ1: What themes emerged from social media discussions of COVID-19 and BLM?

RQ2: How do social media users make sense of the relationship between COVID-19 and BLM?

RQ3: How have social media users discussed the race and health disparity issues of COVID-19 on Twitter?

Theoretical Framework, Research Method, and Research Procedures

The theoretical framework for this study was the public sphere theory (Habermas, 2006). The public sphere is a social place where people can freely identify and express ideas about societal issues, present information, debate, and form a community for developing solutions (Wessler & Freudenthler, 2011). Toepfl and Piwoni (2015) highlighted the importance of the public sphere and counter-public space of user-generated comments on news sites. Analysis of user comments leads to understanding of the support for, and resistance to, issues discussed in the public sphere and how some topics that are not receiving much media attention can be elevated through online discourse (Cranmer & Sanderson, 2018).

The data set for this study was drawn from Twitter with hashtags used as keywords for data collection. It was limited to publicly posted, English-only, original tweets, containing any combination of co-occurring hashtag combinations of #BLM and #Covid-19 (e.g., #Covid #BLM, #Covid #Blacklivesmatter, #Covid19 #BLM, or #Covid19 #Blacklivesmatter). Retweets of initial tweets were not included in the data set. In total, there were 12,206 tweets generated.

These data were obtained corresponding with tweets posted between May 15, 2020 and June 4, 2020, with co-occurring hashtags of BLM and COVID-19. The start and end dates (ten days before and ten days after the May 25, 2020, killing of George Floyd) were used to capture public sentiment for COVID-19 and BLM on Twitter. Floyd's highly publicized and controversial death sparked outrage that reverberated around the world, setting off weeks of daily protests for the arrests of the Minneapolis police officers involved, as well as for police reform in general.

These dates are also significant, as during this period, reports of COVID-19-related deaths revealed striking and disproportionate impacts on African Americans (Yancy, 2020). For example, African Americans in Chicago (who accounted for 30% of the city's population in April 2020) represented 50% of COVID-19 cases and 70% of COVID-19 deaths (Reyes et al., 2020).

Consistent with prior research analyzing a large data set, a sample of 400 tweets were extracted from the initial data set of 12,206 tweets (Ahmed et al., 2019). This sample data set reflected 100 tweets posted ten days before Floyd's murder and 200 tweets posted on May 25, 2020, ten days after Floyd's murder. Researchers selected an additional 100 tweets at random from the last ten days of the data set to determine whether any new themes or categories emerged and to ensure coding saturation.

Researchers coded and analyzed these tweets using the web-based qualitative data analysis software Dedoose (Version 8.3.20). Hyperlinks and images included in the tweets were excluded from this data analysis. An inductive thematic analysis was used to capture emerging themes during data analysis through a six-phase systematic process (Braun & Clarke, 2006).

In the first phase, all tweets in the sample data set were read to identify meaning and patterns related to the research questions. In the second phase, initial codes were assigned during an additional review of the data set. Codes were organized in Dedoose and exported into an Excel spreadsheet for ease in further reorganization of categories. During the third phase, the codes were reviewed and combined to develop overarching themes.

Thematic analysis was used to identify common themes (Kilgo et al., 2018). The constant comparison method was used to compare a case for coding to other cases in the same and different categories (Glaser & Strauss, 1967). As themes emerged, the process of constant comparison facilitated the collapse, elimination, and reorganization of codes and themes. The fourth stage included the refinement and further collapsing and elimination of themes for theme cohesion and inter-theme distinction. This phase included reviewing additional data to ensure coding saturation and theme validity (Braun & Clarke, 2006). The fifth stage included defining and naming themes to reflect the essence of each theme represented in relation to the research questions and reaching the final stage, the report (Braun & Clarke, 2006). The coding process was completed by a single researcher, and two researchers performed member-check to ensure the validity of the coding.

Data Analysis

After carefully coding and reading the tweets, data analysis was arranged in relation to RQs for better understanding. Seventeen themes emerged in total from the sampled tweets.

RQ1: Themes that Emerged Regarding COVID-19 and BLM

Eight prominent themes emerged from the data related to social media discussions of COVID-19 and BLM before Floyd's killing, and two additional themes emerged in tweets posted after Floyd's killing.

Theme 1: Racialized Health Care

Tweets included in this theme expressed a lack of respect for Black and Brown people's health in terms of access to COVID-19 testing and therapeutic treatment. This theme included tweets expressing feelings that those in power view minority groups as disposable because of their race. For example:

> (1) #TrumpAdministration will never care about Black and Brown!!! They are loving the fact, #BlackLivesMatter and #LatinosUnidos are dying from #COVID

Theme 2: Pandemic of Racism

Tweets included in this theme addressed the U.S. pandemic preparedness and response as an institutionalized, structural issue. This theme's tweets also reflected that the pandemic of racism is normalized in the United States and around the world, as expressed by the following tweets:

> (2) Normal is economic, health care, and environmental inequalities that allowed for the disproportionate killing of Black and brown people at the hands of #COVID19.
>
> (3) Because #InstitutionalisedRacism doesn't stop during a global pandemic #CoVid19 #BlackLivesMatter

Theme 3: Economic Injustice

Tweets in this theme reflected a concern with pressure by President Trump to reopen the economy despite the growing rates of COVID-19-related deaths in communities of color. These tweets also reflected the perceived injustices suffered by vulnerable members of society who were not being helped economically, including essential workers, seniors, women, and people who were incarcerated or dealing with mental illness. For example:

> (4) I wonder if we would be so anxious to reopen the economy if the majority of#COVID19 cases and deaths hadn't been in black and brown communities.
>
> #BlackLivesMatter

Theme 4: GOP Leadership

Tweets in this theme explicitly identified President Trump and the Republican Party leadership as complicit in the United States' weak response to the pandemic. This theme included tweets suggesting that Trump's incompetent leadership was responsible for the inadequate pandemic response and American deaths. Furthermore, Grand Old Party, or Republican Party (GOP) leaders and the president were criticized for their silence during the pandemic and accused of abetting genocide. A tweet supporting this theme is:

> (5) How can Trump command a Space Force, he can't even enforce a 6 foot space protocol? #COVID19 #Biden2020 #BlackLivesMatter #TrumpIsAnIdiot
>
> #TrumpLiesAmericansDie

Theme 5: Memorializing the Loss from COVID-19

Tweets reflecting this theme honored the grim milestones of deaths attributed to COVID-19, named specific people lost to COVID-19, and brought attention to Breonna Taylor, an unarmed Black woman who was tragically killed by Louisville police. Tweets reflecting this theme include:

> (6) 100,000 Americans dead & 20,000 of Black people in America dead #BlackLivesMatter #COVID19
>
> (7) #EMT helping with #Covid_19 #Covid19 patients. #ExcessiveForce #BLM #ShotInOwnHome

Theme 6: Role of Media in Covering COVID-19

Tweets categorized in this theme focused on the role of the media in covering the pandemic. In general, tweets were critical of COVID-19 coverage provided by major news outlets (e.g., *CNN*, *Fox News*, and *NBC*). These tweets also suggested mainstream news media should provide coverage on specific topics, including police brutality, as in the following tweet:

> (8) I pretty disgusted by the news media who has basically forgotten about #COVID19. Allow us to prove we can handle two things at once. #BlackLivesMatter, especially considering how deadly the virus is to African Americans. @CNN @MSNBC @NBCNews @ABC @CBSNews fix this!

Theme 7: Information Sharing on COVID-19-Related Issues

Tweets in this theme focused on sharing information to increase public awareness on COVID-19-related issues. This category included tweets that shared statistical data on COVID-19 transmission rates and deaths, information related to infectious disease prevention, and information about specific coronavirus hotspot locations to avoid. For instance:

> (9) As a Black person, sun basking has taken a totally new meaning. It's no longer about enjoying the warmth. Now it's about boosting my vitamin D & immunity – a smart part in avoid the rona #COVID19 #BlackLivesMatter

Theme 8: Solidarity During BLM Movement

This theme was supported by tweets encouraging the public to unite in solidarity behind the BLM movement, to provide mutual support, and to fight against the Trump administration, particularly through the electoral process. For example:

> (10) We have to take some self-responsibility as a community, and not solely for #COVID. We must stop ignoring our own faults and promoting the victim's mentality. #BlackLivesMatter #BLEXIT https://t.co/YteB1if7JH

Themes that emerged from tweets before Floyd's killing were reinforced in tweets that emerged after Floyd's killing. A counter-narrative to the solidarity theme mentioned above emerged from tweets made after Floyd's killing. It questioned the perceived lack of public support for counter-narratives that denounced attacks on Asians; furthermore, Trump's rhetoric of referring to COVID-19 as "the China Virus" was thought to have instigated these attacks on Asian Americans, as in:

(11) How come none of the #BLM came out to support #AsianAmericans or donated millions to Asians when they were harassed, attacked or killed by fellow #Americans this year for #COVID19? Where's our justice? Our peace?

(12) Many kept quiet when #Asians were attacked. Our coverages went unseen, our voices unheard, and the hate was hardly spoken. Racism is as real as its pain, especially when you're on the receiving end. #AsiansForBlackLives #GeorgeFloyd #COVID19 #BlackLivesMatter #CoronaVirus

Two additional themes emerged from tweets posted after Floyd's killing: (a) the risks of protesting during the pandemic and (b) conspiracy theories.

Theme 9: Risks of Protests During the Pandemic

This category of tweets questioned protestors' strategy of participating in mass gatherings during the pandemic because COVID-19 mitigation measures, including social distancing and contact tracing, are difficult to facilitate in large gatherings. Tweets in this theme also offered solidarity and support to those willing to risk their personal health and safety to participate in mass demonstrations, such as:

(13) #BlackLivesMatter. Shouldn't we be concerned about the thousands that will die from #COVID19 after these protests?

(14) How will #COVID19 contact tracing be done after #BlackLivesMatter protests?

Theme 10: Conspiracy Theories

Tweets in this category addressed several theories regarding the BLM movement and COVID-19, including that Floyd was murdered in order to incite riots. Conspiracy theorists implied that this could lead to an increase in citizen arrests and voter disenfranchisement in advance of the 2020 presidential election. Tweets also reflected a theory that police officers chose not to wear masks in order to purposely spread the virus among protestors, like these:

(15) What if: This is being made worse by #police etc. to ensure

1. More blacks & their allies are exposed to #COVID19
2. More blacks & liberals are jailed losing the right to #vote

3. More businesses are destroyed and blighted so big gov/corps can buy them out.

#BlackLivesMatter

(16) All planned by #DeepState. A faux #COVID19 lock down—unemployment, excess idle time, & dependency. Violent offenders released to streets—riots, No bail reform—criminals released. Use of #GeorgeFloyd murder—protests—riots, destruction, looting, violence by #BLM & #ANTIFAN

RQ2: Sense-Making of COVID-19 and BLM

Political differences were apparent in the discussion and debate happening around COVID-19 and the BLM movement. Two themes emerged from the discussion on tweets posted during the days before and after Floyd's death to reflect how COVID-19 exasperated pre-existing inequities in social justice and in public health, respectively.

Theme 11: COVID-19 Exasperated Pre-Existing Inequities in Social Justice

The tweets reflected debate about the public's right to protest against social injustices and to do so in the wake of a resurgence of the virus during a global pandemic. For instance:

(17) Unbelievable. Law enforcement seizes masks meant to protect anti-racist protestors from #COVID19. #BlackLivesMatter

Theme 12: COVID-19 Exasperated Pre-Existing Inequities in Public Health

From the start of the pandemic, the Trump administration controlled the flow of pandemic information and attempted to silence or ignore the advice and expertise of trained public health officials and scientists working with the CDC and National Institutes of Health (Rutledge, 2020). COVID-19 exposed and compounded inequalities in the U.S. public health system. These tensions were evident in tweets that expressed opinions concerning the response of the public health system to the pandemic and Trump's influence on the public information available for informed decision-making. For example:

(18) Black People Need To Create Their Own Media. Whoever Controls Your Information Controls Your Mind #90DaysFianceBeforeThe90Days #BlackLivesMatter #COVID19

(19) Disinformation Counter Measure #WeAreAUnitedPeople Discern Information from all sources Common Sense vs Narrative Control #RussiaGate #MuellerReport #COVID19 #BlackLivesMatter #LawAndOrder is the foundation of #OurRepublic

Theme 13: COVID-19 Is Related to BLM: COVID-19 as State-Sanctioned Violence Against Black and Brown People

Twitter users debated vehemently about the connections between BLM, COVID-19, and state violence against Black and Brown people, such as:

(20) U support police contributing to spreading covid like unarmed peaceful BLM protestors were trying to prevent w/masks?! #BLM

Theme 14: COVID-19 Is Not Related to BLM: Trump Lies/Americans Die

It has been suggested that President Trump's crisis management approach—misdirection, misinformation, divisiveness, and hostility toward science and data-driven assessments—stymied the U.S. pandemic response (Rutledge, 2020). This theme's tweets reflected the belief that President Trump's authoritarian style of governance and his disregard for established American norms of governance contradict a chief executive's expected behaviors. Twitter discussion regarding President Trump also suggested a desire for American society to return to normal. For instance:

(21) This is an important read! WE CANNOT NORMALIZE #TrumpDictatorship Behavior This is #TrumpCult Plan #CorruptGOP #RacistInChief Is a menace to every American! #COVID19 #BlackLivesMatter #VoteBlueTo SaveAmerica2020 #resist Or we will never get out of this!

RQ3: Discussions Among Social Media Users About COVID-19-Related Race and Health Disparity Issues

Most Twitter users believed that COVID-19 disproportionally affected Black and Brown people. Furthermore, Twitter users expressed views that the BLM movement and forthcoming election were important factors in stopping the spread of COVID-19. Three themes emerged.

Theme 15: Voting (Political Participation) Needed to Change COVID-19/System of Racism

While some users believed the 2020 Election could change the course of COVID-19, others believed the problems would remain the same in 2021 (despite a potential change of president or development of an effective vaccine), exampled in the following tweet:

> (22) Pandemics, protests and people in pain. Let's not forget it's Trump who got us here! Take a trip down memory lane in my new music video "TRUMPS AMERICA" out now! #DumpTrump2020 #Covid19 #BunkerBoy #BlackLivesMatter https://t.co/qAe8WB90Z9

Theme 16: Black Unity Needed for Change

Tweets in this theme reflected the call for Black unity by activists from all forces to resist acceptance of the current situation and to believe that change is possible. This theme also captured the sentiment that without change, the future existence of Blacks was at stake, as in this tweet:

> (23) "black people, what do you have to lose?"—@realDonaldTrump is an existential threat to all black Americans. Our lives are at the intersection of death, #COVID19 on one side & endorsed police brutality on the other. #GeorgeFloyd #BlackLivesMatter #ICantBreathe #ohshittheeconomy

Theme 17: Media Framing of BLM Impacting Perceptions of Issues

Tweets in this theme addressed perceptions that media framing was impacting public perceptions on the issues of BLM and COVID-19, including perceptions that the media's attention to BLM protests detracted public attention from the coronavirus. For example:

> (24) And just like that...poof. #COVID19 is now second fiddle to #blacklivesmatter. Interesting how quickly the media can change the narrative. Now no one will remember how wrong they were about the virus, they are too busy being angry at the police. Well done #Soros, well done.

In addition to concerns that media framing used BLM as a smoke screen to COVID-19, users also expressed concern by tweeting about negative media framing of the BLM movement and BLM protests, like:

> (25) Media already seeding the idea of a new COVID-19 spike due to breaches of social distancing/mass gatherings at protests. This will justify 2nd wave restrictions. #covid19 #coronavirustruth #antifa #BlackLivesMatter

Finally, tweets reflected the media's failure both to expose the social inequities fueling BLM protests and to provide the public context to understand the racial disparities of COVID-19, as in this tweet:

> (26) America is sick. #COVID is the least profound illness; the chief one is racism (others include greed). Inequality, an atomized society, low civic education, elite capture of gov't—plus media aimed at increasing cortisol, lowering IQ—are ripping us apart. #BlackLivesMatter

Discussion

Twitter users discuss a wide range of topics around the implications of COVID-19, including politics, race and racism, health disparities, and social injustice. In a time of intense political division, people express varied attitudes toward the impacts of BLM and COVID-19. The implications of this study include the following.

In answering RQ1, ten themes emerged indicating that the race war was intensified because of COVID-19 and, specifically, the death of George Floyd. Twitter is used as an online community to express democratic principles and differences, such as racialized healthcare (Theme 1), pandemic of racism (Theme 2), and economic injustice (Theme 3). Twitter users also debated the risks of protesting during the pandemic (Theme 9) and solidarity during the BLM movement (Theme 8). Twitter users discussed COVID-19 information sharing and media coverage (Themes 5, 6). Users also debated politics and conspiracy theories and memorialized the losses caused by COVID-19 (Themes 5, 10).

With regard to RQ2 (making sense of COVID-19 and BLM), tweets reflected tensions around the right of the public to protest against social injustices, as well as the need to protect public health during a pandemic. When social distancing is mandated, public gatherings are prohibited—but people still have the right to protest. Most protesters took precautions while engaged in public protests, such as wearing facial masks and keeping six feet away from others, which helped these events avert becoming "super spreader" threats as predicted (Dave et al., 2020). Critics spoke out in opposition to protests happening during a pandemic, and some blamed the BLM movement or Democratic party for looting and violence that occurred.

In discussing RQ3 (race and disparities), Twitter users analyzed issues of Black unity, media framing, and the election. In 2020, these issues were inextricably linked to COVID-19 and BLM. Each one of these issues cannot be examined in a vacuum; they are all interrelated.

Limitations and Future Studies

This chapter has discussed the perceptions of COVID-19 and the BLM movement. Thematic analysis was used to identify common themes and offers insights on how social media impacts knowledge regarding public health crises. There are, however, limitations to this study. First, the platform examined (Twitter) attracts a narrow subset of the population, impacting the findings' generalizability. A Pew report found Twitter users in the United States are more likely to be relatively young, be well-educated, identify as Democrats, and earn higher incomes than other U.S. adults. This report also indicates that most Twitter users rarely tweet, suggesting that tweets posted in this study represent a small and narrow segment of the population (Wojcik & Hughes, 2020).

Another limitation was the inability to know the authenticity of tweets analyzed. Data sets were subject to misinformation as authors of the posts may have posted content solely for a reaction on social media. Data sets included English-only tweets, but not all Americans speak English as their primary language, including many Latinx people. Analysis of English-only tweets limited potential opinions of a segment of the United States that uses Twitter and posts about BLM and COVID-19. Future studies may include Spanish language tweets and expand to another platform to gain enhanced understanding of public opinion regarding the topics of BLM and COVID-19.

References

Abd-Alrazaq, A., Alhuwail, D., Househ, M., Hamdi, M., & Shah, Z. (2020). Top Concerns of Tweeters During the COVID-19 Pandemic: Infoveillance Study. *Journal of Medical Internet Research, 22*(4), e19016.

Ahmed, W., Bath, P., Sbaffi, L., & Demartini, G. (2019). Novel Insights Into Views Towards H1N1 During the 2009 Pandemic: A Thematic Analysis of Twitter Data. *Health Information and Libraries Journal, 36*(1), 60–72. https://doi.org/10.1111/hir.12247

APM Research Lab. (2020, December 10). COVID-19 Deaths Analyzed by Race and Ethnicity—APM Research Lab. Retrieved from www.apmresearchlab.org/covid/deaths-by-race-december2020

Blevins, J. L., Lee, J. J., McCabe, E. E., & Edgerton, E. (2019). Tweeting for Social Justice in #Ferguson: Affective Discourse in Twitter Hashtags. *New Media &Society, 21*(7), 1636–1653.

Bolsen, T., Palm, R., & Kingsland, J. T. (2020). Framing the Origins of COVID-19. *Science Communication, 42*(5), 562–585.

Braun, V., & Clarke, V. (2006). Using Thematic Analysis in Psychology. *Qualitative Research in Psychology, 3*(2), 77–101.

Castells, M. (2015). *Networks of Outrage and Hope: Social Movements in the Internet Age.* Cambridge, UK: Polity Press.

Centers for Disease Control and Prevention. (2019, March 8). 2014-2016 Ebola Outbreak in West Africa. www.cdc.gov/vhf/ebola/history/2014-2016-outbreak/index.html

Centers for Disease Control and Prevention. (2020a, May 1). Weekly Updates by Select Demographic and geographic Characteristics. Retrieved from www.cdc.gov/nchs/nvss/vsrr/covid_weekly/

Centers for Disease Control and Prevention. (2020b, July 24). Health Equity Considerations and Racial and Ethnic Minority Groups. Retrieved from www.cdc.gov/coronavirus/2019-ncov/community/health-equity/race-ethnicity.html

Centers for Disease Control and Prevention. (2020c, October 23). Race, Ethnicity, and Age Trends in Persons Who Died from COVID-19—United States, May–August 2020. *Morbidity and Mortality Weekly Reports, 69*(42), 1517–1521. www.cdc.gov/mmwr/volumes/69/wr/mm6942e1.htm

Chen, E., Lerman, K., & Ferrara, E. (2020). Tracking Social Media Discourse About the COVID-19 Pandemic: Development of a Public Coronavirus Twitter Data Set. *JMIR Public Health and Surveillance 6*(2), e19273. doi: **10.2196/19273**

Cranmer, G. A., & Sanderson, J. (2018). "Rough Week for Testosterone": Public Commentary Around the Ivy League's Decision to Restrict Tackle Football in Practice. *Western Journal of Communication, 82*(5), 631–647. doi:10.1080/10570314.2018.1441431

Das, S., & Dutta, A. (2020). Characterizing Public Emotions and Sentiments in Covid-19 Environment: A Case Study of India. *Journal of Human Behavior in the Social Environment, 31*(1–4), 154–167. doi.org/10.1080/10911359.2020.1781015

Dave, D. M., Friedson, A. I., Matsuzawa, K., Sabia, J. J., & Safford, S. (2020, June 18). Black Lives Matter Protests, Social Distancing, and COVID-19. *NBER*. Retrieved from www.nber.org/papers/w27408

Egede, L. E., & Walker, R. J. (2020). Structural Racism, Social Risk Factors, and Covid-19— A Dangerous Convergence for Black Americans. *The New England Journal of Medicine, 383*, e77.

Fuchs, C. (2015). *Culture and Economy in the Age of Social Media.* New York, NY: Routledge.

Glaser, B. G., & Strauss, A. (1967). *The Discovery of Grounded Theory.* Chicago, IL: Aldine.

Glenn, C. L. (2015). Activism or "Slacktivism?": Digital Media and Organizing for Social Change. *Communication Teacher, 29*(2), 81–85. https://doi.org/10.1080/17404622.2014.1003310

Grinberg, N., Joseph, K., Friedland, L., Swire-Thompson, B., & Lazer, D. (2019). Fake News on Twitter During the 2016 US Presidential Election. *Science, 363*(6425), 374–378. pmid:30679368

Habermas, J. (2006). Political Communication in Media Society: Does Democracy Still Enjoy an Epistemic Dimension? The Impact of Normative Theory on Empirical Research. *Communication Theory, 16*(4), 411–426. doi:10.1111/j.1468-2885.2006.00280.x

Ince, J., Rojas, F., & Davis, C. A. (2017). The Social Media Response to Black Lives Matter: How Twitter Users Interact with Black Lives Matter Through Hashtag Use. *Ethnic and Racial Studies, 40*(11), 1814–1830.

Jo, W., & Chang, D. (2020). Political Consequences of COVID-19 and Media Framing in South Korea. *Frontiers in Public Health, 8*, 1–10. doi.org/10.3389/fpubh.2020.00425

Khazanchi, R., Evans, C. T., & Macelin, J. R. (2020). Racism, Not Race, Drives Inequity Across the COVID-19 Continuum. *JAMA Network Open, 3*(9), e2019933. doi:10.1001/jamanetworkopen.2020.19933

Kidd, D., & McIntosh, K. (2016). Social Media and Social Movements. *Sociology Compass*, *10*(9), 785–794. https://doi.org/10.1111/soc4.12399

Kilgo, D. K., Yoo, J., & Johnson, T. J. (2018). Spreading Ebola Panic: Newspaper and Social Media Coverage of the 2014 Ebola Health Crisis. *Journal of Health Communication*, *34*(8), 811–817. https://doi.org/10.1080/10410236.2018.1437524

Lazard, A., Scheinfeld, E., Bernhardt, J., Wilcox, G., & Suran, M. (2015). Detecting Themes of Public Concern: A Text Mining Analysis of the Centers for Disease Control and Prevention's Ebola Live Twitter Chat. *AJIC: American Journal of Infection Control*, *43*(10), 1109–1111. https://doi.org/10.1016/j.ajic.2015.05.025

Lee, P. S., So, C. Y., & Leung, L. (2015). Social Media and Umbrella Movement: Insurgent Public Sphere Information. *Chinese Journal of Communication*, *8*(4), 356–375.

Meyer, R. (2020, June 1). The Protests Will Spread the Coronavirus. *The Atlantic*. www.theatlantic.com/health/archive/2020/06/protests-pandemic/612460/

Miller, M., Banerjee, T., Muppalla, R., Romine, W., & Sheth, A. (2017). What Are People Tweeting about Zika? An Exploratory Study Concerning Its Symptoms, Treatment, Transmission, and Prevention. *JMIR Public Health and Surveillance*, *3*(2), e38. https://doi.org/10.2196/publichealth.7157

Mundt, M., Ross, K., & Burnett, C. M. (2018). Scaling Social Movements Through Social Media: The Case of Black Lives Matter. *Social Media + Society*, 4(4),1–14. doi.org/10.1177/2056305118807911

Nania, R. (2020, May 8). Blacks, Hispanics Hit Harder by the Coronavirus. *AARP*. Retrieved from www.aarp.org/health/conditions-treatments/info-2020/minority-communities-covid-19.html

Ogbodo, J. N., Onwe, E. K., Chukwu, J., Nwasum, C. J., Nwakpu, E. S., Nwankwo, S. U., Nwamini, S., Elem, S., & Ogbaeia, N. I. (2020). Communicating Health Crisis: A Content Analysis of Global Media Framing of COVID-19. *Health Promotion Perspectives 10*(3), 257–269. doi:10.34172/hpp.2020.40

Perrin, A. (2020, October 16). 23% of Users in U.S. Say Social Media Led Them to Change Views on an Issue; Some Cite Black Lives Matter. *Pew Research*. Retrieved from www.pewresearch.org/fact-tank/2020/10/15/23-of-users-in-us-say-social-media-led-them-to-change-views-on-issue-some-cite-black-lives-matter/

Poirier, W., Ouellet, C., Rancourt, M.-A., Béchard, J., & Dufresne, Y. (2020). (Un)Covering the Covid-19 Pandemic: Framing Analysis of the Crisis in Canada. *Canadian Journal of Political Science*, *53*, 365–371. https://doi.org/10.1017/S0008423920000372

Ray, R., Brown, M., Fraistat, N., & Summers, E. (2017). Ferguson and the Death of Michael Brown on Twitter: #BlackLivesMatter, #TCOT, and the Evolution of Collective Identities. *Ethnic and Racial Studies*, *40*(11), 1797–1813.

Reyes, C., Husain, N., Gutowski, C., Clair, S. S., & Pratt, G. (2020, April 7). *Chicago's Coronavirus Disparity: Black Chicagoans Are Dying at Nearly Six Times the Rate of White Residents, Data Show*. Retrieved from www.chicagotribune.com/coronavirus/ct-coronavirus-chicago-coronavirus-deaths-demographics-lightfoot-20200406-77nlylhiavgjzb2wa4ckivh7mu-story.html

Rutledge, P. E. (2020). Trump, Covid-19, and the War on Expertise. *The American Review of Public Administration*, *50*(6–7), 505–511. doi:10.1177/0275074020941683

Toepfl, F., & Piwoni, E. (2015). Public Spheres in Interaction: Comment Sections of News Websites as Counterpublic Spaces. *Journal of Communication*, *65*(3), 465–488. doi:10.1111/jcom.12156

University of Southern California. (2020, May 20). Covering Coronavirus: The Pandemic's Unequal Toll Webinar. *USC Annenberg Center for Health Journalism*. NIHCM Foundation and Commonwealth Fund.

Van Beusekom, M. (2020, September 25). Studies Spotlight COVID Racial Health Disparities, Similarities. *CIDRAP (Center for Infectious Disease Research and Policy) News.* www.cidrap.umn.edu/news-perspective/2020/09/studies-spotlight-covid-racial-health-disparities-similarities

Wen, L. S., & Sadeghi, N. B. (2020, July 20). Addressing Racial Health Disparities in the Covid-19 Pandemic: Immediate and Long-Term Policy Solutions. *Health Affairs.* www.healthaffairs.org/do/10.1377/hblog20200716.620294/full

Wessler, H., & Freudenthler, R. (2011). Public Sphere. *Oxford Bibliographies.* Retrieved from www.oxfordbibliographies.com/view/document/obo-9780199756841/obo-9780199756841-0030.xml

Wicke, P., & Bolognesi, M. M. (2020). Framing COVID-19: How We Conceptualize and Discuss the Pandemic on Twitter. *PLOS ONE, 15*(9), e0240010. https://doi.org/10.1371/journal.pone.0240010

Wilkens, D. J., Livingstone, A. G., & Levine, M. (2019). Whose tweets? The Rhetorical Functions of Social Media in Developing Black Lives Matter Movement. *British Journal of Social Psychology, 58,* 786–805.

Wojcik, S., & Hughes, A. (2020, May 30). How Twitter Users Compare to the General Public. Retrieved from www.pewresearch.org/internet/2019/04/24/sizing-up-twitter-users/

Yancy, C. W. (2020, May 19). COVID-19, African Americans, and Health Disparities. Retrieved from https://jamanetwork.com/journals/jama/fullarticle/2764789

6

SAME PANDEMIC, DIFFERENT PLIGHTS

The Conjoined Effects of Socioeconomic Status and Ethnoracial Identity on Psychological Distress at the Dawn of COVID-19

Tyson D. King-Meadows, Abigail Timbol, and Priscilla Nalubula

Introduction

While scholars and health practitioners have long recognized the impact of ethnoracial identity and socioeconomic status on wellness in the United States, it was not a foregone conclusion at the onset of the COVID-19 outbreak that either factor would significantly affect COVID's trajectory within communities. On the one hand, it was easy to imagine that COVID-19 would illuminate pre-existing disparities. Speaking to this at the 2021 meeting of the American Council on Education, African American Policy Forum Executive Director Kimberlé Crenshaw remarked that the COVID-19 pandemic was akin to an "MRI" (magnetic resonance imaging) on structural racism. For Crenshaw, the pandemic revealed the need for policymakers to acknowledge that structural racism shapes disease prevention, mitigation, and treatment. Others also saw the psychological distress expressed by minorities as evidence of their unique vulnerability to the pandemic's economic shocks and social upheaval. These shocks, scholars argued, translated into more virulent forms of cumulative disadvantage and adverse health outcomes for minorities (Novacek et al., 2020).

On the other hand, previous research on the social determinants of health had shown that neither ethnic/racial identity nor socioeconomic status could fully explain disparities in mental health outcomes, like distress. Some observers argued that racial disparities in distress could be due to the types of public-facing wage-based jobs generally held by racial and gender minorities. Scholars also suggested that other factors could explain differences in distress, like attitudes about health maintenance, ideology, and news attentiveness. Therefore, for some observers, two things were plausible about the trajectory of distress for different groups at the onset of the COVID-19 outbreak: first, that socioeconomic status could provide a

DOI: 10.4324/9781003268710-6

prophylactic barrier against stress for certain ethnoracial groups; and second, that there would be a minimal relationship, if any, between gender, ethnoracial identity, socioeconomic status, and psychological distress. In other words, for some, the onset of the COVID outbreak did not necessarily provide enough clues to how ethnoracial groups might fare differently under that specific health crisis.

The purpose of this chapter is to estimate the separate and interactive effects of ethnoracial identity, income, and news consumption on psychological distress. Specifically, we look for clues about the plight trajectory of groups by analyzing early COVID-related mental health outcomes as reported by U.S. adults in two large surveys conducted by the Pew Research Center. These surveys were fielded shortly after the World Health Organization had declared the COVID-19 outbreak to be a pandemic.

The chapter proceeds as follows. First, cumulative disadvantage, ethnoracial health disparities, and health news briefly summarizes the extant literature on health disparities. This is followed by sections on data and methods and results that detail our analytical strategy and findings. The final section places our findings in the context of actions in early 2021 to expand vaccine distribution. Overall, we argue that the early COVID surveys from the Pew Research Center should help scholars further contextualize the ethnoracial dimensions of infection rates, hospitalizations, and deaths.

Cumulative Disadvantage, Ethnoracial Health Disparities, and Health News

Scholars and health practitioners underscore that there are multiple shapers of health inequality. Disparities between White and non-White communities, for example, result from "cumulative disadvantage," which occurs early in life, grows over time across the life course, and differentiates cohorts. DiPrete and Eirich (2005) write, "[T]he advantage in question is typically a key resource [essential] to the stratification process, for example, cognitive development, career position, income, wealth, or health." Other items related to the stratification process include family financial difficulties, parental divorce, neglect, life-threatening childhood illness, and maladjustments such as mental illness, substance abuse, and criminality (Green et al., 2010). The aforementioned outcomes are linked to racial categorization because race and class shape how people navigate life, including where people live. Resulting disparities are also further exacerbated by political under-representation, segregation, and economic isolation. Scholars also note that health disparities left unchecked enhance citizen distrust in the healthcare system and in the political structure. This distrust invariably undermines relief initiatives and disease mitigation plans, a feedback loop that reinforces cumulative disadvantage (Loeb et al., 2021).

Individuals in predominantly non-White communities are often the most vulnerable because they have lower levels of socioeconomic status than Whites. Race-based data show that minorities report higher levels of depression, anxiety, victimization from violent crimes, and abuse than do Whites (Loeb et al., 2021). Individuals with significant long-term exposure to poverty, joblessness, or inadequate housing have also been shown to have a greater likelihood of experiencing mental and physical distress. For instance, neighborhood residents affected by accumulated disadvantages have been found to be more likely to develop major chronic health conditions and to limit their pro-health physical activities (Shin et al., 2019). For some scholars, like Crenshaw, the trauma inflicted by inequality highlighted the need for policymakers to guide COVID-19 relief through race-conscious interventions that specifically addressed the psychological distress of vulnerable communities (Novacek et al., 2020).

Relatedly, the multifaceted nature of health disparities also implicates news consumption practices due to a possible relationship between social identity, psychological reactions to public calamities, and mental health. In a study of media influence, Sell et al. (2017) found that "risk-elevating messages" from Ebola virus news stories in the United States emphasized harm over prevention and scientific knowledge. The authors write, "The high frequency of risk-elevating messages in news coverage may have contributed to increased public concern about EVD in the United States, which was greater than the situation warranted." They also concluded, "Consumers of news media would have been exposed to risk-elevating messages more often than risk-minimizing messages, potentially increasing their perception of risk for EVD." Jennifer Jerit et al. (2019) offer an analogous claim about the role of local and national news reporting on the Zika outbreak. Tian and Stewart (2005) report similar findings about how the news characterized the risks associated with severe acute respiratory syndrome (SARS-Cov). In short, scholars investigating public reaction to health-related stories suggest that adverse mental health outcomes related to extreme health calamities, like the COVID-19 pandemic, could result from both inputs (i.e., the content of news reports) and outputs (i.e., the attention audiences pay).

The COVID-19 Magnifier

As a magnifying event, which drew heightened attention to a specific infectious disease and to the consequences of contracting the said disease, the COVID-19 pandemic did more than enhance the predictive variables associated with certain social determinants of health disparities. Not only did the pandemic decrease access to specific preventive measures and to a quality education, the pandemic also increased overall social precarity. The impact of COVID-19 on the African American community was of note in this regard. Some early studies found African Americans comprising most of the COVID-19 hospitalizations despite making up only 13% of the U.S. population (Kullar et al., 2020). Other early studies found infection rates in majority-black counties to be three times higher than their majority-White counterparts (Kullar et al., 2020). Undoubtedly, systems of oppression that predated COVID-19 led to the increased vulnerability faced by African Americans during the pandemic (Kullar et al., 2020).

The COVID-19 pandemic also affected pre-existing health disparities in the Hispanic/Latinx community. Scholars have shown that the cumulative impact of coexisting medical conditions as well as other factors, like concentration in low-wage service jobs, increased the vulnerability of Hispanics to the pandemic (Gil et al., 2020). These impacts increased the risk of exposure by reducing access to healthcare, to information about COVID-19 mitigation measures, and to telework opportunities (Gil et al., 2020).

The COVID-19 pandemic also enhanced health disparities among Asian Americans. However, unlike the pandemic's early impact on African American and Hispanic/Latinx communities, the early negative impact on Asian Americans was also associated with a "dramatic increase in discrimination against Asian individuals worldwide" (Chen et al., 2020). The rise in anti-Asian American sentiment and the rise in hate crimes against Asians/Asian Americans unleashed a barrage of harmful effects on community health (Chen et al., 2020). These communities were already under-resourced: Studies done prior to COVID had shown that Asian Americans were among the lowest demographic utilizing mental health services (Chen et al., 2020). In all, the COVID outbreak was certainly able to magnify the emotional distress of individuals who lacked the resources to withstand the pandemic-related socioeconomic upheaval.

Data and Methods

To assess how much the onset of COVID-19 magnified health disparities in the early weeks of the pandemic, we turn to survey data from two consecutive waves of the Pew Research Center's American Trends Panel (ATP). We use these surveys to measure the relationship between ethnoracial identity, news consumption practices, and disparities in psychological distress. Begun in 2014, the ATP is a web-based "nationally representative panel of U.S. adults who answer self-administered questions" about various topics. The first survey, ATP Wave 64 ($N = 11,537$), was conducted on March 19–24, 2020. The second survey, ATP Wave 66 ($N = 10,139$), was conducted on April 20–26, 2020. We examine the weighted samples in Wave 64 (7,297 White non-Hispanics, 1,306 Black non-Hispanics, 1,810 Hispanics of any race, and 979 Other Racial Minorities) and in Wave 66 (6,450 White non-Hispanics, 1,155 Black non-Hispanics, 1,550 Hispanics of any race, and 860 Other Racial Minorities). Respondents answered questions about their mental health, perceptions about the outbreak, and evaluation of leaders. Respondents also answered standard sociodemographic questions. For ease of presentation, we refer to our analysis of Wave 64 and Wave 66 as Study 1 and Study 2, respectively. As a comparison, we also analyze the weighted data from Wave 65 ($N = 4,917$), conducted on April 7–12, 2020, which contained 3,167 White non-Hispanics, 570 Black non-Hispanics, 688 Hispanics of any race, and 420 Other Racial Minorities.[1]

We employ two quantitative methods to ascertain the relationship between ethnoracial identity, socioeconomic status, and mental health outcomes. We first attend to the bivariate relationship between ethnoracial identity and five measures of psychological distress. Next, we utilize ordinary least squares (OLS) regression to model the drivers of aggregate psychological distress. Afterwards, we use k-means cluster analysis to categorize respondents based upon their answers to the five measures. We follow the procedure outlined by Makles (2012) to determine the optimal number of clusters. We then apply a hierarchical cluster analysis to stress test our initial findings.

Dependent Variable

Following conventions utilized by the Pew Research Center, we use responses to five mental health questions from Wave 64 and from Wave 66 to serve as our dependent variables. The first four questions asked how often a respondent experienced something in the past seven days: anxiety, depression, loneliness, and trouble sleeping. The fifth question asked, "In the past 7 days, how often have you had physical reactions, such as sweating, trouble breathing, nausea, or a pounding heart, when thinking about your experience with the coronavirus outbreak?" The response options were "rarely, some or little of the time, occasionally, most or all of the time, and no answer." Respondents were restricted to one response and were able to skip any question.

We replicate and expand upon the methodology used by the Pew Research Center (March 2020) to examine the five questions as one measure of psychological distress. Rather than use a raw additive index, we normalize our additive index between 0 and 1 (*Psychological Distress*). We conducted a series of tests to ascertain the viability of combining the five measures into one scale. We were satisfied by the results.[2] Moreover, each response option also provided both numerical and semantical differentiation. We take this as additional justification for our treatment of the five psychological distress measures as one interval measure.[3]

Independent Variables (Study 1)

Our primary variables of interest are respondent socioeconomic status (*Education* and *Income*), gender, and racial/ethnic identity. We combine gender and ethnoracial identity into eight dichotomous variables: *White Male, White Female, Black Male, Black Female, Hispanic Male, Hispanic Female, Other Minority Male*, and *Other Minority Female*. This strategy enables us to model the effects of a respondent's conjoined experiences on the probability of reporting an adverse COVID-related mental health outcome.

Our second set of independent variables address experience with the COVID-19 crisis: wage/job loss due to the outbreak, news attentiveness, perception of the threat posed by the outbreak, confidence in the healthcare system, and evaluation of policymakers' response to COVID. To ascertain *COVID News Attention*, we utilize the following question: "How closely have you been following news about the outbreak of the coronavirus strain known as COVID-19?" The response option was the standard four-point "not at all closely" to "very closely." We expect a positive association between news consumption and adverse mental health. To measure threat perception, we use answers to "How much of a threat, if any, is the coronavirus outbreak for" the following four areas: the health of the U.S. population (*U.S. Health*), your personal health (*Personal Health*), the U.S. economy (*U.S. Economy*), and your personal financial situation (*Personal Finances*). We expect respondents who view COVID-19 as major threats to their personal well-being to be more likely to report higher levels of psychological distress. Because perceptions of the COVID-19 threat may have been influenced by attitudes about the U.S. healthcare system, we include answers to the question "How confident, if at all, are you that each of the following will be able to handle the medical needs of people who are seriously ill during the coronavirus outbreak?" Respondents were prompted to address three areas—"Hospitals and medical centers in your area," "Hospitals and medical centers around the country," and "Nursing homes in your area." We utilized a four-point response option of "not at all confident" to "very confident." We then normalized each response to a 0 to 1 scale, and we averaged the three results. Respondents at "1" express the most amount of confidence and respondents at "0" express the least amount of confidence in the capacity of the system to deal with the outbreak (*Heath System Confidence*).[4] We expect lower levels of confidence to be associated with higher levels of distress. Likewise, we expect wage/job loss due to the outbreak (*Job Loss*) to be associated with higher distress. Finally, we measure the evaluation of the response to COVID by opinion leaders and policymakers. We use the question "How would you rate the job each of the following is doing responding to the coronavirus outbreak?" We coded responses about the Centers for Disease Control and Prevention (CDC), President Trump, and the news media as follows: 1 = Excellent; 2 = Good; 3 = Only fair; 4 = Poor. We expect higher numbers to be associated with higher distress.

A third set of independent variables serve as controls. We expect younger respondents, unmarried respondents, and less educated respondents to express higher distress levels. We expect conservatives, Republicans, and Republican-leaning Independents to express lower distress levels. Furthermore, we expect beliefs in interpersonal dynamics to affect mental health. We follow the Pew Research Center methodology by differentiating respondents according to their answers to three questions measuring trust (Rainie and Perrin, 2020). Respondents with optimistic answers to all questions are categorized as *High Trusters*. Respondents with optimistic answers and pessimistic answers are *Medium Trusters*. Respondents with pessimistic answers to all questions are *Low Trusters*. Relatedly, we expect higher distress levels to be reported by individuals who felt unhopeful in the seven days preceding the interview (*Hopeful*). Finally, we control for mental health status before COVID (*Prior Diagnosis*) with "Has a doctor or other healthcare provider ever told you that you have a mental health condition?"

Independent Variables (Study 2)

We use two batches of questions in Wave 66 to ascertain the impact of COVID-related news consumption practices and attitudinal dispositions on mental health.

The first batch asks respondents to identify how closely they followed "national news and information" about various topics related to the pandemic: economic impact of the outbreak (*Economic Impact*); actions and statements by the federal government (*Fed Actions*); number of confirmed U.S. cases and deaths (*Cases and Deaths*); advice from national health organizations, such as the CDC (*CDC Advice*); ability of hospitals across the country to treat patients (*Hospital Ability to Treat*); the health impact of the coronavirus on people like me (*Impact on People Like Me*).[5] Respondents were provided the traditional four-point response option of "very closely" to "not at all closely." We reverse code each answer so that higher numbers equal greater attentiveness. We expect distress-inducing attentiveness to be offset by comfort-inducing attentiveness. Nonetheless, we incorporate a respondent's feelings about "keeping up with news about the coronavirus outbreak" with *Emotional Response* (1 = Makes Me Feel Better emotionally; 2 = Does not change my emotions; 3 = Makes Me Feel Worse emotionally). Similarly, we account for the impact of futuristic orientation (*Hopeful*) on mental health. We utilize the coding scheme from Study 1 to measure socioeconomic status, gender, and racial/ethnic identity.

The second batch of questions pertain to perceptions and dispositions. Respondents were asked, "Thinking about the coronavirus outbreak, how in general do you think ... has responded?" Respondents answered about President Trump, the CDC, and the news media. We coded the response options so higher numbers reflect a perception that leaders overestimated the coronavirus risk (1 = not taken the risks seriously at all; 5 = greatly exaggerated the risks). We hypothesize that respondents who believe opinion leaders exaggerated the COVID-19 risk will be less likely to be distressed by the outbreak. Moreover, we hypothesize politically astute respondents will report less distress than their non-astute counterparts. As such, we include a measure developed by the Pew Research Center (*Political Knowledge*).[6] Finally, we account for religious beliefs (*Born Again*) and expect Evangelical Christians to report less psychological distress.

Results

We first examine descriptive statistics from the two waves. Using the scale of 1 ("rarely") to 4 ("most or all of the time"), we find average anxiety levels in March (2.342) had declined by April (2.119). However, respondents reported higher levels of "not sleeping" in April (Mean = 2.136, SD = 1.080) than they did in March (Mean = 2.066, SD = 1.068). Respondents also had higher levels of depression in April (Mean = 1.814, SD = 0.950) than in March (Mean =1.807, SD = 0.992). Higher levels of loneliness were reported in April (Mean = 1.781, SD = 0.973) than in March, with an increase of 0.074 from the baseline.

We found other noteworthy differences across the two waves. For example, in March (Wave 64), respondents who viewed the COVID-19 pandemic as a threat to the U.S. population's health had a 1.359 mean (out of scale from 1 to 3, where 3 was defined as "not a threat"), while those who thought the pandemic posed a major threat to their personal health had a 1.755 mean. Additionally, individuals who believed that the pandemic posed a threat to the U.S. economy had a mean of 1.131, while those who thought that it posed a threat to their personal finances had a mean of 1.628. Respondents were more concerned about the impact of COVID on their personal health and finances than on the nation's overall health and economy. Relatedly, we also find that respondents were confident in area hospitals and medical centers (a mean of 2.86) but were less confident in U.S. hospitals and medical centers (a mean of 2.78) and in area nursing homes (a mean of 2.56). Lastly, we find that individuals thought differently about how Trump, the CDC, and the news responded to COVID in March and April. Respondents in Wave 64 gave a high rating to the CDC (1.96) but gave a low rating to Trump (2.60) and to the media (2.52). Respondents in Wave 66 expressed similar sentiments: Respondents were more likely to report that Trump had not taken the risk quite seriously (2.26), that the news had exaggerated the risks (3.57), and that the CDC had gotten the risk about right (3.17).

Table 6.1 shows reported levels of psychological distress across five measures per ethnoracial identity group for Wave 64 and Wave 66. Overall, we find that all four racial categories reported high levels of anxiety and of not sleeping. However, we also find specific differences across the racial groups. Results from an ANOVA test show that race was a significant predictor of anxiety in Wave 64 ($F = 12.43$, $p < .001$). For example, Whites and Hispanics in Wave 64 had a 0.46 level of anxiety that was 0.02 higher in comparison to Other Racial Minorities. Whites were also more anxious than Blacks ($p < .001$). In Wave 66, anxiety levels were generally lower but Other Minorities were the most anxious (0.40). Self-reported depression had little variance across all racial categories in both waves. However, while Blacks and Hispanics expressed high depression in both waves, Hispanics and Other Minorities expressed the highest levels of depression in Wave 66. The ANOVA results for depression in Wave 64 were significant ($F = 3.51$, $p < .01$) as were the results for loneliness ($F = 24.36$, $p < .001$). Loneliness was prevalently higher in

TABLE 6.1 Ethnoracial Identity and Mean Distress Across Five Measures of Mental Health

	Wave 64				Wave 66			
	White	Black	Hispanic	Other	White	Black	Hispanic	Other
Anxiety	0.46	0.39	0.46	0.44	0.37	0.34	0.39	0.40
Depression	0.26	0.29	0.29	0.27	0.26	0.27	0.30	0.30
Loneliness	0.22	0.29	0.25	0.27	0.24	0.30	0.28	0.31
Not Sleeping	0.35	0.38	0.35	0.34	0.38	0.37	0.40	0.37
Physical Reaction	0.08	0.10	0.11	0.09	0.07	0.11	0.10	0.09

Source: Pew Research Center, ATP Wave 64, March 19–24, 2020 and ATP Wave 66, April 20–26, 2020.

Notes: Distress measured on 0 to 1 scale.

Table 6.1 shows five mental stressors among various racial and ethnic groups.

Blacks and Hispanics in comparison to Whites. The White–Black difference (0.07) was significant ($p < .01$). Not sleeping also had little variation across all racial categories in both waves, although Blacks reported the highest average amount of restlessness. By comparison, the results for "physical reaction" were close to zero, with minimal differences across the groups.

In Figure 6.1, we examine experiences with COVID economic displacement within eight different ethnoracial identity and gender groups. Results for Panel A show that wage/job loss was highest among Hispanics and least among Whites. Except for wage/loss among Black males, we also see that wage/job loss among men was generally lower than among women. Hispanic women and Hispanic males reported the greatest wage/job loss in their respective gendered ethnoracial categories. White males and White females hovered at the lowest percentage rate with a 3% difference in reported wage/job loss. The results for Panel B show a similar pattern for the eight groups. Hispanics experienced the most amount of economic displacement, while Whites reported the least displacement.

In analyzing data for Wave 66, we also find that aggregate psychological distress among respondents varied based on ethnoracial identity and income level. For instance, Other Racial Minorities with less than $30,000 in income reported the highest aggregate distress level (0.39) compared to their income bracket counterparts. By contrast, lower income Whites reported a distress level (0.34) that was close to the level reported by lower income Blacks (0.33). Moreover, Blacks and Whites with incomes of greater than $75,000 reported the lowest distress level (0.22), while Hispanics of that income bracket reported the highest (0.27).

We examine the drivers of early COVID-related psychological distress in Table 6.2. On average, we found limited evidence that the effect of minoritized race or gender identity was significant when controlling for multiple factors. The OLS regression results for Wave 64 are shown on the left side of Table 6.2. Respondents in the 30–49 age group reported less distress than respondents in the youngest age group. The only exception was for White women. We also found that individuals with higher levels of education were less likely to report experiencing distress than were individuals who only had a high school diploma. Moreover, respondents who were high trusters in the healthcare system reported a lower distress level compared to medium trusters. Hopeful respondents reported lower distress levels. Furthermore, compared to individuals who believed the pandemic posed no threat to their personal health, individuals who believed the pandemic posed a major threat reported higher stress levels.

The OLS regression results for Wave 66 also showcase the varied impact of sociodemographics, ethnoracial identity, and perception on psychological distress. Higher levels of education and being married decreased distress levels. Respondents in the upper and medium income brackets reported lower distress than did the baseline (less than $30,000). Moreover, respondents with greater degrees of hope for the future and with higher levels of political knowledge reported less distress. As expected, we found that emotional response to COVID-related news had the strongest impact on distress. Respondents who reported that keeping up with the

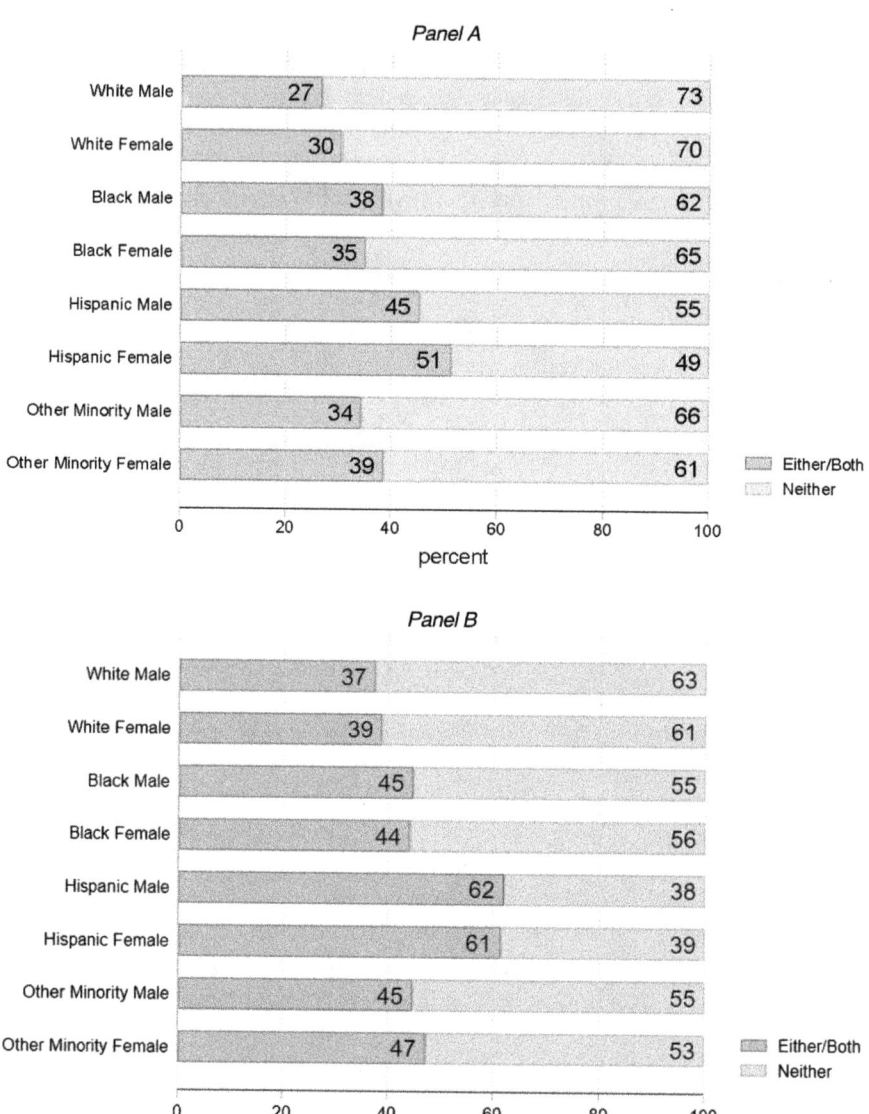

FIGURE 6.1 Experience with Early COVID-19 Job Loss at Intersection of Race and Gender

The figure shows the percentage of individuals who lost their jobs based on race and gender.

Sources: Authors' analysis of ATP, Wave 64, March 19–24, 2020; authors' analysis of ATP, Wave 65, April 7–12, 2020.

TABLE 6.2 Estimated OLS Regression Coefficients for Psychological Distress at Onset of COVID-19 Crisis by Ethnoracial Identity, SES, and Attitudinal Dispositions

Wave 64			Wave 66		
Variable	β	SE	Variable	β	SE
Age: 18–29	0.052***	(0.012)	Age: 18–29	0.068***	(0.017)
Age: 30–49	0.040***	(0.009)	Age: 30–49	0.064***	(0.012)
Age: 50–64	0.033**	(0.008)	Age: 50–64	0.037***	(0.011)
Education	-0.007*	(0.003)	Education	-0.010*	(0.004)
Democrat/Lean Democrat	0.000	(0.012)	Democrat/Lean Democrat	-0.014	(0.014)
White Female	0.057***	(0.008)	White Female	0.039***	(0.010)
Black Male	0.001	(0.028)	Black Male	0.000	(0.035)
Black Female	-0.021	(0.016)	Black Female	-0.019	(0.020)
Hispanic Male	-0.032*	(0.015)	Hispanic Male	-0.007	(0.020)
Hispanic Female	0.017	(0.014)	Hispanic Female	-0.001	(0.022)
Other Minority Male	-0.021	(0.016)	Other Minority Male	-0.027	(0.024)
Other Minority Female	0.035*	(0.016)	Other Minority Female	0.030	(0.022)
Income: $75,000 +	-0.021*	(0.011)	Income: $75,000 +	-0.054***	(0.014)
Income: $30,000–$74,999	-0.020*	(0.010)	Income: $30,000–$74,999	-0.038**	(0.013)
Married	-0.030***	(0.007)	Married	-0.032**	(0.010)
Ideology	0.003	(0.005)	Ideology	0.007	(0.008)
COVID Job Loss: Either/Both	0.012	(0.008)			
COVID News Attentiveness	0.010	(0.006)			
Hopeful about the Future	-0.083***	(0.012)	Hopeful about the Future	-0.096***	(0.014)
Health Confidence Index	-0.083***	(0.016)	Political Knowledge Index	-0.020***	(0.006)
Trust: High	-0.068***	(0.009)	Born Again Christian	-0.017	(0.010)
Trust: Medium	-0.053***	(0.009)			

(continued)

TABLE 6.2 Cont.

Wave 64			Wave 66		
Variable	β	SE	Variable	β	SE
Prior Mental Health Diagnosis	0.147***	(0.010)	News: Economic Impact	-0.001	(0.007)
Threat (Major): U.S. Health	-0.039	(0.032)	News: Federal Government actions	-0.001	(0.006)
Threat (Minor): U.S. Health	-0.047	(0.031)	News: Cases and Deaths	0.004	(0.006)
Threat (Major): Personal Health	0.089***	(0.012)	News: CDC Advice	-0.002	(0.008)
Threat (Minor): Personal Health	0.038***	(0.011)	News: Hospital Ability to Treat	0.010	(0.008)
Threat (Major): U.S. Economy	0.032	(0.046)	News: Impact on People Like Me	0.008	(0.007)
Threat (Minor): U.S. Economy	0.028	(0.047)	Response to News: Feel Better	0.040*	(0.018)
Threat (Major): Personal Finance	0.035**	(0.011)	Response to News: Feel Worse	0.124***	(0.009)
Threat (Minor): Personal Finance	-0.000	(0.010)	Properly Estimated Risk:Trump	-0.021***	(0.007)
Rating:Trump Response	0.020***	(0.005)	Properly Estimated Risk: CDC	0.002	(0.007)
Rating: CDC Response	0.012*	(0.005)	Properly Estimated Risk: News	-0.009	(0.005)
Rating: News Response	-0.001	(0.004)	Constant	0.319***	(0.069)
Constant	0.185*	(0.074)			
Observations	9936		Observations	5523	
R-Squared	0.279		R-Squared	0.208	

Notes: Omitted baselines and Geography variables not reported ($p > .1$), $*p < .05$, $**p < .01$, $***p < .001$.

Table 6.2 describes the psychological distress at Onset of COVID crisis by demographics.

news "made them feel worse emotionally" reported different distress levels than did respondents who had no emotional reaction to the news. Finally, a belief that Trump properly responded to the outbreak reduced overall distress.

In Figure 6.2, we display the average marginal effects (AME) of the covariates on aggregate psychological distress as computed from the OLS results for Wave 64 reported in Table 6.2. On average, being a Democrat compared to being a Republican increased the probability of aggregate psychological distress, a change of 0.023 ($p < .001$). Compared to being a White male (omitted baseline), being a White female was associated with a significant increase in distress. Obtaining a higher education level compared to being only a high school graduate decreased the overall distress level from 0.283 to 0.277. Furthermore, going from the lowest level to the highest level of confidence in the healthcare system lessened the degree of psychological distress by 0.107. Being the most hopeful about the future reduced distress (0.090). Having a prior health diagnosis increased distress (by 0.145). In contrast to being single, being married reduced distress (going from 0.298 to 0.266, a change of 0.032).

Our analysis of AMEs for the covariates in Wave 66 (April), depicted in Figure 6.3, reveals a similar pattern to what was seen in Figure 6.2. As shown, age had an impact on overall psychological distress whereby on average, relative to the lowest age group, being 65 and over decreased psychological distress, a change of −0.068 ($p < .001$). Being a White female compared to being a White male increased distress (going from 0.240 to 0.279, $p < .001$). Being married decreased psychological distress from 0.269 to 0.238, $p < .001$. On average, moving from the lowest level to the highest level of income also reduced distress, a change of 0.054 ($p < .001$). Likewise, moving to the highest level of political knowledge reduced distress ($p < .001$). Being the most hopeful about the future also decreased distress (a change of −0.096, $p < .001$). On average, attentiveness to COVID-related news had no statistically significant impact. However, having an emotional reaction to COVID-related news increased psychological distress: respondents who felt worse after engaging the news reported the highest levels of distress.

We perform our multivariable regression analysis on the White, Black, and Hispanic subsamples across each wave to ascertain a finer analysis of factors shaping early stage COVID-related psychological distress. Five noteworthy findings emerge from the estimates reported in Table 6.3. First, the impact of age and news attentiveness was not uniform across groups in either wave. Second, on average, age mattered only for Whites. Third, threat perceptions, evaluations of policymakers, and hopefulness were more impactful in shaping the distress of White respondents than the distress of Black and Hispanic respondents in Wave 64. Fourth, on average, distress reported by Blacks in Wave 66 was more likely to be shaped by income and evaluation of policymakers than was distress reported by Whites and by Hispanics. Fifth, perceptions of COVID as a threat to the U.S. economy in Wave 64 was a significant predictor of psychological distress for Hispanics but not for other respondents.

Results from our k-means cluster analysis, as reported in Table 6.4, confirm findings from our regression analysis.[7] We report select variables to highlight five

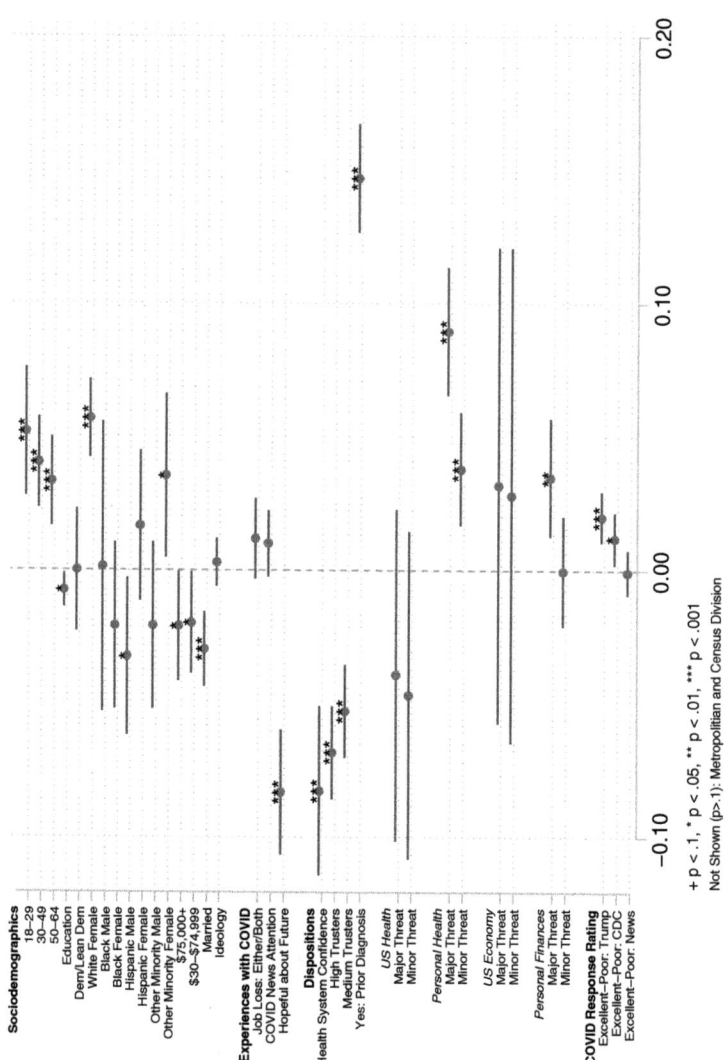

FIGURE 6.2 Average Marginal Effects of Variables Predicting Psychological Distress, Wave 64

Notes: Effects generated from OLS regression results shown in Table 6.2. Metropolitan and Census Divisions not shown.

The Figure shows the effects of psychological distress, Wave 64.

Source: ATP, March 19–24, 2020, Pew Research Center.

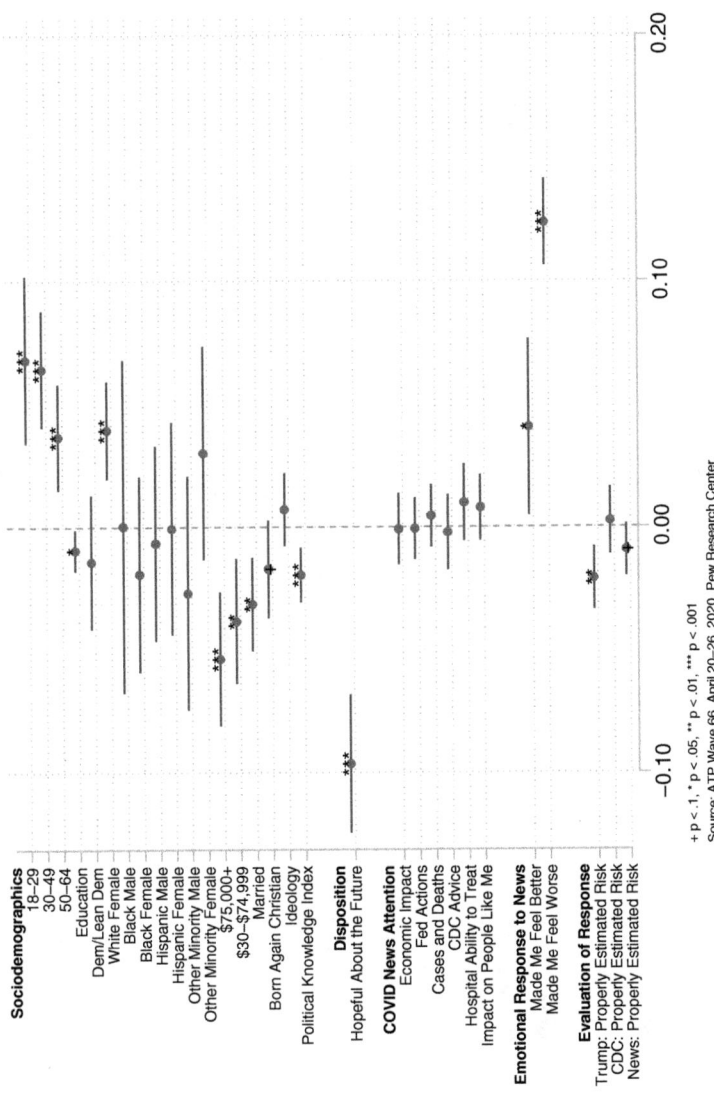

FIGURE 6.3 Average Marginal Effects of Variables Predicting Psychological Distress, Wave 66

Effects generated from OLS regression results shown in Table 6.2

The figure shows the effects of psychological distress, Wave 66.

Source: ATP, April 20–26, 2020, Pew Research Center.

TABLE 6.3 Estimated OLS Regression Coefficients for Psychological Distress by Ethnoracial Group, Wave 64 and Wave 66

Wave 64	Whites		Blacks		Hispanics	
Variable	β	SE	β	SE	β	SE
Age: 18–29	0.05***	(0.01)	0.01	(0.01)	0.05	(0.04)
Age: 30–49	0.05***	(0.01)	−0.01	(0.01)	0.02	(0.03)
Age: 50–64	0.04***	(0.01)	0.01	(0.01)	0.02	(0.03)
Education	−0.01	(0.00)	−0.03*	(0.00)	−0.00	(0.01)
Democrat/Lean Dem	−0.01	(0.00)	0.03	(0.00)	−0.02	(0.06)
Female	0.06***	(0.01)	−0.01	(0.01)	0.04*	(0.02)
Income: $75,000 +	−0.02	(0.01)	−0.06	(0.01)	0.01	(0.03)
Income: $30,000–$74,999	−0.01	(0.01)	−0.07*	(0.01)	−0.01	(0.03)
Married	−0.02**	(0.01)	−0.03	(0.01)	−0.05*	(0.03)
Ideology	0.00	(0.01)	−0.01	(0.01)	0.02	(0.01)
Hopeful about the Future	−0.13***	(0.01)	0.03	(0.01)	0.01	(0.04)
COVID Job Loss: Either/Both	0.01	(0.01)	−0.00	(0.01)	0.02	(0.03)
COVID News Attentiveness	0.01	(0.01)	0.01	(0.01)	0.02	(0.02)
Health Confidence Index	−0.07***	(0.02)	−0.06	(0.05)	−0.13**	(0.04)
Trust: High	−0.07***	(0.01)	−0.09**	(0.01)	−0.08***	(0.03)
Trust: Medium	−0.06***	(0.01)	−0.05	(0.01)	−0.04*	(0.03)

Wave 66	Whites		Blacks		Hispanics	
Variable	β	SE	β	SE	β	SE
Age: 18–29	0.06**	(0.02)	0.09	(0.03)	0.07	(0.04)
Age: 30–49	0.06***	(0.01)	0.08*	(0.03)	0.03	(0.04)
Age: 50–64	0.03**	(0.01)	0.02	(0.03)	0.08*	(0.04)
Education	−0.01	(0.00)	−0.02	(0.01)	−0.00	(0.01)
Democrat/Lean Democrat	−0.02	(0.02)	0.01	(0.04)	0.01	(0.03)
Female	0.04***	(0.01)	−0.04	(0.03)	0.01	(0.02)
Income: $75,000 +	−0.05**	(0.02)	−0.13***	(0.03)	−0.02	(0.03)
Income: $30,000–$74,999	−0.03	(0.02)	−0.14***	(0.03)	−0.00	(0.03)
Married	−0.03**	(0.01)	0.01	(0.03)	−0.05*	(0.02)
Ideology	0.01	(0.01)	−0.01	(0.02)	0.01	(0.02)
Hopeful about the Future	−0.15***	(0.02)	0.06	(0.04)	0.00	(0.04)
Political Knowledge Index	−0.01	(0.01)	−0.02	(0.02)	−0.04*	(0.02)
Born Again Christian	−0.02	(0.01)	−0.02	(0.03)	−0.02	(0.03)
News: Economic Impact	−0.00	(0.01)	−0.03	(0.02)	0.02	(0.02)
News: Federal Government Actions	−0.00	(0.01)	−0.00	(0.02)	0.01	(0.02)
News: Cases and Deaths	0.00	(0.01)	0.02	(0.02)	0.01	(0.02)

	(1)	(2)	(3)
Prior Mental Health Diagnosis	0.13*** (0.01)	0.17*** (0.04)	0.21*** (0.03)
Threat (Major): U.S. Health	-0.05 (0.03)	-0.17 (0.13)	-0.02 (0.05)
Threat (Minor): U.S. Health	-0.07* (0.03)	-0.12 (0.12)	0.00 (0.05)
Threat (Major): Personal Health	0.10*** (0.01)	0.04 (0.04)	0.08** (0.03)
Threat (Minor): Personal Health	0.04*** (0.01)	0.00 (0.04)	0.05 (0.03)
Threat (Major): U.S. Economy	0.02 (0.06)	0.03 (0.12)	0.14** (0.05)
Threat (Minor): U.S. Economy	0.01 (0.06)	0.10 (0.12)	0.11* (0.05)
Threat (Major): Personal Finance	0.02 (0.01)	0.10* (0.04)	0.08** (0.03)
Threat (Minor): Personal Finance	-0.01 (0.01)	0.03 (0.04)	0.02 (0.03)
Rating: Trump Response	0.02*** (0.01)	0.03* (0.01)	0.03** (0.01)
Rating: CDC Response	0.02** (0.01)	-0.03 (0.01)	0.01 (0.01)
Rating: News Response	-0.00 (0.00)	0.01 (0.00)	0.01 (0.01)
Constant	0.20** (0.07)	0.30 (0.24)	-0.04 (0.11)
Observations	6265	1074	1462
R-Squared	0.3238	0.2338	0.3046

	(4)	(5)	(6)
News: CDC Advice	-0.00 (0.01)	0.03 (0.02)	-0.02 (0.02)
News: Hospital Ability to Treat	0.00 (0.01)	-0.00 (0.02)	0.03 (0.02)
News: Impact on People Like Me	0.01 (0.01)	-0.00 (0.03)	0.02 (0.03)
Response to News: Feel Better	0.08*** (0.02)	-0.00 (0.04)	-0.01 (0.04)
Response to News: Feel Worse	0.13*** (0.01)	0.13*** (0.03)	0.09*** (0.03)
Properly Estimated Risk: Trump	-0.02* (0.01)	-0.05*** (0.01)	-0.01 (0.01)
Properly Estimated Risk: CDC	-0.00 (0.01)	0.04* (0.01)	-0.01 (0.02)
Properly Estimated Risk: News	-0.00 (0.00)	-0.05** (0.00)	-0.00 (0.01)
Constant	0.31** (0.06)	0.40* (0.17)	0.19 (0.15)
Observations	3410	631	818
R-Squared	0.2694	0.2630	0.1527

Notes: Baseline categories not shown. Other Minorities group excluded from analysis. Geography variables not reported ($p > .1$), *$p < .05$, **$p < .01$, ***$p < .001$.

Table 6.3 provides a description of psychological distress among various racial and ethnic groups.

TABLE 6.4 Results of *k*-Means Cluster Analysis and Distribution on Select Sociodemographic and Attitudinal Variables

Wave 64					Wave 66				
Variable	Response Option	Low	Moderate	High	Variable	Response Option	Low	Moderate	High
Age	18–29	33	35	32	Age	18–29	39	45	16
	30–49	38	38	24		30–49	48	39	13
	50–64	45	34	21		50–64	55	35	10
	65 and above	52	35	13		65 and above	63	31	6
Gender	Male	48	33	19	Gender	Male	58	34	8
	Female	36	39	26		Female	45	40	15
Race	White	42	38	20	Race	White	52	38	10
	Black	43	30	27		Black	51	34	15
	Hispanic	41	32	28		Hispanic	50	38	13
	Other Racial Minority	42	34	24		Other Racial Minority	50	38	12
Income	$75,000 + Above	43	41	16	Income	$75,000 + Above	60	32	8
	$30,000–$74,999	43	37	20		$30,000–$74,999	51	38	11
	Less Than $30,000	37	30	34		Less Than $30,000	40	44	16
Area Hospitals	Not at All Confident	23	40	38	Political Knowledge	Low	45	40	15
	Not too Confident	31	40	29		Middle	54	37	1
	Somewhat Confident	42	38	19		High	57	35	8
	Very Confident	57	25	18	COVID News:	Made Me Feel Better	47	36	17
Area Nursing Homes	Not at All Confident	28	41	31		No Change	65	30	5
	Not too Confident	35	40	25		Made Me Feel Worse	36	46	17
	Somewhat Confident	46	35	19	Trump Response	Not Taking Risks Seriously at All	43	52	15

Social and General Trust				
	Very Confident	57	24	19
	High	50	36	14
	Medium	43	37	19
	Low	34	34	32
Threat: Personal Health				
	Major Threat	32	37	31
	Minor Threat	44	37	18
	Not a Threat	59	25	16
Ratings: Trump Response				
	Excellent	59	26	15
	Good	45	37	18
	Only Fair	34	39	27
	Poor	31	40	29

Not Taking Risks Quite Seriously	50	38	12
Gotten the Risks about Right	59	33	8
Slightly Exaggerated the Risks	53	39	9
Greatly Exaggerated the Risks	54	36	10
CDC Response			
Not Taking Risks Seriously at All	36	43	21
Not Taking Risks Quite Seriously	46	34	19
Gotten the Risks about Right	50	39	11
Slightly Exaggerated the Risks	57	35	8
Greatly Exaggerated the Risks	58	34	8

Note: Row percentages may add up to more than 100% due to rounding. See Appendix for full table of cluster membership by all variables.

Table 6.4 provides a select sociodemographic and attitudinal variables.

noteworthy impacts of ethnoracial identity, sociodemographic character, and attitudinal disposition on distress. First, in Wave 64, there was a greater proportion of individuals classified as falling in the Low Distress Cluster (42%, N = 4,734) and the Moderate Distress Cluster (36%, N = 4,080) than in the High Distress Cluster (22%, N = 2,555). Second, we find a relatively even spread across the clusters for ethnoracial groups. Third, confidence in the health system differentiated cluster memberships. A greater percentage of respondents who were "very confident" (57%) in their area hospitals were classified as being in the Low Distress Cluster. Respondents who were "not at all confident" (40%) were more likely to be in the Moderate Distress Cluster. Fourth, we find variation in cluster membership for respondents who felt that COVID-19 posed a threat to their personal health. A similar pattern emerged for those who believed that the outbreak posed a major threat to their personal finances (see Appendix for full table).[8] A large percentage of respondents who believed the pandemic posed "no threat" to their personal health were in the Low Distress Cluster (59%), while the remaining respondents indicating "no threat" or "minor threat" were spread across the other two clusters. Fifth, respondents with high social trust and with favorable impressions of Trump were more likely to be in the Low Distress Cluster.

As displayed in Table 6.4, our *k*-means cluster analysis of psychological distress reported in Wave 66 parallel patterns from Wave 64. A supermajority of respondents was classified in either the Low Distress Cluster (51%, N = 5,113) or in the Moderate Distress Cluster (37%, N = 3,735), with a low proportion being classified in the High Distress Cluster (11%, N = 1,129). Most males fell into the Low Distress Cluster (58%), while most females fell into the High Distress Cluster (45%). Respondents with incomes of $75,000 or greater were more likely to be represented in the Low Distress Cluster. Perceptions of Trump also differentiated cluster membership: Most respondents who perceived the Trump Response as "not taking the risks seriously at all" were in the Moderate Distress Cluster (52%), while most who believed Trump "greatly exaggerated the risks" were in the Low Distress Cluster (54%). A bit more than a third of respondents who reported that keeping up with the news "made them feel better" fell in the Low Distress Cluster (36%), while a larger proportion fell into the Moderate Distress Cluster. Income, knowledge, and marital status were also important.[9]

As a complementary analysis, we turned to two questions in Wave 65 (April 7–12, 2020) to document the extent to which differences in ethnoracial identity shaped fears about perpetuating COVID and being hospitalized. The first question asked, "How concerned, if at all, are you that you might spread the coronavirus to other people without knowing that you have it." The second question asked, "How concerned, if at all, are you that you will get the coronavirus and require hospitalization."

Figure 6.4 depicts our results. The greatest proportion of those "very concerned" about spreading COVID were Hispanics (50%) and Blacks (38%). Whites were less somewhat concerned (33%) and not too concerned (37%). The differences across the groups about proliferating COVID was statistically significant ($F = 20.37, p <$

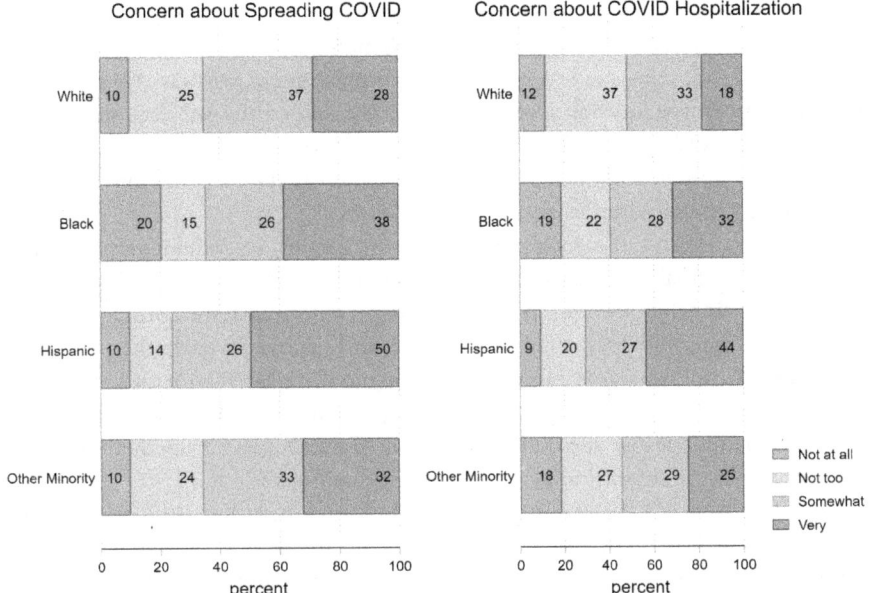

FIGURE 6.4 Racial Differences in Concerns about COVID-19 Spread and Hospitalization, Wave 65

The figure shows bar charts of the COVID-19 spread and hospitalization among various racial and ethnic groups.

Source: ATP, Wave 65, April 7–12, 2020, Pew Research Center.

.001). The racial differences in concerns about being hospitalized due to COVID were strikingly similar ($F = 45.20$, $p < .000$). For example, Hispanics and Blacks had the highest percentage of respondents who were very concerned (44% and 32%, respectively). When combining the last two categories of concern, all three racial minority groups outpaced Whites: Blacks (60%), Hispanics (70%), and Other Minorities (57%). A similar racial cleavage emerged when looking at whether respondents indicated that they knew a COVID patient ($F = 27.92$, $p < .000$). Twenty-eight percent of Blacks reported in the affirmative, compared to only 13% of Whites and Hispanics and 14% of Other Racial Minorities. In sum, we found significant racial cleavages in perceptions about COVID and the response of leaders to the outbreak across three consecutive waves of surveys conducted at the onset of the pandemic.

Discussion and Conclusion

Our analysis underscores four takeaways about the mental health ramifications of the onset of the coronavirus pandemic as shown in surveys by the Pew Center. First, our findings provide evidence for both positions about the prophylactic effects of socioeconomic status on the emergence (and eventual cessation) of pandemic-related psychological distress. We found that Whites experienced the lowest aggregate distress levels compared to other racial groups. Yet distress was also associated with differences in education levels, affluence, age, and attitudinal dispositions. But we acknowledge that these differences are not disconnected from racialized social stratification. We conclude that perception of the COVID-19 pandemic amplified pre-existing vulnerabilities in certain communities.

Second, we found the intersection of race, gender, sociodemographic character, and attitudinal disposition to shape the impact of COVID experiences. Our findings support other research showing that experiences with the coronavirus pandemic varied by individual, ethnoracial group, and gender. As such, the perceptual differences we found across groups were not merely related to experience with COVID or with socioeconomic status. The pandemic clearly exaggerated racial health disparities because the outbreak intensified everyone's engagement with the social, economic, and political factors shaping overall quality of life.

Third, fighting COVID-related health disparities between Whites and non-Whites, and between the poor and the affluent, cannot be separated from the campaigns to stymie cumulative disadvantage. In the aftermath of COVID-19, all Americans have rightly amplified their attention to the social determinants of health. However, we assert that this amplified attention sidestepped the initial outrage of minority groups. We argue that circumstances were clear long before the COVID crisis that minoritized communities *would* experience and report different trajectories of pandemic-related psychological distress.

Lastly, our findings suggest that the pandemic and its aftermath will have a long-lasting negative impact on efforts to thwart health inequalities in minority populations. Our concerns are driven, in part, by the unequal distribution of COVID vaccinations in the early months of 2021, where White and affluent communities reportedly received a disproportionate share of the vaccine. We contend that many vaccine distribution plans failed to address racial disparities in psychological distress and in pre-existing health inequities. We hope policymakers and medical professionals utilize our findings and other findings about COVID to support more robust treatment and mitigation plans that attend to the different trajectories of psychological distress. Failure to do this, we contend, will prolong, if not make nearly permanent, the negative effects of COVID-related psychological distress.

Notes

1 We treat the waves as independent cross-sectional samples and set aside the panel design aspects of the data.
2 Our tests results supported creating an index: Cronbach's alpha (α = 0.762), Raykov's reliability coefficient (RRC = 0.786), and Kaiser–Meyer–Olkin statistic (KMO = 0.775) indicating the items' correlations were compact.
3 For example, "Rarely or none of the time (less than 1 day)."
4 Weighted Cronbach's alpha (α = 0.8645) and Raykov's reliability coefficient (RRC = 0.867).

5 A diagnostic test confirmed these variables could be combined into an index (α = 0.855, weighted). However, given our analytical interests, we chose to leave the variables individualized.

6 The Political Knowledge Index variable included in Wave 66 is comprised of nine questions asked of respondents in Wave 57 (October 29 to November 11, 2019). The Pew Research Center created the index: low (0–5 correct answers), medium (6–7 correct answers), and high (8–9 correct). We acknowledge the limitations of this variable and that some Wave 66 respondents may have increased their political knowledge between November 2019 and March 2020.

7 To assess the predictive validity of our cluster analysis of Wave 64 data, we computed an adjusted rand index (ARI) using the grouping variable identified by Pew Research Center. Our ARI statistic (0.5773) suggested comparability between our cluster groupings and the grouping variable created by Pew. We could not compute an ARI for Wave 66 because the diagnostic requires an externally provided cluster membership variable.

8 Appendix available from website of first author.

9 Educational attainment and party affiliation also differentiated respondents. Most postgraduates fell into the Low Distress Cluster (57%), whereas a small proportion of respondents with a high school degree or less fell into the High Distress Cluster (13%). A large percentage of Republicans were classified in the Low Distress Cluster (58%), while a smaller percentage of Democrats (45%) were in the same cluster.

References

Chen, Justin A., Emily Zhang, and Cindy H. Liu. (2020). Potential Impact of COVID-19-Related Racial Discrimination on the Health of Asian Americans. *American Journal of Public Health, 110*(11): 1624–1627.

DiPrete, Thomas A., and Gregory M. Eirich. (2006). Cumulative Advantage as a Mechanism for Inequality: A Review of Theoretical and Empirical Developments. *Annual Review of Sociology, 32*(1): 271–297.

Gil, Raul Macias, Jasmine R. Marcelin, Brenda Zuniga-Blanco, Carina Marquez, Trini Mathew, and Damani A. Piggott. (2020). COVID-19 Pandemic: Disparate Health Impact on the Hispanic/Latinx Population in the United States. *Journal of Infectious Diseases, 222*(10): 1592–1595.

Green, Jennifer Greif, Katie A. McLaughlin, Patricia A. Berglund, Michael J. Gruber, Nancy A. Sampson, Alan M. Zaslavsky, and Ronald C. Kessler. (2010). Childhood Adversities and Adult Psychiatric Disorders in the National Comorbidity Survey Replication I: Associations with First Onset of DSM-IV Disorders. *Archives of General Psychiatry, 67*(2): 113–123.

Jerit, Jennifer, Yangzi Zhao, Megan Tan, and Munifa Wheeler. (2019). Differences Between National and Local Media in News Coverage of the Zika Virus. *Health Communication, 34*(14): 1816–1823.

Kullar, Ravina, Jasmine R. Marcelin, Talia H. Swartz, Damani A. Piggott, Raul Macias Gil, Trini A. Mathew, and Tina Tan. (2020). Racial Disparity of Coronavirus Disease 2019 in African American Communities. *Journal of Infectious Diseases, 222*(6): 890–893.

Loeb, Tamra B., Megan T. Ebor, Amber M. Smith, Dorothy Chin, Derek M. Novacek, Joya N. Hampton-Anderson, Enricka Norwood-Scott, Alison B. Hamilton, Arleen F. Brown, and Gail E. Wyatt. (2021). How Mental Health Professionals Can Address Disparities in the Context of the COVID-19 Pandemic. *Traumatology, 27*(1) , 60–69.

Makles, Anna. (2012). Stata tip 110: How to get the optimal *k*-means cluster solution. *The Stata Journal, 12*(2): 347–351.

Novacek, Derek M., Joya N. Hampton-Anderson, Megan T. Ebor, Tamra B. Loeb, and Gail E. Wyatt. (2020). Mental Health Ramifications of the COVID-19 Pandemic for Black Americans: Clinical and Research Recommendations. *Psychological Trauma: Theory, Research, Practice, and Policy, 12*(5): 449–451.

Pew Research Center. (2020). Most Americans Say Coronavirus Outbreak Has Impacted Their Lives. Accessed on January 10, 2021. www.pewsocialtrends.org/2020/03/30/most-americans-say-coronavirus-outbreak-has-impacted-their-lives/

Rainie, Lee and Andrew Perrin. (2020). The State of Americans' Trust in Each Other Amid the Covid-19 Pandemic. *Pew Research Center.* Accessed on January 10, 2021. www.pewresearch.org/fact-tank/2020/04/06/the-state-of-americans-trust-in-each-other-amid-the-covid-19-pandemic

Sell, Tara Kirk, Crystal Boddie, Emma E. McGinty, Keshia Pollack, Katherine Clegg Smith, Thomas A. Burke, and Lainie Rutkow. (2017). Media Messages and Perception of Risk for Ebola Virus Infection, United States. *Emerging Infectious Diseases, 23*(1): 108–111.

Shin, Eun Kyong, Youngsang Kwon, and Arash Shaban-Nejad. (2019). Geo-Clustered Chronic Affinity: Pathways from Socio-Economic Disadvantages to Health Disparities. *Journal of the American Medical Informatics Association (JAMIA), 2*(3): 317–22.

Tian, Yan and Concetta M. Stewart. (2005). Framing the SARS Crisis: A Computer-Assisted Text Analysis of CNN and BBC Online News Reports of SARS. *Asian Journal of Communication, 15*(3): 289–301.

7

THE AUTO-IMMUNIZATION OF BLACK LIFE IN PANDEMIC AMERICA

Mark Martinez

Introduction

Biopolitics, in curtailed definition, means phenomena that illustrate times and places where "life" itself becomes the foundational object of politics. Michel Foucault, seen as giving the first explicit conception of this phenomena, saw biopolitics as illustrating a marked shift from an ancient sovereignty or governance with the power to take life to a modern form that administered life to the point of disallowing other forms of life (Foucault, 1990, pp. 138–139). Biopower, or this new capability to govern, has both a positive (administering) and a negative (disallowing) "valence" on forms of, in this case, human life[1] (Mills, 2018, p. 3).

Importantly, Foucault noted another positive and negative distinction in biopower, the management and deployment of sex (including genetics of populations) represents the novel form of biopower that administers life, while the ancient form of power, which Foucault notes is still inherited by the modern nation-state, is that of the symbolics of blood, or race (Foucault, 1990, p. 149). As Foucault noted, it was true that with biopower came increasingly productive forms of governance, of producing and managing new forms of life, particularly economically viable life forms.[2]

However, neither the economy nor the state let go of the old form of sovereignty, that being race war for protection of sovereign borders. This idea of modern (even postmodern) race war, which necessitates the biopolitical production of life today, is a crucial underpinning of this chapter. It discusses the observations of an America today, exacerbated by the COVID-19 pandemic that needs to produce American citizens who are meant to be race enemies. Biopolitics gives us an illustration of the contradiction of American sovereignty, a government, economy, and culture that actively produces people of color (POC) life precisely in order to strip that life of rights and violate it—this is done in order to continually define and manage

DOI: 10.4324/9781003268710-7

the difference between mere American life and "good" American life. The later work of Jacques Derrida encapsulates this problematic of American governance and power over race, particularly in his description of an "auto-immunity" at work. Auto-immunity is a turning in on itself by American democracy, a turning inward to thwart off perceived enemies of democracy who live within democracy—and whose deaths guarantee continued democracy.

This chapter uses Jacques Derrida's biopolitics to engage media representations during the COVID-19 pandemic and the subsequent resurgent Black Lives Matter (BLM) protests. The pandemic has illustrated that his biopolitical metaphor of auto-immunization has materialized in the acts of violence against POC in America. While touching on the various ways that auto-immunization generally affects non-Whites in America, I focus on the Black experience from which current protest movements have emerged. I discuss the repercussions of the extraordinary social conditions set by COVID-19, particularly in urban areas, as the recognition that POC have been produced in ways by state and economy that assumes their own separation from the fully formed, right-bearing American Life.

Life Taking Hold of the Political

On February 23, 2020, the Director General of the World Health Organization (WHO), Dr. Tedros Adhanom Ghebreyesus, gave a media briefing in which he quickly claimed that what should "give all countries hope, courage and confidence is that this virus can be contained" (WHO who.int, February 24). By June 30, he publicly claimed that "the worst is yet to come" (Global News, June 29, 2020), and also, in a striking warning he pleaded to "quarantine covid politics," because "it can exploit division" (Global News, June 29, 2020). What is fascinating about this public plea is how easily Ghebreyesus, a biologist, could conflate a biological phenomenon with the language of politics, specifically political conflict or partisanship.

Importantly for America, Ghebreyesus was publicly wrestled into quarantining a virus' politics because of the position of then president Donald Trump on COVID-19. President Trump himself proclaimed that COVID-19 itself was political. He publicly decried that the virus was unidirectionally politicized by Democrats and that COVID-19 was in fact the party's latest hoax (The Telegraph, 2020). We should note here the complex rhetorical conflation he makes to his supporters here. He infused Democratic Americans' concerns about COVID-19 with concern for it by the global scientific community, and a "hysterical" media, all within the figure of a "hoax." The final conflation made was of a long-standing nightmarish picture in America's history—that of a country and people with open borders (The Telegraph, 2020). It was the complex of Democrats/global scientists/media perpetuating a virus hoax that obfuscated the real threat to the security and health of American lives—the letting in and free movement of Un-American bodies.

In making this conflation, Trump inadvertently stumbled upon an insight from the theory of biopolitics. There is no limit and no sacrosanct object or idea that modern politics cannot take hold of and manage. Even something as void of humanity, of the social, as a particular virus strain, becomes a political subject. He also illustrated how inextricably linked the language of biology and medicine is with American politics, and how these metaphors have material power. Trump's was a position that was a sort of inversion of Ghebreyesus and a repudiation of WHO, and scientific knowledge in general. This battle against expert knowledge in general, and science specifically was part and parcel of Trump's policy making and rhetoric to his constituency.[3] Scientific knowledge that did not lead to an expansive unregulated market economy was anathema to American way of life, and the WHO, a *foreign* scientific body, exacerbated that threat to American lives.

There are two reasons why the melding of biological life with political discourse gleans insight into our ongoing moment of pandemic and the struggle between fully recognized protected lives and lives that are unprotected and marginalized. First, when the sacrosanct liberal democratic charge for unity, for an "us in this together," is broken, COVID will exploit the disagreement and will thrive in the division. Second, that the virus can exploit life in political conflict implies that COVID has some form of agency, an abject form of agency, that can impinge on political life as severely or more than it can on biological life. What becomes clear is that there is an inextricable link between the biological and the political that we reproduce and circulate through language and media. However, using the lens of biopolitical theory, we observe that this division, which is a connection between biological and political life, goes beyond organicist metaphor or mere representation.

The language and media of COVID have been materially productive of new forms of life, in POC, that at the same time produce repetitions of older forms that have been made abject in America. As abject Americans, POC are reproduced, persecuted, and violated in novel ways—whether representationally in media as ungrateful celebrity activists, as disruptive, coddled protestors across campuses, or as Black bodies that serve a function to be detained and prosecuted in particular spaces. COVID as an abject agency has helped to produce a repetition of a former BLM movement with new populations and communities that spread ideologic-ally and physically into American life. What begins to be visible is a repetition of representation and bodily domination, a circular movement. It is a democracy that has built in it the need to violate parts of its own citizenry that leads to new activated and resistant citizens. The object of biopolitical analysis is Life and its very limits—not only Death, but the limits that are set by government and law that daily manage some lives and preclude others. While this may result in seemingly grim or pessimistic prose, the upshot of biopolitics is that it also illuminates the future and possibilities of new life. After historical and political treatments of biopolitics, particularly aspects of colonialism, exploitation, and racism, theorists have made a prescriptive turn in biopolitics, thinking and writing of an "affirmative" biopolitics that can engender social change. This chapter, acknowledging the gravity of the term "race war," seeks to foreground possibilities, affirmation, and empathy for his-torically embattled POC life in America.

Good American vs. Mere American Life

Derrida refers to the concept of aporia in much of his writing. An aporia is a contradiction, a confusion, or an absolute impasse to a metaphysical idea that he connects with the idea of a death (Wortham, 2010, pp. 14–15). In the case of Democracy, aporias arise from the absolute belief and/or devotion to ideals repeated and circulated, such as, "under God, indivisible, with liberty and justice for all." There is, as I discuss below, a contradiction between the sovereignty of the State and the sovereignty of the free citizen in American democracy. For the fully realized citizen of rights, the ideal of democracy has long since been in doubt based upon material conditions of an unfettered capitalism and the perceived reality of economic and cultural elites. For the POC, a citizen neither fully recognized nor represented, that same doubted ideal materializes into severe poverty, urban food deserts, and life-threatening policing to mention a few.

In terms of democracy, the term "auto-immunity" marks a turning inward that is self-violence, or a symbolic suicide, "but, more seriously still, it threatens always to rob suicide itself of its meaning and supposed integrity" (Derrida, 2005, p. 45). Part of the subtle insight here for POC is that we have been witnessing and talking about violence and murder done to others, not to self, in America. So why think in terms of killing of self? America, its policy, infrastructure, rule of law, deference to capitalism—all of these systems that fail POC on a daily basis—are killing American democracy. To the extent that any of us as citizens believe in the ideal of freedom, we witness the continual suicidal death of that ideal in the treatment of POC, not to mention women, and LBGTQ+ (lesbian, bisexual, gay, transgender, queer, and others) citizens. American democracy is suicidal in that it has two foundational desires:

> to welcome only men, and on the condition that they be citizens, brothers, and compeers [semblables] , excluding all the others, in particular bad citizens, rogues, noncitizens, and all sorts of unlike and unrecognizable others, and, on the other hand, at the same time or by turns, it has wanted to open itself up, to offer hospitality, to all those excluded.
>
> *Derrida, 2005, p. 63*

Biopolitics, points to the ways that politics, including policy and law making, political culture and social mores, and crucially law enforcement, continue to encroach on the basic processes of human biology and reproduction, all while killing their purported intention of democratic process. Redlining, gentrification, disenfranchisement, neighborhood criminalization, all enforced through the violence of policing, are the biopolitical elements that produce certain POC subjects—certain forms of raced lives in America. Regardless of the reality of their actual economic or social status, POC are determined by American hegemony to be economically unviable, socially unruly, and violent on a daily basis. White America responds to the dangers of POC through an auto-immunization, specifically of Black Americans in urban areas, that is both symbolic and material. An auto-immune response is the attacking of a body by itself, and in America, safe spaces for commerce, tourism, and a "public," are created through the concerted attack on its own citizenry, its most marginalized form of citizenry, POC. The auto-immunization culminates in spectacle of police detaining or killing Black and Brown Americans in public as a sacrifice to the inevitability of safe spaces in America.

Biopolitics and Race War

Slavery is often deemed the original sin of America as a democratic project. It was the impetus for the breaking away of American colonies and the penning of a document by men who, to varying degrees, were complicit in the new democracy's continuation of it. Slavery has at the same time transplanted and circumscribed those of African descent into the American democratic context. The burden of violence that Black Americans have been subject to in this sense is that their existence in America preceded its existence as a sovereignty. The ideologies or movements that have recognized Black difference to the perceived detriment of (White) unity, from X, to the Black Panthers, to BLM, are taken as mortal wounds to the Democracy. Perhaps, referring to the original sin of slavery, the resistive and emancipated slaves were the first instance of this contradiction, where Africans wanting to be other than in bondage, to share in the freedoms of White men, were taken as the ultimate threat to a way of life.

We see in this contradiction between unity and difference the conditions of possibility for race wars to emerge and reproduce in America, as White America's response to Black difference against "we the people" results in a more radical form of separation, that being the identification of a mortal enemy. In line with this radical separation, Michel Foucault speaks of an entire historical thread of race struggle as opposed to mere racist thought that has existed. This race struggle is what defines the protection of a society itself. Black Americans are then,

> not the race that came from elsewhere or that was, for a time, triumphant and dominant, but that it is a race that is permanently, ceaselessly infiltrating the social body, or which is, rather, constantly being re-created in and by the social fabric.
>
> *Foucault, 2008, p. 61*

Derrida's metaphor of an auto-immune response also illustrates this fear in White Americans that Blacks are doing violence, particularly cultural and political, to the governance of society, to the promise of its continued existence. Race war is then the reaction to the dissolution of White civilization (Euro-American), which leads to the biological result of White genocide. If biopolitics marks the time and place where the realm of politics takes hold of and manages life itself, then race war is when Black life is put under attack by all the resources and infrastructures of politics. What emerges is all out destruction of Black life, biological and social, by

White citizens on the one hand and a White supremacist state on the other—race war as state racism,

> a racism that society will direct against itself, against its own elements and its own products. This is the internal racism of permanent purification, and it will become one of the basic dimensions of social normalization.
>
> *Foucault, 2008, p. 62*

A biopolitical term for the war against Black lives is what Achille Mbembe calls a necropolitics, or the management and subjugation of some forms of life by only one political (State) power, to put to death (Mbembe, 2003, p. 39). Or as Ta-Nahe Coates frames it, the power of American citizens and sovereignty is "the right to break the Black body as the meaning of their sacred equality" (Coates, 2015, p. 150). Race war has historically been the attempt by White America/ns to assert a unified sovereignty, a power to decide and act, through the social, symbolic, and biological killing of Black life. It should be noted that this is the framework by which some biopolitical theorists "see" race relations and conflict through the lens of sovereignty and the apparatus of law enforcement. It is in terms of inclusion/exclusion that the stakes for race in America get elevated and forms not only of resistance but racial solidarity and ally-ship among White Americans and POC get obfuscated. So, it should again be acknowledged that through the ostensible political divisiveness in America and devastation of COVID, there has been an antidote to race war—in the forms of activism, protest, and community building.

American Representation

In one of his last publications, Jacques Derrida wrote, as an admission of sorts, "at the end of a long detour, right near the end, it will perhaps become clear that democracy in America or, more precisely, democracy and America will have been my theme" (Derrida, 2005, p. 14). Derrida felt an ambivalence toward America as a rhetorical figure of international sovereignty and perceived rule of the people domestically.

The problem was inherent in the "representational" character of America's signs, of both its State and its People, both, as it were, independent. It is the "good people" who declare themselves free and independent by the relay of their representatives and of their representatives of representatives. One cannot decide, and that's the interesting thing, the force and the coup of force of such a declarative act, whether independence is stated or produced by this utterance (Derrida, 1986, p. 9). The problem emerges from the double declaration, the two separate declarations of independence.

On the one hand, the sovereign people are represented in as unadulterated a manner as possible by the pen of the representatives of government. On the other, the representatives of government, being wholly different from any form of sovereignty that came before, represent their own independence—the independence of a State founded on and embodying individual sovereignty. Derrida astutely noted the "force and the coup of force," within this double declarative act. The violence of representation from State to citizen produces violence of bodies between them.

The overall aporia in American democracy, but also in liberalism generally, what in Giorgio Agamben's analysis as an "inner solidarity between liberalism and totalitarianism" (Agamben, 1998, p. 10)—has been laid bare through the Trump presidency and the pandemic. The aporia is evident in the disbelief of many Americans today, in the utterance, "how could this have happened?" It is disbelief itself, that a transgressive event like Charlottesville, or George Floyd's and Breonna Taylor's killings, or the siege on Capitol Hill, could perpetrate our democratic way of life. Certainly, the long list of political pundits and journalists uttering, "I'm shocked but not surprised,"[4] embodies in speech this contradiction in thought between a sovereign democratic nation and sovereign individuals making up a free people.

Living Dead Machines and Biopolitical Possibilities

I want to emphasize here the role of the machine that risks certain forms of American life when those machines are brought into precarious spaces and interact between perceived fully acknowledged right bearing citizens and those suspected of violating the Law. I state again that biopolitics has a positive valence (Mills, 2018, p. 3), and it is productive of new forms of life. "Power is not negative and repressive but positive and productive" (Mills, 2018, p. 24), and law enforcement, the most concrete, visual and visceral form of governing power, is precisely a point of biopolitics where citizens can transform into more than mere perpetrators—and where police can become agents that question violent policy and offer dignity to encounters with fellow citizens that they serve and protect. The biopolitics of race war is not an end point of violence but a starting point for the ways in which both White Americans and POC are capable of creating forms of citizenship that resist and escape the forms of violence being described. However, first we need to observe, or witness—and the term "witness" will be crucial in what follows—what forms of power and violence have persisted in the encounters between the Law and POC in America.

I specifically refer here to machines of law enforcement and of domestic militaristic acts upon our citizenry. The deployment of National Guard as well as private security (former military personnel, commonly referred to as mercenaries) was a discourse part and parcel with the national protests against police brutality in 2020–2021. This status of death for and by machines is what Derrida describes as a "machinalité," or a "cutting off from or independence from any living subject—the psychological, sociological, transcendental, or even human subject, and so forth" (Derrida, 2002, p. 136).

The, "republic, state, commonwealth, civitas" (Derrida, 2009, p. 28), only ever come into existence based on the fear-driven animal-machine sovereignty.

> The fear that the beast instills is also the fear of the machine, the combined power of the animal-machine is the power, to amplify the power of the living,

the living man that it protects, that it serves, but like a dead machine, or even a machine of death, a machine which is only the mask of the living, like a machine of death can serve the living.

Derrida, 2009, p. 28

Fellow POC have seen all too clearly—the power of the animal-machine encounter between police officer and Black male.

The amalgam emerges from the various machines of arrest that the officer deploys—handcuffs, night sticks, Tasers, handguns, riot gear, shields—in contact with the animalistic responses the civilian is left with. One either takes flight or freezes in the face of a machine of death with arms risen. I have also seen the representational power of wearable policing technologies as documenting or witnessing eyes and their effects on the status quo of American authority. Wearable video cameras have, in the light of recent civilian killings, gotten much publicity as a means of visual documentation and for police to "self-police" and to curb excessive force.

However, police forces are also poised to use a battery of other wearable technologies, including smart watches and tactical headset computers—all functional because they are hands-free tech used in the heat of an altercation when police hands are occupied with other low-tech wearables, namely Tasers, pepper spray, or handguns. This wearable police officer is a subject of the State, a prosthetic of U.S. law and order, and an animal-machine designed to symbolically legitimate a form of sovereignty that, as Derrida describes it, is a machine of death meant to protect the living. While police perform incapacitating and lethal violence to certain bodies, wearable technologies identify, document, and informationalize citizen lives that are racially and ideologically marked as improper.

The discussion of biopolitics as a mode of analysis quickly turns to a matter of ethics. Can we begin to think about moving "beyond biopolitics" (Mills, 2018, p. 181) as a feature of modern/postmodern life where the stakes are an entire population of citizens of color whose lives are daily marginalized toward non-existence? The strength of biopolitical analysis, as well as the social change we have witnessed through protest and organization through the pandemic, claims a resounding "yes."

Giorgio Agamben calls this a "form of life," or a "happy" life that can only begin when we collectively stop creating a severe separation in the form of dichotomy, between a good life and bad life, human and inhuman (Mills, 2018, p. 139). In America, this division persists as the citizen vs. the non-citizen and the law abider vs. the criminal. However, Agamben recognizes that this division continues to put lives in the latter of the dichotomies and repeats the violence done to those lives. So something else must be done: "... an ethics of a new form of life begins where dignity ends" (Agamben, 1999, p. 69). To witness or to bear witness[5] is to suffer and to survive human indignity, to view an act of inhumanity, knowing that there is no strict distinction between that inhumanity and our own sense of being human.

Based in no small part on the (digital) machines we have derided for bringing fake news, an era of post-truth, and a divisive American populace, we have all been made witness to the truth of an inhuman act in the event of George Floyd's death. An urgent witnessing of George Floyd's final moments becomes infused with possibilities for new life and new treatment of POC when,

> being human is fundamentally conditioned by an indefinite potentiality for being non-human, for being capable of everything and of enduring the inhuman. Being human is a question of enduring, of "bearing all that one could bear," and surviving the inhuman capacity to bear everything.
>
> *Mills, 2018, p. 53*

As Agamben sees it, the possibility for human dignity and happiness lay in exploding the distinction between good and bad life, human and inhuman—and then giving testimony of that truth to others (Mills, 2018, pp. 53–54). In this way, we are not only witnesses to George Floyd's truth but testimonials that circulate throughout the body politic. The discourse productively moves beyond the anger and indignity, to empathy, different informed and activated citizens, and different outcomes.

American Rogue

According to Derrida, American democracy shifted from being the "proper name of deconstruction in progress," in the 1980s, to an object illustrating brutal sovereignty and animality in a post-9/11 world. In his opening of *The Beast and the Sovereign: Vol. I*, Derrida charged America as the "first accused accuser" in the debate on modern rogue nations (Derrida, 2009, p. 41). For him, the United States, possibly the original or at least most brash modern rogue, who accuses others of participating in rogue sovereignty, actually defines the very rules and stakes that a rogue may violate and escape consequence for doing so. For America, the symbolic violence of the rule breaker or risk taker has long been embraced as panacea to the corruption of status quo politics. The styles of frontier figures—cowboys, mavericks, outlaws—have been injected into individual personas as well as the character of parties. Throughout Donald Trump's presidency and this pandemic, we are faced with a political and cultural moment where a rogue style has engendered and produced ideologies of misogyny, xenophobia, and White supremacy that are articulated to citizens whose organizing culminated in direct physical violence at the Capitol on January 6, 2021.

In impressing the centrality of animality, which has been discussed above, in American political rhetoric, Derrida notes the definition of "rogue" from a prominent American publication,

> the *Chronicle of Higher Education* notes, "in the animal kingdom, a rogue is defined as a creature that is born different. It is incapable of mingling with the herd, it keeps to itself, and it can attack at any time, without warning."
>
> *Derrida, 2005, p. 94*

The point to emphasize here is that, while American democracy produces POC life forms as violable, killable animal-machines, it is also productive of a kind of animal citizen that is afforded the status and rights of a "good" American—likely more so than citizens who play by the rules of democratic law.

When speaking of rogues, beasts, and sovereigns, Jacques Derrida more than once turned inward on himself and referred to his own roguish behavior. He spoke personally about what seemed a fond memory of being charged as rogue, or voyou in French:

> "Voyou!" which, I neglected to say, can be turned with the right intonation into something tender, affectionate, maternal (when I was little, my maternal grandmother would sometimes say, pretending to be angry with me, "Voyou, va!" [You little rascal!]).
>
> *Derrida, 2005, p. 78*

I was particularly struck by his anecdote, mainly because it caused me to remember the rogue in me. When I was a boy, and I ever disobeyed, intentionally, broke rules, thought that I or my feelings were most important, my mother had a name for me, "condenado," or condemned. This utterance, or interpellation—being charged as a rogue subject, with humor, acceptance, and affection—gave me a sense of individuality. I remember that feeling more than I remember any time that I had brazenly disobeyed parental or legal authority. All too common still is the adage, "boys will be boys."

Popular images of the acceptable or proper rogue abound with, for example, The Cowboy, a rugged individualist. The production of the rogue in America is, of course, ever-evolving into what can be more roguish and transgressive. There is a story from Hollywood, where John Wayne, the rugged individualist icon of the mid-20th century, feels the winds of rogue change in the emergence of Clint Eastwood.

> "Well, now, when you get behind him, then you shoot him." There was a long pause, and then John Wayne says, "I don't shoot anyone in the back." And then Don made the worst mistake he could have possibly made. He said, "Clint would shoot him in the back."
>
> *Leydon, 2005*

I mention this shift in the figure of the rogue representationally because first, the Republican Party, champion of rugged individualism, has historically touted the figure of the Cowboy as a right and just rogue. The maverick as well, picked from the lexicon of the old west, has represented the "independent" and unpredictable thinking of those in the Republican Party. Second, the party was taken aback at the winds of change throughout its base leading to the election and continued transgressive behavior of Donald Trump.

The utterance of racialized statements produced by this president was unprecedented even to his party. Trump's verbal harangue against his public enemies in terms of race and of war have been well documented in political and popular outlets, as *The Atlantic* did in its piece, "An Oral History of Trump's Bigotry," in which the authors found examples, "of bigotry involving Donald Trump span more than four decades" (Graham et al., 2019). Trump continued to declare himself the president of "law and order," in direct response to the nation and worldwide protests for the murders of George Floyd and Breonna Taylor, and as a reassurance to law enforcement/his base. He threatened anti-racist protestors gathered at the White House with, "the most vicious dogs, and most ominous weapons, I have ever seen. That's when people would have been really badly hurt, at least" (Haberman, 2020). A portend of what was to occur later on Capitol Hill via White Americans, it has been clear that throughout his presidency his handlers and the center of power for the Republican Party have struggled immensely and awkwardly to justify Trump based on the history and codification of what kind of subject the President of the United States should be vs. what they want(ed) as men. The men (and women) who continued to support the rogue as president did so because of the auto-immunitary response to power. Did they want the power of the State and the Law to themselves, with the responsibility that they would act in accordance with them, or did they want that acceptable, excusable rogue to have that power instead, destroying all pomp and deference to the rule of law and promise of democracy? Derrida likens the rogue to a seducer, where, "the libidinal connotation remain[s] ineffaceable in the accusation" (Derrida, 2005, p. 66). President Trump exited, having two failed attempts by the State to censure/impeach him for his actions, and today still seduces crowds and politicians with consistent talks of reemerging.[6]

Many Americans take note of the more benign instances of rogue behavior in America (any fellow citizen succumbing to road rage), or citizens fighting and stealing in a Walmart on Black Friday, for example. Even these occurrences suggest an auto-immune character when POC are involved and the level of violence has increased since the pandemic. However, we have been living in a moment in America where there are frightening displays of rogue sovereignty that call for nothing save condemnation. The rogue White serial shooter with his AR15 style weapon. This rogue subject, a uniquely American one, is perhaps a manifestation of the deadly sovereignty, discussed before as "animal-machine." This is the abject combination of the uncivilized beast Derrida reads as opposing the sovereign, what in America is the rogue male, and the "machinality," the dead machine, as in lifeless, or the machine that brings death.

The latest horrific instantiations of this rogue figure, as I write this, include a shooting spree at three different spas in Atlanta, killing eight people, seven of whom were women and six of whom were Asian. This is yet another murderous event that sheds light on the production of those Americans whose lives then become forfeit in relation to a White male citizen (the killer). Reports are that the killer is claiming his own victimhood, that he was addicted to sex, that his life was in shambles (Berman et al., 2021; Luscombe, 2021). Regardless of his intentions, the rogue shooter reproduced a consistent event in America in the killing of marginalized American life. In doing so, he reproduced himself as a rogue and made certain that new rogue shooter subjects will be produced in the future. The rogue male shooter is the logical extension of an America that needs protection from itself. It is an auto-immunitary response to its democracy, to its Janus face desire to take in all the tired, poor, homeless, and wretched refuse as its own.[7] The promise of democracy is the peril of democracy's most vulnerable and least akin to its center (White maleness). The auto-immunitary rogue action of our country has produced a question for the general American public, "how does our government protect our way of life?" The baldly authoritarian and racist answer has beamed across media outlets, through our presidency, and onto our policed streets—an answer that continues to fuel the activist and public responses today. Provided by Derek Chauvin choking George Floyd to death for a period of 8 minutes and 47 seconds—the answer has ostensibly been to deploy and repeat an apparatus of dichotomy and division between two kinds of life—fully realized and protected on the one hand, and marginalized on the other.

Auto-immunity. Suicidal tendency. The dichotomy is structured from within, and we have witnessed our citizens against our citizens in seeming acts of war impinged on by race, geography, and foreignness. Derrida notes that there is "no worse war than that between enemy brothers" (Weber, 2013, p. 17). We are first compelled to substitute citizens (of all identities) for "brothers." Second, perhaps the above is an incorrect and unethical question. Our way of life as Americans should not be protected, it should be risked. In order to break from the cycle and repetition of biopolitical violence in race war, we must communicate, as Derrida calls it, an "absolute hospitality," in this case to the (POC) other, in which liberty and democracy are not a home that I own and offer to the foreigner, the other (Weber, 2013, p. 100).

The Democracy to Come for Black Life

When speaking of America as the last Rogue State, Derrida continuously mentions the "democracy to come." In Derrida fashion, he explains that this phrase has two different meanings. One, it is a disbelief or rejection of the current state of things, "… a militant and interminable political critique. A weapon aimed at the enemies of democracy, it protests against all naïveté and every political abuse …" (Derrida, 2005, p. 86). The "democracy to come" rejects the ideology of equality that has obfuscated so much pain and death in the ongoing race war. Certainly, both Black activists and allies have not been heartened or even fooled into thinking that Trump replaced by a democratic president will bring paradigmatic shifts to police brutality or the prison-industrial complex. Nor will the continuing stimulus relief/welfare funds do anything to correct structural and historical financial disparity or speak to the reparations owed to the Black community from generations of race war through economics. The Republicans continued kowtowing to Trump for his racially incensed base, recent reports of online calls to violence like the Capitol riot on January 6, 2021, and, as I write, the mobilizing of citizens and politicians against "critical race theory"—all of these characteristics reveal why we reject the very idea that there is a "democracy that is now."

However, "democracy to come" has another significant sense in which it can speak to desires for resistance, community building, and social movements by Black Americans. For, if there is an auto-immune response, a suicidal attack within American democracy, Derrida sees an inversion of that as an opportunity. Democracy is the system that allows, even engenders, an attack on itself from within, a critique of "everything publicly, including the idea of democracy, its concept, its history" (Derrida, 2005, p. 87). This other sense of the phrase relies on the "to come" and is future oriented, aspirational not of the reform but of the revolution toward a new form of governance. "Democracy to come" becomes performative as well when we (Black Americans, other POC, allies, and accomplices of all sorts) act out our critique and resistance to our current moment because of the imperative of our belief that there will be a form of American democracy we could welcome.

In the struggle to end race war, it is not the positive outcome of inclusion that propels us into the future but rather the continual process of our resistance. Likewise, it is not our desire to extricate this auto-immune or suicidal paradigm within American democracy, but rather our recognition that the inverse of this paradigm is a power for racial justice. When we buy into the "democracy to come," we continue to attack the lie that is *democracy now* from within all of its institutions that purport to destroy Black life. Inside the status quo State that pushes marginalization and dehumanization of Black Americans to the logical conclusion of social and biological death, we continue to live against its will. All the while, we recognize that ideas of risk, altruism, and hospitality to the Other remain strong in America. America, not a nation-state, but a community, is that which "constitutes us without belonging to us" (Esposito, 2010, p. 134). We continue the violence of race war through holding on to these notions of patriotism, and good or proper (law abiding and rights bearing) American citizens, at our peril. We foster and engender new liberated and courageous forms of American life by risking them.

Notes

1 Biopolitical theory has been picked up to include nonhuman life and posthuman studies.
2 Foucault names, "homo economicus" that new subject that is not hampered or punished by laws but is rather free and incentivized to contribute to the economy. See Foucault (2003) *"Society Must Be Defended."*
3 Nature, Scientific American.
4 See for examples, Stephen L. Carter, "Shocked But Not Surprised: A Mantra for the Trump Era," (2020) *Bloomberg, www.bloomberg.com/opinion/articles/2020-11-12/shocked-but-not-surprised-a-mantra-for-the-trump-era,* and, Jane C. Timm, "Election workers weren't surprised by the Capitol riot. Trump's supporters targeted them first." (2021) *NBC News,* www.nbcnews.com/politics/elections/election-workers-weren-t-surprised-capitol-riot-trump-s-supporters-n1256535
5 Agamben notes that witness derives from the Greek "martis, martyr."

6 "I think people are going to be very, very happy when I make a certain announcement …" (The Hill).
7 Emma Lazarus, "The New Colossus."

References

Agamben, G. (1998). *Homo Sacer: Sovereign Power and Bare Life*. (D. Heller-Roasen, Trans.). Stanford, California: Stanford University Press.

Agamben, G. (1999). *Remnants of Auschwitz: The Witness and the Archive*. (D. Heller-Roasen, Trans.). New York: Zone Books.

Berman, M., Shammas, B., Armus, T., and Fisher M. (2021, March 19). The Atlanta Spa Shooting Suspect's Life Before Attacks. *The Washington Post*. Retrieved from www.washingtonpost.com/national/atlanta-shooting-suspect-robert-aaron-long/2021/03/19/9397cdca-87fe-11eb-8a8b-5cf82c3dffe4_story.html

Coates, N. (2015). *Between the World and Me*. New York: One World.

Derrida, J. (1986). Declarations of Independence. *New Political Science, 15*(9), 7–15.

Derrida, J. (2002). *Without Alibi*. (P. Kamuf, Trans.). Stanford University Press.

Derrida, J. (2005). *Rogues: Two Essays on Reason*. (P. Ann-Brault and M. Nass, Trans.). Stanford University Press.

Derrida, J. (2009). *The Beast and the Sovereign, vol. 1*. In Michel Lisse, Marie-Louise Mallet, and Ginette Michaud (Eds.). (G. Bennington, Trans.). University of Chicago Press.

Esposito, R. (2010). *Communitas: The Origin and Destiny of Community*. (T. Campbell, Trans.). Stanford University Press.

Foucault, M. (1990). *The History of Sexuality: An Introduction, vol. 1*. (R. Hurley, Trans.). New York: Picador.

Foucault, M. (2008). *Society Must Be Defended: Lectures at the Collège de France, 1975–1976*. (D. Macey, Trans.). New York: Picador.

Foucault, M. (2010). *The Birth of Biopolitics: Lectures at the Collège de France, 1978-1979*. (G. Burchell, Trans.). New York: Picador.

Global News. (2020, June 29). *Coronavirus: WHO Director-General Says "The Worst Is Yet to Come" Regarding Pandemic, Pleads to "Quarantine COVID Politics."* Retrieved from https://globalnews.ca/video/7120797/coronavirus-who-director-general-says-the-worst-is-yet-to-come-regarding-pandemic-pleads-to-quarantine-covid-politics/

Graham, D. A., Green, A., Murphy, C., and Richards, P. (2019). An Oral History of Trump's Bigotry. *The Atlantic*. Retrieved from www.theatlantic.com/magazine/archive/2019/06/trump-racism-comments/588067/

Haberman, M. (2020). Trump Threatens White House Protesters With "Vicious Dogs" and "Ominous Weapons." *The New York Times*. Retrieved from www.nytimes.com/2020/05/30/us/politics/trump-threatens-protesters-dogs-weapons.html

Kurtz, J. (2021, May 4). Trump Teases 2024 Decision: Supporters Will Be "Very Happy." *The Hill*. Retrieved from https://thehill.com/blogs/in-the-know/in-the-know/551704-trump-teases-2024-decision-supporters-will-be-very-happy

Leydon, J. (2005). Clint Eastwood. *Cowboys & Indians*. Retrieved from www.cowboysindians.com/2005/04/clint-eastwood/

Luscombe, B. (2021, March 21). What an Expert on Evangelicals and Sex Says About the Atlanta Shooter's Claim He Had a Sex Addiction. *Time*. Retrieved from https://time.com/5948362/atlanta-shootings-sex-addiction/

Mbembe, A. (2003). Necropolitics. (L. Meintjes, Trans.). *Public Culture, 15*(1), 11–40. https://warwick.ac.uk/fac/arts/english/currentstudents/postgraduate/masters/modules/postcol_theory/mbembe_22necropolitics22.pdf

Mills, C. (2018). *Biopolitics*. New York: Routledge.

The Telegraph. (2020, February 29). *Trump: Coronavirus Is Democrats' "New Hoax"* [video]. www.youtube.com/watch?v=G5TZ6fTYrsE

Waytz, A., Hoffman, K. M., and Trawalter, S. (2015). A Superhumanization Bias in Whites' Perceptions of Blacks. *Social Psychological and Personality Science, 6*(3), 352–359.

Weber, E. (Ed.) (2013). *Living Together: Derrida's Communities of Violence and Peace*. New York: Fordham University Press.

World Health Organization. (2020, February 23). *WHO Director-General's Opening Remarks at the Media Briefing on COVID-19*. Retrieved from www.who.int/director-general/speeches/detail/who-director-general-s-opening-remarks-at-the-media-briefing-on-covid-19---24-february-2020

Wortham, S.M. (2010). *The Derrida Dictionary*. New York: Continuum.

8

FIGHT THE VIRUS, FIGHT THE BIAS

Asian Americans' COVID-19 Racism Experience, Health Impact, and Activism

Jungmi Jun and Nanlan Zhang

Introduction

Asian Americans ("AsAms" hereafter) have been the target of racial discrimination and hate crimes during national crises throughout U.S. history (Lee, 2016). The global pandemic of COVID-19 has exposed AsAms to violent and hostile discrimination and isolation from their own country because of their race/ethnicity and physical appearance. Nearly three-in-ten AsAms (31%) reported that they have been subject to racial slurs or jokes since the outbreak began. Four-in-ten U.S. adults (39%) agreed that it is more common for people to express racist or racially insensitive views about Asians than it was before the outbreak, according to the Pew Research Center (Ruiz et al., 2020). As of June 2021, more than 9,000 incidences of COVID-19-related discrimination have been reported to STOP AAPI Hate (Jeung et al., 2021). The U.S. Federal Bureau of Investigation (FBI) warned that hate crimes against AsAms will increase across the country as the pandemic continues (Margolin, 2020).

The U.S. news media's early reporting of COVID-19 played a substantial role in affecting how the public attributed the cause of the virus to Asia, which further impacted how they view Asians and AsAms. Extant studies suggested that most COVID-19 cases of the first U.S. outbreak in the New York City area were imported from Europe (Fauver et al., 2020; Gonzalez-Reiche et al., 2020). However, the frequent portrayals of Asians in masks and the focus on Asians' wild animal consumption or the hygiene of the Wuhan seafood market as the causes of the virus in COVID-19 news coverage have constructed implicit assumptions about China as the origin of the coronavirus; this coverage resulted in fears and suspicions of AsAms being the carriers of the disease (Ellerbek, 2020; Tessler et al., 2020). Consequently, one-third of U.S. adults (32%) have witnessed someone blaming Asian people for

DOI: 10.4324/9781003268710-8

the COVID-19 pandemic in the United States, according to the Center for Public Integrity (Ellerberk, 2020).

In addition, many American political figures, including the former U.S. president, Donald Trump, have consistently used improper terms in referring to COVID-19, such as "Kung flu," "Chinese virus," "Chinese flu," and "Wuhan virus," citing the first report of the outbreak in Wuhan, China, as justification (Rogers, 2020; White House, 2020). These stigmatizing and racist labels have influenced public discourse regarding the virus as shown in social media analytics (The Atlantic Council, 2020). The racist rhetoric has been accompanied by increasing racist/xenophobic attacks and discrimination against not only Chinese or Chinese Americans but also the entire AsAm population or anyone who looks East Asian (Ma & McLaughlin, 2020; Oung, 2020). Racism and xenophobia are not a "natural" reaction to the threat of the virus; rather, they are outcomes of the American history of discrimination, stereotypes, and biases, placing AsAms outside the boundaries of Whiteness and U.S. citizenship (Tessler et al., 2020).

This chapter aims to capture the racist rhetoric and explore AsAms' real-life experiences of COVID-19 racism with four sections. First, we discuss the racist rhetoric of the U.S. politics and its impact on public discourse. Second, we present the type and prevalence of anti-Asian COVID-19 racism based on our recent survey and Asian advocacy groups' incident reports in conjunction with the history of anti-Asian racism in the U.S. society. Third, we discuss the impact of COVID-19 racism on AsAms' mental and physical well-being and report our survey findings regarding the population's anxiety and behaviors during the pandemic. Fourth, we introduce various activism movements to combat anti-Asian racism and to advance the AsAm community. In conclusion, we summarize scholars' future directions to assist AsAms to cope with COVID-19 racism and its detrimental impacts.

"Kung-flu" and "Chinese Virus"—Racist and Stigmatizing Rhetoric in American Politics and Its Impacts

The World Health Organization (WHO) guidelines for disease taxonomy mandate that new human infectious disease names should not refer to a specific geographic location, animal, individual, or group of people as that can be inaccurate and stigmatizing (Fukuda et al., 2015; WHO, 2015). This was the reasoning behind the WHO's official designation of the virus as "COVID-19" on February 2020 (Mansoor, 2020; WHO, 2020). Despite such guidelines, many political figures in the United States have used improper terms in referring to COVID-19. The former U.S. president, Donald Trump, has consistently used the terms "the Chinese virus" or "China virus" in his tweets and during news conferences (Gover et al., 2020), and even used a racist term "Kung-flu" (Nakamura, 2020; White House, 2020).

Trump's misleading rhetoric is better understood within the context of the White House's disagreements with WHO as well as the government of the People's Republic of China, from whom the White House has demanded greater accountability for the pandemic (White House, 2020). As shown in an official statement released by the White House, the decision to revoke the U.S. funding for WHO in April 2020 was based on what the White House perceived as a "dangerous bias toward the Chinese government." Specifically, the White House has criticized WHO for "[parroting] the Chinese government's claims that the coronavirus was not spreading between humans, despite warnings by doctors and health officials that it was" (White House, 2020). Furthermore, both governments have traded diplomatic blows, accusing each other of starting the pandemic with respective conspiracy theories (Feng & Cheng, 2020; Miller, 2020). Other U.S. politicians, including, but not limited to, Secretary of State Mike Pompeo, Senator Tom Cotton, Representative Paul Gosar, and House Minority Leader Kevin McCarthy have followed suit by using the terms "Wuhan virus" or "Chinese coronavirus" in public forums (Rogers, 2020). John Cornyn, U.S. Senator for Texas, stated that the "Chinese virus" originated from a "culture where people eat bats, snakes, and dogs," which reflects the reinvigoration of old stereotypes of Chinese people and a phobia of Chinese food (Gee et al., 2020).

Research suggests that such improper labeling of COVID-19 has significant influences on public discourse regarding the virus. According to the Atlantic Council's digital forensic research, Representative Gosar's tweet that labeled COVID-19 as the "Wuhan virus" was trending on Twitter in the subsequent days, and tweets using the term "Wuhan virus" were shared more than 24,000 times within the first hour of Gosar's tweet being published. After Secretary Pompeo referred to COVID-19 as the "Chinese coronavirus" on the news networks *CNBC* and *Fox* on March 7, 2020, online usage of the term increased by 800%. Furthermore, the former president Trump's usage of the term "foreign virus" during an Oval Office speech on March 11 saw an immediate spike in usage of the term on Twitter, with impressions (i.e., number of times a term is seen on Twitter) rising from negligible levels to the tens of millions on March 13 (The Atlantic Council, 2020). Following this trend, insulting memes and jokes about bats, China, and Chinese people flooded social media platforms (Tessler et al., 2020).

The increase of such racially charged and scientifically incorrect rhetoric has been accompanied by a number of physical and verbal racist attacks against AsAms, isolation of AsAm people during the outbreak, and a significant decrease of AsAm businesses, as reported in news media (Ma & McLaughlin, 2020; Oung, 2020). The increasing anti-Asian COVID-19 racism has impacted many lives in the United States. The AsAm population is the fastest growing racial group in the United States, which increased 72% between 2000 and 2015 (López et al., 2017). A total of 22.2 million people or 6% of the U.S. population identified themselves as being Asian or Asian in combination with another race, as of 2019 (U.S. Census, 2019). The proportion of AsAms in the United States is expected to reach 14% by 2065 (Cohn, 2015). The AsAm population was recently noted to be the fastest growing group of eligible voters increasing 139% from 2000 to 2020 due to the influx of naturalized citizens immigrated from East-, Southeast-, and South Asia (Budiman, 2020). With the addition of Asians residing in the United States without U.S. citizenship, the Asian population consists of an even greater number. For instance, international students from Asia account for more than 65% of over one million international students in the United States (Institute of International Education, 2019), and Asians accounted for one-quarter of the U.S. foreign-born labor force in 2019 (U.S. Department of Labor, 2019).

Anti-Asian COVID-19 racism occurs in a context of historically entrenched attitudes toward the Asian race and racial hierarchy within U.S. society (H. A. Chen et al., 2020). The act of interpreting the current national crisis as an external threat and ascribing this danger to Chinese or Asian bodies should not be a surprise to the scholars who study AsAms given the long history of cognitive association of AsAms to Asia and to diseases (Tessler et al., 2020). Therefore, it is necessary to review the context of historical racial dynamics and typical forms of anti-Asian racism and biases to fully understand the AsAm experience during the COVID-19 pandemic. We suggest at least two types of anti-Asian biases—"invalidation of interethnic differences among Asians" and "Asians as perpetual foreigners" are reinforced and overtly expressed during the pandemic. In the next section, we discuss the historical precedents of these two anti-Asian biases and relevant incidents during the pandemic.

Anti-Asian Biases and COVID-19 Attacks

Invalidation of Interethnic Differences

Asia comprises of nearly 50 countries, and the AsAms in the United States are correspondingly heterogeneous in terms of ethnicity, language, culture, religion, and immigration history. Nonetheless, many Americans of Asian ancestry have been uniformly assumed to be Chinese or Japanese (H. A. Chen et al., 2020), and the diversity within AsAms is often disregarded, as identified in a number of anti-Asian racism studies (e.g., Cheryan & Monin, 2005; Jun, 2012; Liang et al., 2004). A social-psychologist, Sue, who has long studied racism and microaggressions targeting Asians suggested a term "invalidation of interethnic differences" to describe this phenomenon of assuming AsAms as a unified racial group and eradicating the visibility and perspectives of other Asian communities (Sue, Bucceri, et al., 2007). AsAms frequently hear the statement, "All Asians look alike" or the question "Are you Chinese or Japanese?"

Although racist/xenophobic attacks against Chinese or Americans of Chinese ancestry cannot be justified because of the location of the first COVID-19 outbreak, many current attacks against AsAms occur in a context of the invalidation of interethnic differences. For instance, Burmese American family members, including a 2-year-old girl and a 6-year-old boy, were stabbed at a Sam's Club store in Midland, Texas, and the attacker indicated that he did so because he thought the family was Chinese and infecting people with COVID-19 (Margolin, 2020). On March 10, 2020, a Korean American woman was grabbed by the hair, shoved, and punched in the face by an assailant in midtown Manhattan, while the perpetrator yelled at the victim, "You've got coronavirus, you Asian" and "Where's your mask?" (H. A. Chen et al., 2020).

Asians as Perpetual Foreigners

Anti-Asian racist attacks during COVID-19 reflect another pervasive bias toward Asians—"Asians as perpetual foreigners"—regardless of where they were born or how long they have lived in the United States, Asians are perceived as eternal "others" in American society (Lee, 1999). AsAms live with the questions, "Where are you really from?" or "Do you speak English?" that represent the typical assumption about Asians as outsiders in America (Cheryan & Monin, 2005; Wu, 2002). American media and pop-culture, which define what is American, have stereotyped Asians as "others" or "not Americans" regardless of their nativity or citizenship (Suzuki, 2002; Wu, 2002; Zhang, 2010). An overt instance of the perpetual foreigner bias is the *MSNBC* headline at the 1998 Winter Olympics "American beats out Kwan" to refer to the victory of Tara Lipinski over Michelle Kwan, who was born and raised in California (Wu, 2002). This bias has been an overwhelming threat to AsAms' identity and interracial relationships. In an experiment on facial recognition based on race and ethnicity, Asian faces were seen as the least American followed by White, Blacks, and Hispanics (Cheryan & Monin, 2005), and Americans from other races were least likely to initiate friendships with Asians as compared to people of other racial groups (Zhang, 2010). To deal with the denial of their national identity and social marginalization, AsAms have to present their American cultural knowledge more often and claim greater participation in traditional American practices (Cheryan & Monin, 2005).

The *perpetual foreigners* bias is long-standing in American history and has forcefully re-emerged during the COVID-19 crisis. During this crisis, AsAms have been treated as the physical embodiment of foreignness and disease (Tessler et al., 2020). Even AsAms healthcare workers were marginalized as dangerous foreigners who brought the disease into the United States, rather than the front-liners. An AsAm doctor was told to "go back to f--- China" on his way to work, and an Asian nurse delivering medicine to a sick patient was spat on. Parents at a children's hospital refused care from healthcare staff with "Asian appearances" (H. A. Chen et al., 2020).

Historically, racial minorities were depicted as less clean or immune and more harmful as compared to their White counterparts, and minority group members have felt that they have been erroneously blamed and feared by others who perceived them to be "dirty" or "sickly" (Roberto et al., 2020). A White-supremacy ideology consistently recurred during the previous public health crises. When the bubonic plague swirled around America in the 19th century, the belief that Asians could be infected due to their unhygienic lifestyles, resulted in some extreme measures taken by the authorities toward the Asian population; officials and authorities quarantined Chinatown as a precautionary measure to control bubonic plague (Mohr, 2006; Trauner, 1978). AsAms were stereotyped as bloodthirsty and sneaky immigrants who spread diseases in the 20th and 21st centuries (Kawai, 2005; Lee,

1999). More recently, there was an increase in discourse on Chinatowns as the epicenters of SARS in 2003. Consequently, AsAms and their businesses suffered from the racism and discriminations during the epidemic, even though the negative impact of COVID-19 on AsAms has been far more severe than that of SARS (Tessler et al., 2020).

Patterns of Anti-Asian COVID-19 Racism

Prior to COVID-19, some scholars stated that racist expressions have evolved from the "old fashion" form in which overt racial hatred is consciously and publicly displayed to a modern and symbolic form that is more ambiguous (Dovidio et al., 2002; Sue, Capodilupo, et al., 2007). Previous research suggested that covert discrimination (subtle unfair treatment and messages with less courtesy or respect from others) was more prevalent than overt discrimination (direct and hostile harassment/attack), as experienced by older AsAms (Chan, 2020). However, since the COVID-19 outbreak, more AsAms may face overt discrimination; the vast majority of reported incidents were overt discrimination, including verbal harassment and physical assaults (Jeung & Nham, 2020). Another minority group in the United States, Muslim Americans reported experiencing a similar increase of overt discrimination and Islamophobia after the September 11 attacks (Bleich, 2011).

An AsAm reporter at *CNN* who was verbally harassed by a racist passerby while preparing a live newscast on COVID-19 stated, "*I have seen racial slurs on social media, but it has been a while to hear a racial slur directly at my face, probably since elementary school. It is now happening*" (CNN, 2020). A number of hate crimes targeting AsAms involving physical violence, harassment, and death threats during COVID-19 were reported (OCA, 2020) or published on social media in the form of bystander videos (Gover et al., 2020). In March 2020, an AsAm man wearing a mask in Brooklyn was stabbed 13 times by another man in a mask; meanwhile, an AsAm woman was attacked at a crosswalk in San Francisco. In April 2020, a man in New York poured acid on an AsAm woman, hospitalizing her with serious burns. During the completion of this manuscript, six Asian women were murdered in the Atlanta area shootings (Holcombe, 2021).

Anti-Asian hate crimes have varied in weapons use including acid, an umbrella, and a log as well as locations, such as bus stops, subway stations, convenience stores, and on the street (Jeung & Nham, 2020; Tessler et al., 2020). Death threats have been made against owners of Asian restaurants and Asian passersby (Parascandola, 2020). Multiple cases of vandalism and property damage to Asian businesses have been reported and documented by the police. More explicit references to COVID-19 were documented in some vandalism cases with phrases including "take the corona back to you ch★nk" and "watch out for corona" (Goodell & Mann, 2020; Wang, 2020).

While the discrimination against AsAms during COVID-19 has become more overt and violent, countless instances of verbal and nonverbal discrimination may still continue. Given the literature on microaggressions against AsAms (Liang et al.,

2004; Sue, Bucceri, et al., 2007), racial discrimination during the pandemic can include explicit verbal attacks intended to hurt AsAms as well as nonverbal discrimination, such as avoidant behavior, rejection, and unfair evaluation directed at AsAms. As the nature of discrimination experienced by AsAms is expected to change since the COVID-19 outbreak, we conducted an online survey to investigate various forms of anti-Asian COVID-19 racism.

In our analysis of survey responses from 858 people who identified themselves as being of Asian descent, 283 people (33.1%) reported to have experienced discrimination due to their race or ethnicity since the COVID-19 outbreak. Of those targeted AsAms, more than 85% reported to having experienced ignorance by others (87.2%) followed by being walked away from (84.7%), racial slurs (74.4%), verbal harassment (74%), bullying (72.3%), being told to go back to their country (71.1%), social isolation (59.1%), rejection for service (57.9%), unfair evaluation, (51.7%), and physical attacks (46.7%). Reports of covert discrimination (i.e., being ignored or being walked away from) during the pandemic significantly increased compared to before the pandemic. A majority of participants also reported that they have experienced overt discrimination (i.e., racial slurs, verbal harassment, and being told to go back to your country) during the pandemic. These results reveal the level of aggravated discrimination against AsAms during the pandemic (see Figures 8.1 and 8.2).

Some of our results are aligned with patterns of anti-Asian attacks during COVID-19 that were identified by Asian advocacy groups and scholars. According to Stop AAPI Hate, there are five trends of COVID-19 discrimination against AsAms that emerged from 2,583 incidents across the United States from March to August, 2020 (Jeung & Nham, 2020). First, verbal attacks are rampant; seven out of ten incidents involved verbal harassment, including racial slurs, name calling, and profanities. Second, civil rights are being violated; potential civil rights violations, including workplace discrimination and being barred from establishments and transportation, comprised 8% of the incidents. Third, incidents at businesses are prevalent; nearly 40% of the hate incidents took place at places of business, followed by public streets (20%) and public parks (11%). Online incidents comprised 11% of the incidents. Fourth, there are gender disparities in incidents; women reported

33%

of Asian Americans have experienced COVID-19 racism

FIGURE 8.1 Percentage of Asian Americans Who Reported Experiencing Racism During the COVID-19 Pandemic ($N = 858$)

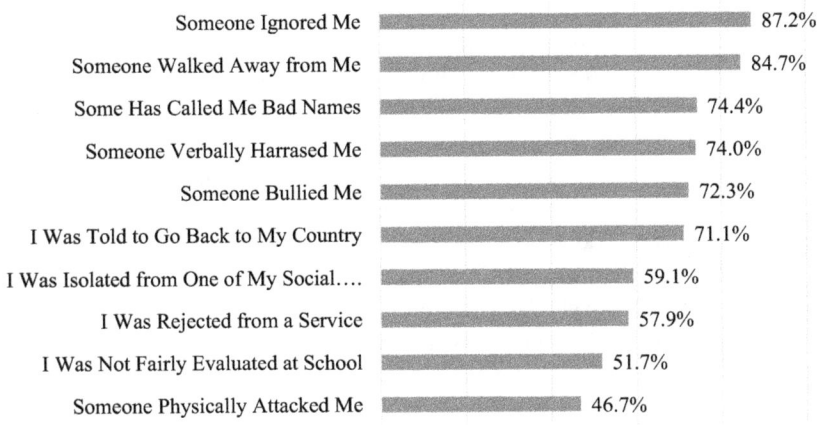

FIGURE 8.2 Asian Americans' Experience of Different Types of Discrimination in the United States During the COVID-19 Pandemic ($N = 858$)

discrimination 2.4 times more than men. Fifth, discrimination affects people of all ages; one in seven of those reporting were young people under 20 years old (14%) and elderly made up 7.5% of the respondents. Of the hate incidents reported by youth (aged 12–20), over eight out of ten (81.5%) reported being bullied or verbally harassed, one out of four (24%) were involved in face-to-face shunning and social isolation, and 24 cases of physical assaults (8%) were reported (Jeung et al., 2020).

In our survey, AsAms were aware of COVID-19 racism incidents even if they have not been directly targeted. A majority of AsAm bystanders were aware of the increase of discrimination targeting AsAms since the COVID-19 outbreak (83%), physical attacks on streets across the country (75%), suffering of AsAm businesses (73%), or school bullying of AsAm students (63%). Most had heard about Trump's labeling of COVID-19 as a "Chinese Virus" (90%) and nearly two-thirds (65%) were aware of FBI's warning on an increase of hate crimes against AsAms. In addition, more than half of them had heard about a hate crime involving the stabbing of AsAm family members in Texas (55%) and another stabbing of an AsAm man for wearing a mask in Brooklyn (57%). These results reveal AsAms' awareness of their marginalized social status and challenges presented by the pandemic. In the next section, we discuss the impact of COVID-19 racism on AsAms' mental and physical well-being and present AsAms' anxiety and pandemic behaviors identified from our survey.

The Impact of COVID-19 Racism on AsAms' Health

Racism is a chronic social stressor that negatively impacts targeted individuals' psychological, physiological, and subjective health and well-being, as evidenced by a number of studies (e.g., Suzuki, 2002; Watkins et al., 2009; Williams et al., 2008). Historical precedents and previous research suggest that COVID-19 racism exerts harmful effects on AsAms' mental and physical health. Japanese Americans who were confined to internment camps during World War II exhibited nearly twice greater rates of both suicide and cardiovascular disease as compared to their counterparts who were not interned (Nagata et al., 2019). Following the 9/11 attacks, increased Islamophobia, anti-Muslim rhetoric, and hate crimes were associated with greater psychological distress and health problems among Arab and Muslim Americans (Padela & Heisler, 2010). Racial discrimination has been a robust and consistent predictor of diminished well-being and increased mental problems, such as reduced life satisfaction, lower self-esteem, and increased symptoms of anxiety, depression, and suicidal ideation (Bernstein et al., 2017; Hwang & Goto, 2008; Nadal et al., 2015). The literature to date also suggests that discrimination exacerbates a range of chronic health conditions, including cardiac disease, respiratory conditions, and pain among AsAms (Gee et al., 2007).

Emerging evidence supports detrimental health impacts of COVID-19 on AsAms. The news media has reported increased anxiety among AsAms, such as fear for their physical safety when running everyday errands, being self-conscious about coughing or being ill, and concern about being targeted for hate crimes. Some AsAms attempt to hide their Asian identity or emphasize their American citizenship so as to avoid potential hate crimes (Buscher, 2020; Cheung et al., 2020; Tang, 2020). AsAms' use of an anxiety screening tool by Mental Health America has increased at 39% since the beginning of the pandemic, surpassing a 22% total increase of all users (Campbell & Ellerbeck, 2020). Choi et al. (2020) found that experiencing everyday discrimination and perceiving that the discrimination targets Asians has increased during the COVID-19 pandemic, and such experience and perceptions were powerful predictors of psychological distress among Korean Americans in the United States.

Anxiety, Depression, and Health Behaviors During the Pandemic

Many AsAms reported stress, anxiety, and increased substance use in our analysis of 520 survey responses collected in March 2020. In particular, about 45% of them answered that they felt more anxious than before the pandemic, and more than 30% said that they are not as confident about themselves. In addition, many showed worry of being attacked by a racist (31%), going outside because of their race/ethnicity (28%), and being discriminated at work/school (26%). Little less than one-fifth reported to having thought about killing themselves (18%).

Some respondents in our survey indicated a greater level of substance use and self-protective behaviors; more frequent use of alcohol (19%), tobacco (14%), and medicine/drugs (14%) during the pandemic. In addition, more than one-fifth answered to having improved home security (21%) and considered buying a weapon to protect themselves (22%). Nearly one-fourth (23%) reported to having limited interactions with people of other races (see Figure 8.3).

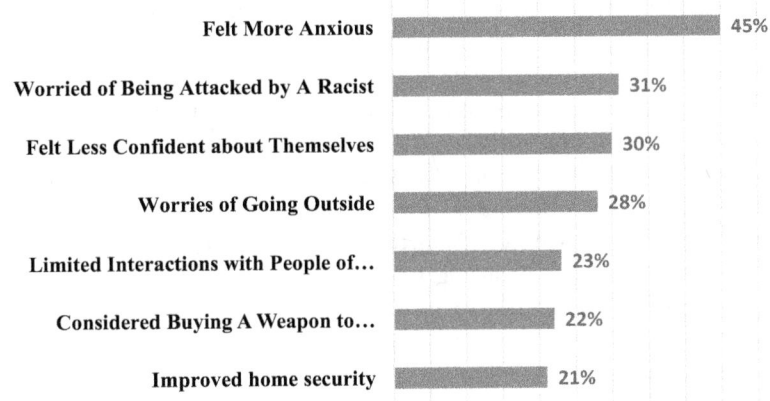

FIGURE 8.3 Asian Americans' Substance Use and Self-Protective Behaviors During the COVID-19 Pandemic (N = 520)

Source: Data come from a survey conducted by the researcher's team in March 2020.

We assessed depressive symptoms of AsAms who reported exposure to COVID-19 racism using the 20-item Center for Epidemiologic Studies of Depression (CES-D) Scale (Radloff, 1977). Examples of the items included how often the respondent "thought [their] life had been a failure" and how often the respondent "felt that everything [they] did was an effort." Our study participants, on average, had either at least 11 of the 20 symptoms in the CES-D scale with a moderate persistence one week after the experience or most of the symptoms for shorter periods of time. We found that AsAms who reported severe exposure to COVID-19 racism were more likely to experience stronger depressive symptoms. Specifically, COVID-19 racial discrimination was a significant social stressor, even when considering previous experience of racial discrimination before the pandemic. There were no ethnic differences in the detrimental mental effects of COVID-19 discrimination, indicating that COVID-19 racism negatively impacts all AsAms—not only Chinese Americans. In the next section, we describe and discuss AsAms' actions to combat COVID-19 racism.

AsAm Advocacy Actions to Combat COVID-19 Racism

Although experiencing racial discrimination is a stressful life event, it can trigger targeted individuals to increase the willingness to undertake social change efforts (Simon et al., 1998). Studies have found support for this relationship between discrimination experience and activism for their own group (e.g., Duncan, 1999; Tran & Curtin, 2017). Social- psychology research explains this relationship with the development of structural awareness through racial discrimination experiences (Duncan, 1999; Tran & Curtin, 2017). Structural awareness is the attribution of inequality to social structures rather than to abilities or traits of individuals or groups

(Curtin et al., 2015). Increased structural awareness also prompts more salient group identity and eventually leads to activism (Duncan, 1999).

AsAm activists began organizing pan-ethnic AsAm communities to combat anti-Asian racism and resist Western imperialism in response to the radical politics in the late 1960s and early 1970s in the United States (Kurashige, 2000). AsAm activists or advocacy groups lead or ally with others for various racial/social justice movements, the rights of sexual minorities, victims of domestic violence, and environmental justice (Aguirre & Lio, 2008; Sze, 2004). In response to the rise of anti-Asian racism during the COVID-19 outbreak, AsAm advocacy groups have taken joint actions to monitor incidents against AsAms, announce public statements, implement COVID-19 relief and communication campaigns to increase awareness of COVID-19 biases against Asians, and provide resources for AsAms' management and coping of COVID-19 racism (e.g., Ascend COVID-19 Resource Guide, AsAm Federation's COVID-19 resource guide, Asian Pacific American Advocate's COVID-19 Toolkit, #IAMNOTVIRUS campaign). Asian Pacific Policy and Planning Council (A3PCON), Chinese for Affirmative Action, and San Francisco State University's AsAm Studies Department established a national coalition, STOP AAPI Hate, to address anti-Asian discrimination amid the pandemic.

In the fight against anti-Asian biases, social media have served as the key arena where Asians can speak out about their own encounters and launch various counter campaigns (Abidin & Zeng, 2020). Nearly 1,200 new messages were posted during the pandemic on a Facebook group "Subtle Asian Traits," which is one of the largest online Asian communities with more than 1.7 million members (Abidin & Zeng, 2020). Personal experiences of hate crimes during COVID-19 were published on social media in the form of bystander videos (Gover et al., 2020). Asians around the world utilized social media communities to speak out about everyday encounters of COVID-19 racism as well as to engage in mutual care, discursive activism, and collective coping amid the rise of anti-Asian racism and xenophobia during the pandemic (Abidin & Zeng, 2020). Social media also become an important tool for AsAms' coping with discrimination as scholars suggested private messaging and posting/commenting are associated with better well-being through perceived social support (Yang et al., 2020).

The considerable reports of anti-Asian crimes on the news media drew public attention on the issue, and limited but some departmental responses were commissioned at both community and federal levels. The *BBC* has documented 120 distinct news articles covering alleged incidents of anti-Asian racism during the pandemic (Cheung et al., 2020). Advocates and activists have initiated online campaigns, such as #washthehate, #hateisavirus, and #fightthevirusfightthebias, to combat biases and racism. OCA—Asian Pacific American Advocate, STOP AAPI Hate, and Racismiscongtagious.com operate a platform where people can report incidents of racism and discrimination associated with COVID-19. The Commission on Civil Rights agreed on taking actions to respond to the anti-Asian hate crimes and discriminations during COVID-19 (Campbell & Ellerbeck, 2020).

Conclusion

Socially constructed racism and discrimination toward AsAms are rooted from individual-level prejudiced attitudes and behaviors and are amplified and reinforced by institutional-level support during public health crisis or difficult times, such as the COVID-19 pandemic (Gover et al., 2020). While racial inequality is a continuing problem in the United States, this public health crisis made it evident for advocates and activists to be aware of the rights and well-being of minority groups, including AsAms (Roberto et al., 2020). There are three major ways to address anti-Asian racism during the pandemic—policy, research, and practice—as suggested by Misra et al. (2020); we suggest inclusion of another component—activism.

Policy. A group of well-known AsAm officials, including Rep. Grace Menge (District of New York), who is also the vice chair of the Congressional Asian Pacific American, and Rep. Judy Chu (Southern California), led discussions of anti-Asian sentiment and racially motivated attacks during the COVID-19 pandemic. In particular, Rep. Grace Menge proposed resolutions for denouncing the spike in anti-Asian violence, including (1) all public officials to condemn such discriminatory deeds; (2) federal law enforcement to address COVID-19-related hate crimes through data collection, documentation, and investigation; (3) a state-level correspondence to racial bias cases concerning retail access, fair employment, and quality mental health services in educational settings and other social settings (Gover et al., 2020; Jeung et al., 2021). This proposal was signed by more than 130 House lawmakers and urged the administration to better track anti-Asian hate crimes, aligned with the U.S. Commission on Civil Rights, suggesting Congress pass legislation that would give states an incentive to better track and report hate crimes (Campbell & Ellerbeck, 2020).

The leading scholars of STOP AAPI, Jeung et al. (2021) called for a robust response from law enforcement and the federal and state governments where hate crimes occur, including schools, workplaces, businesses, and public spaces. However, federal and local governments' responses to prevent and address the inequity in terms of policy decisions, public communications, and community mitigation have been limited (Campbell & Ellerbeck, 2020; Roberto et al., 2020). Although President Biden signed the "COVID-19 Hate Crimes Act" into law in May 2021, during the completion of this chapter (Sprunt, 2021), neither the Justice Department nor the Centers for Disease Control and Prevention (CDC) have announced efforts to prevent the public targeting of Asians, which ranges from bias incidents to hate crimes. Both agencies were quick to act in similar situations: the CDC during the 2003 severe acute respiratory syndrome outbreak and the Justice Department after the 9/11 terrorist attacks (Campbell & Ellerbeck, 2020).

Research, practice, and activism. The spikes of anti-Asian racism during the COVID-19 pandemic and the lack of concerted effort from federal and local agencies call for more research and resources to support AsAm communities to mitigate negative health impacts as well as to empower communities to take action to fight against racial injustice and influence policymakers. Previous research documented that African Americans with low socioeconomic status showed elevated risk for high blood pressure when they have a tendency to actively cope with psychosocial stressors (Fernander et al., 2003; James et al., 1987). These findings highlight the importance of adequate coping resources (e.g., civic and legal protections; salient ethnic identity) accompanied with the efforts to communicate and promote activism to fight against racism. Thus, it is critical to provide adequate coping resources that can help such civic actions that lead to positive health and wellness of the participants in addition to the efforts to encourage activism. Health professionals and researchers should continue to develop specific interventions mitigating detrimental health effects of COVID-19 racism for AsAms, building on previous innovations such as cognitive behavioral therapy for individuals facing oppression (J. A. Chen et al., 2020).

Gee et al.'s (2020) seven recommendations to stop anti-Asian racism provided implications for relevant research and intervention practices to discontinue COVID-19-related racism: (1) avoiding the connection of diseases to social groups, (2) developing infrastructure to track discrimination and establish antiracist countermeasures, (3) enhancing science-based education, (4) reevaluating current racialized practices, (5) monitoring and fact-checking biases on social media, (6) overcoming nationalism and strengthening global collaboration on research and policies, and (7) requiring more research on racism. Roberto et al. (2020) emphasized communicative strategies and training of employees, public servants, and organizations to minimize stigmatization, overcome stereotypes, and reduce aggressive behaviors as well as to incorporate cultural competence and social equity in leading diverse communities (Roberto et al., 2020).

Despite many challenges presented by the COVID-19 pandemic, there are also reasons for optimism. Notwithstanding their long history of fighting for racial and social justice (Aguirre & Lio, 2008; Sze, 2004), the model minority myth has limited AsAms' ability to partner with other racial minority groups in dealing with racial justice (H. A. Chen et al., 2020). COVID-19 racism may have facilitated AsAms' increased structural awareness of their vulnerable and marginalized social hierarchy and detrimental impacts of racial inequality, which are important predictors of activism (Duncan, 1999). Scholars suggested the possibility of COVID-19 racism experience as a trigger for reinvigoration of a pan-ethnic AsAm identity and social movement (Tessler et al., 2020). In fact, AsAms have mobilized to participate in Black Lives Matter movements following the death of George Floyd, and scholars noted AsAm communities' increased motivation to tackle discrimination and intent to engage in cross-racial political and civic engagement (H. A. Chen et al., 2020). Researchers, advocacy groups, and educators should continue developing and providing more resources and toolkits for targeted AsAms as well as bystanders to provide communication strategies to challenge biases, to raise critical consciousness of racism, and to create strategic alliances across diverse AsAm ethnic communities and other racial minority groups.

References

Abidin, C., & Zeng, J. (2020). Feeling Asian Together: Coping With #COVIDRacism on Subtle Asian Traits. *Social Media + Society, 6*(3), 205630512094822. https://doi.org/10.1177/2056305120948223

Aguirre, A., & Lio, S. (2008). Spaces of Mobilization: The Asian American/Pacific Islander Struggle for Social Justice. *Social Justice, 35*(2 (112)), 1–17. JSTOR.

Bernstein, K., Park, S.-Y., & Nokes, K. M. (2017). Resilience and Depressive Symptoms Among Korean Americans with History of Traumatic Life Experience. *Community Mental Health Journal, 53*(7), 793–801. https://doi.org/10.1007/s10597-017-0142-7

Bleich, E. (2011). What Is Islamophobia and How Much Is There? Theorizing and Measuring an Emerging Comparative Concept. *American Behavioral Scientist, 55*(12), 1581–1600. https://doi.org/10.1177/0002764211409387

Budiman, A. (2020). Asian Americans Are the Fastest-Growing Racial or Ethnic Group in the U.S. Electorate. *Pew Research Center.* www.pewresearch.org/fact-tank/2020/05/07/asian-americans-are-the-fastest-growing-racial-or-ethnic-group-in-the-u-s-electorate/

Buscher, R. (2020). Reality Is Hitting Me in The Face: Asian Americans Grapple with Racism Due to COVID-19. *WHYY.* https://whyy.org/articles/reality-is-hitting-me-in-the-face-asian-americans-grapple-with-racism-due-to-covid-19

Campbell, A., & Ellerbeck, A. (2020). Federal Agencies Are Doing Little About the Rise in Anti-Asian Hate Crime. *San Francisco Chronicle.* www.nbcnews.com/news/asian-america/federal-agencies-are-doing-little-about-rise-anti-asian-hate-n1184766

Chan, K. (2020). The Association of Acculturation with Overt and Covert Perceived Discrimination for Older Asian Americans. *Social Work Research, 44*(1), 59–71. https://doi.org/10.1093/swr/svz023

Chen, H. A., Trinh, J., & Yang, G. P. (2020). Anti-Asian Sentiment in the United States: COVID-19 and History. *The American Journal of Surgery, 220*(3), 556–557. https://doi.org/10.1016/j.amjsurg.2020.05.020

Chen, J. A., Zhang, E., & Liu, C. H. (2020). Potential Impact of COVID-19–Related Racial Discrimination on the Health of Asian Americans. *American Journal of Public Health, 110*(11), 1624–1627. https://doi.org/10.2105/AJPH.2020.305858

Cheryan, S., & Monin, B. (2005). Where Are You Really from? Asian Americans and Identity Denial. *Journal of Personality and Social Psychology, 89*(5), 717–730. https://doi.org/10.1037/0022-3514.89.5.717

Cheung, H., Feng, Z., & Deng, B. (2020). Coronavirus: What Attacks on Asians Reveal About American Identity. *BBC News.* www.bbc.com/news/world-us-canada-52714804

Choi, S., Hong, J. Y., Kim, Y. J., & Park, H. (2020). Predicting Psychological Distress Amid the COVID-19 Pandemic by Machine Learning: Discrimination and Coping Mechanisms of Korean Immigrants in the U.S. *International Journal of Environmental Research and Public Health, 17*(17), 6057. https://doi.org/10.3390/ijerph17176057

CNN. (2020). *CNN's Kyung Lah Describes Racist Encounter with Passerby—CNN Video.* www.cnn.com/videos/us/2020/03/20/california-coronavirus-racial-slur-kyung-lah-tapper-lead-sot-vpx.cnn

Cohn, D. (2015). Future Immigration Will Change the Face of America by 2065. *Pew Research Center.* www.pewresearch.org/fact-tank/2015/10/05/future-immigration-will-change-the-face-of-america-by-2065/

Curtin, N., Stewart, A. J., & Cole, E. R. (2015). Challenging the Status Quo: The Role of Intersectional Awareness in Activism for Social Change and Pro-Social Intergroup Attitudes. *Psychology of Women Quarterly, 39*(4), 512–529. https://doi.org/10.1177/0361684315580439

Dovidio, J. F., Gaertner, S. L., Kawakami, K., & Hodson, G. (2002). Why Can't We Just Get Along? Interpersonal Biases and Interracial Distrust. *Cultural Diversity & Ethnic Minority Psychology, 8*(2), 88–102.

Duncan, L. E. (1999). Motivation for Collective Action: Group Consciousness as Mediator of Personality, Life Experiences, and Women's Rights Activism. *Political Psychology, 20*(3), 611–635. https://doi.org/10.1111/0162-895X.00159

Ellerberk, A. (2020). *More Than 30 Percent of Americans Have Witnessed COVID-19 Bias Against Asians.* https://publicintegrity.org/health/coronavirus-and-inequality/survey-majority-of-asian-americans-have-witnessed-covid-19-bias/

Fauver, J. R., Petrone, M. E., Hodcroft, E. B., Shioda, K., Ehrlich, H. Y., Watts, A. G., Vogels, C. B. F., Brito, A. F., Alpert, T., Muyombwe, A., Razeq, J., Downing, R., Cheemarla, N. R., Wyllie, A. L., Kalinich, C. C., Ott, I., Quick, J., Loman, N. J., Neugebauer, K. M., … Grubaugh, N. D. (2020). *Coast-to-Coast Spread of SARS-CoV-2 in the United States Revealed by Genomic Epidemiology* [Preprint]. Public and Global Health. https://doi.org/ 10.1101/2020.03.25.20043828

Feng, E., & Cheng, A. (2020). *In Coronavirus War of Words With the U.S., China Pulls no Punches.* www.npr.org/2020/05/11/852645612/in-coronavirus-war-of-words-china-pulls-no-punches

Fernander, A. F., Dura'N, R. E. F., Saab, P. G., Llabre, M. M., & Schneiderman, N. (2003). Assessing the Reliability and Validity of the John Henry Active Coping Scale in an Urban Sample of African Americans and White Americans. *Ethnicity & Health, 8*(2), 147–161. https://doi.org/10.1080/13557850303563

Fukuda, K., Wang, R., & Vallat, B. (2015). Naming Diseases: First Do No Harm. *Science, 348*(6235), 643. https://doi.org/10.1126/science.348.6235.643

Gee, G. C., Ro, M. J., & Rimoin, A. W. (2020). Seven Reasons to Care About Racism and COVID-19 and Seven Things to Do to Stop It. *American Journal of Public Health, 110*(7), 954–955. https://doi.org/10.2105/AJPH.2020.305712

Gee, G. C., Spencer, M. S., Chen, J., & Takeuchi, D. (2007). A Nationwide Study of Discrimination and Chronic Health Conditions Among Asian Americans. *American Journal of Public Health, 97*(7), 1275–1282. https://doi.org/10.2105/AJPH.2006.091827

Gonzalez-Reiche, A. S., Hernandez, M. M., Sullivan, M. J., Ciferri, B., Alshammary, H., Obla, A., Fabre, S., Kleiner, G., Polanco, J., Khan, Z., Alburquerque, B., van de Guchte, A., Dutta, J., Francoeur, N., Melo, B. S., Oussenko, I., Deikus, G., Soto, J., Sridhar, S. H., … van Bakel, H. (2020). Introductions and Early Spread of SARS-CoV-2 in the New York City area. *Science, 369*(6501), 297–301. https://doi.org/10.1126/science.abc1917

Goodell, E., & Mann, D. (2020). Take the Corona Back You ******:Yakima Police Investigate Racist Graffiti at Asian Buffet. *Yaktri News.*

Gover, A. R., Harper, S. B., & Langton, L. (2020). Anti-Asian Hate Crime During the COVID-19 Pandemic: Exploring the Reproduction of Inequality. *American Journal of Criminal Justice, 45*(4), 647–667. https://doi.org/10.1007/s12103-020-09545-1

Holcombe, M. (2021). Atlanta Shooting Victims: A Trip to the Spa That Ended in Death: These Are Some of The Victims of the Shootings. *CNN.* www.cnn.com/2021/03/18/us/atlanta-spa-shootings-victims/index.html

Hwang, W.-C., & Goto, S. (2008). The Impact of Perceived Racial Discrimination on the Mental Health of Asian American and Latino College Students. *Cultural Diversity and Ethnic Minority Psychology, 14*(4), 326–335. https://doi.org/10.1037/1099-9809.14.4.326

Institute of International Education. (2019). *International Students in the United States.* OpenDoors. file:///Users/jungmijun/Downloads/Open%20Doors%202019%20Fast%20Facts.pdf

James, S. A., Strogatz, D. S., Wing, S. B., & Ramsey, D. L. (1987). Socioeconomic Status, John Henryism, and Hypertension in Blacks and Whites. *American Journal of Epidemiology*, *126*(4), 664–673. https://doi.org/10.1093/oxfordjournals.aje.a114706

Jeung, R., Horse, A., Lau, A., Kong, P., Shen, K., Cayanan, C., Xiong, M., & Lim, R. (2020). *Stop AAPI Hate Youth Report*. STOP AAPI. www.asianpacificpolicyandplanningcouncil. org/wp-content/uploads/Stop-AAPI-Hate-Youth-Report-9.14.20.pdf

Jeung, R., Horse, A., Popovic, T., & Lim, R. (2021). *Stop AAPI Hate National Report*. https:// secureservercdn.net/104.238.69.231/a1w.90d.myftpupload.com/wp-content/uploads/ 2021/03/210312-Stop-AAPI-Hate-National-Report-.pdf

Jeung, R., & Nham, K. (2020). *Incidents of Coronavirus-Related Discrimination*. Asian Pacific Policy and Planning Council. www.asianpacificpolicyandplanningcouncil.org/wp-content/uploads/STOP_AAPI_HATE_MONTHLY_REPORT_4_23_20.pdf

Jun, J. (2012). Why Are Asian Americans Silent? Asian Americans' Negotiation Strategies for Communicative Discriminations. *Journal of International and Intercultural Communication*, *5*(4), 329–348. https://doi.org/10.1080/17513057.2012.720700

Kawai, Y. (2005). Stereotyping Asian Americans: The Dialectic of the Model Minority and the Yellow Peril. *Howard Journal of Communications*, *16*(2), 109–130. https://doi.org/ 10.1080/10646170590948974

Kurashige, S. (2000). Pan-Ethnicity and Community Organizing: Asian Americans United Campaign Against Anti-Asian Violence. *Journal of Asian American Studies*, *3*(2), 163–190. https://doi.org/10.1353/jaas.2000.0018

Lee, J. H. X. (Ed.). (2016). *Chinese Americans: The History and Culture of a People*. ABC-CLIO.

Lee, R. (1999). *Orientals: Asian Americans in Popular Culture*. Temple University Press.

Liang, C., Li, L., & Kim, B. (2004). The Asian American Racism-Related Stress Inventory: Development, Factor Analysis, Reliability, and Validity. *Journal of Counseling Psychology*, *51*(1), 103–114. https://doi.org/10.1037/0022-0167.51.1.103

López, G., Ruiz, N., & Patten, E. (2017). Key Facts About Asian Americans, a Diverse and Growing Population. *Pew Research Center*. www.pewresearch.org/fact-tank/2017/09/ 08/key-facts-about-asian-americans/

Ma, A., & McLaughlin, K. . (2020). The Wuhan Coronavirus Is Causing Increased Reports of Racism and Xenophobia Against Asian People at College, Work, and Supermarkets. *Business Insider*. www.businessinsider.com/wuhan-coronavirus-racism-asians-experience-fears-outbreak-2020-1

Mansoor, S. (2020). The WHO Has Declared a Formal Name for The New Coronavirus Disease. Why Does the Name Matter? *Time*. https://time.com/5782284/who-name-coronavirus-covid-19/

Margolin, J. (2020). FBI Warns of Potential Surge in Hate Crimes Against Asian Americans Amid Coronavirus. *ABC News*. https://abcnews.go.com/US/fbi-warns-potential-surge-hate-crimes-asian-americans/story?id=69831920

Miller, Z. (2020). Trump Speculates That China Released Virus in Lab "Mistake." *AP NEWS*. https://apnews.com/c9499f7b8ab2ae7097c8588f1ccdddea

Misra, S., Le, P. D., Goldmann, E., & Yang, L. H. (2020). Psychological Impact of Anti-Asian Stigma Due to the COVID-19 Pandemic: A Call for Research, Practice, and Policy Responses. *Psychological Trauma: Theory, Research, Practice, and Policy*, *12*(5), 461–464. https://doi.org/10.1037/tra0000821

Mohr, J. C. (2006). *Plague and Fire: Battling Black Death and the 1900 Burning of Honolulu's Chinatown*. Oxford University Press.

Nadal, K. L., Wong, Y., Sriken, J., Griffin, K., & Fujii-Doe, W. (2015). Racial Microaggressions and Asian Americans: An Exploratory Study on Within-Group Differences and Mental

Health. *Asian American Journal of Psychology*, 6(2), 136–144. https://doi.org/10.1037/a0038058

Nagata, D. K., Kim, J. H. J., & Wu, K. (2019). The Japanese American Wartime Incarceration: Examining the Scope of Racial Trauma. *The American Psychologist*, 74(1), 36–48. https://doi.org/10.1037/amp0000303

Nakamura, D. (2020). With 'kung flu,' Trump Sparks Backlash Over Racist Language—and a Rallying Cry for Supporters. *The Washington Post*. Retrieved from www.washingtonpost.com/politics/with-kung-flu-trump-sparks-backlash-over-racist-language--and-a-rallying-cry-for-supporters/2020/06/24/485d151e-b620-11ea-aca5-ebb63d27e1ff_story.html

OCA. (2020). COVID-19 Toolkit. *Asian Pacific American Advocates*. https://drive.google.com/file/d/1_WiXOHHIP0RsqmtJMRcePOXuyh-e48C0/view

Oung, K. (2020). Coronavirus Racism Infected My High School. *The New York Times*. www.nytimes.com/2020/03/14/opinion/Racism-coronavirus-asians.html

Padela, A. I., & Heisler, M. (2010). The Association of Perceived Abuse and Discrimination After September 11, 2001, With Psychological Distress, Level of Happiness, and Health Status Among Arab Americans. *American Journal of Public Health*, 100(2), 284–291. https://doi.org/10.2105/AJPH.2009.164954

Parascandola, R. (2020). Asian Man Spit On, Threatened in NYC Coronavirus Hate Crime. *New York Daily News*. www.nydailynews.com/coronavirus/ny-coronavirus-hate-crime-brooklyn-subway-spit-20200325-h4w4nzb74fbadpx6li4f7xdoc4-story.html

Radloff, L. S. (1977). The CES-D Scale: A Self-Report Depression Scale for Research in the General Population. *Applied Psychological Measurement*, 1(3), 385–401.

Roberto, K. J., Johnson, A. F., & Rauhaus, B. M. (2020). Stigmatization and Prejudice During the COVID-19 Pandemic. *Administrative Theory & Praxis*, 42(3), 364–378. https://doi.org/10.1080/10841806.2020.1782128

Rogers, K. (2020). Politicians' Use of "Wuhan Virus" Starts a Debate Health Experts Wanted to Avoid. *The New York Times*. www.nytimes.com/2020/03/10/us/politics/wuhan-virus.html

Ruiz, N., Horowitz, J., & Tamir, C. (2020). Many Black and Asian Americans Say They Have Experienced Discrimination Amid the COVID-19 Outbreak. *Pew Research Center*. www.pewsocialtrends.org/2020/07/01/many-black-and-asian-americans-say-they-have-experienced-discrimination-amid-the-covid-19-outbreak/

Simon, B., Loewy, M., Stürmer, S., Weber, U., Freytag, P., Habig, C., Kampmeier, C., & Spahlinger, P. (1998). Collective Identification and Social Movement Participation. *Journal of Personality and Social Psychology*, 74(3), 646–658. https://doi.org/10.1037/0022-3514.74.3.646

Sprunt, B. (2021). Here's What the New Hate Crimes Law Aims to Do as Attacks on Asian Americans Rise. *NPR. Org*. www.npr.org/2021/05/20/998599775/biden-to-sign-the-covid-19-hate-crimes-bill-as-anti-asian-american-attacks-rise

Sue, D., Bucceri, J., Lin, A., Nadal, K. L., & Torino, G. C. (2007). Racial Microaggressions and the Asian American Experience. *Cultural Diversity and Ethnic Minority Psychology*, 13(1), 72–81. https://doi.org/10.1037/1099-9809.13.1.72

Sue, D., Capodilupo, C. M., Torino, G. C., Bucceri, J., Holder, A. M. B., Nadal, K. L., & Esquilin, M. (2007). Racial Microaggressions in Everyday Life: Implications for Clinical Practice. *American Psychologist*, 62(4), 271–286. https://doi.org/10.1037/0003-066X.62.4.271

Suzuki, B. (2002). Revisiting the Model Minority Stereotype: Implications for Student Affairs Practice and Higher Education. *New Directions for Student Services*, 97, 21–33.

Sze, J. (2004). Asian American Activism for Environmental Justice. *Peace Review*, 16(2), 149–156. https://doi.org/10.1080/1040265042000237680

Tang, T. (2020). From Guns to GoPros: Asian Americans Seek to Deter Attacks. *WGME*. https://wgme.com/news/nation-world/from-guns-to-gopros-asian-americans-seek-to-deter-attacks-04-24-2020

Tessler, H., Choi, M., & Kao, G. (2020). The Anxiety of Being Asian American: Hate Crimes and Negative Biases During the COVID-19 Pandemic. *American Journal of Criminal Justice*, *45*(4), 636–646. https://doi.org/10.1007/s12103-020-09541-5

The Atlantic Council. (2020). *U.S. Politicians Exploit Coronavirus Fears With Anti-Chinese Dog Whistles*. https://medium.com/dfrlab/u-s-politicians-exploit-coronavirus-fears-with-anti-chinese-dog-whistles-ff61c9d7e458

Tran, J., & Curtin, N. (2017). Not Your Model Minority: Own-Group Activism Among Asian Americans. *Cultural Diversity and Ethnic Minority Psychology*, *23*(4), 499–507. https://doi.org/10.1037/cdp0000145

Trauner, J. B. (1978). The Chinese as Medical Scapegoats in San Francisco, 1870-1905. *California History*, *57*(1), 70–87. https://doi.org/10.2307/25157817

U.S. Census. (2019). *Asian-American and Pacific Islander Heritage Month: May 2019*. The United States Census Bureau. www.census.gov/newsroom/facts-for-features/2019/asian-american-pacific-islander.html

U.S. Department of Labor. (2019). *Labor Force Characteristics of Foreign-Born Workers Summary*. www.bls.gov/news.release/forbrn.nr0.htm

Wang, J. (2020). *Vandals Tag Downtown Asian Restaurant With Racist Message*. www.kob.com/coronavirus/vandals-tag-downtown-asian-restaurant-with-racist-message/5677160

Watkins, D. C., Walker, R. L., & Griffith, D. M. (2009). A Meta-Study of Black Male Mental Health and Well-Being. *Journal of Black Psychology*, *36*(3), 303–330. https://doi.org/10.1177/0095798409353756

White House. (2020). *President Donald J. Trump Is Demanding Accountability from the World Health Organization*. www.whitehouse.gov/briefings-statements/president-donald-j-trump-demanding-accountability-world-health-organization

Williams, D. R., Neighbors, H.W., & Jackson, J. S. (2008). Racial/Ethnic Discrimination and Health: Findings from Community Studies. *American Journal of Public Health*, *98*(9 Suppl), S29–37.

World Health Organization. (2015). *World Health Organization Best Practices for the Naming of New Human Infectious Diseases*. Retrieved from https://apps.who.int/iris/bitstream/handle/10665/163636/WHO_HSE_FOS_15.1_eng.pdf;jsessionid=2CF63A67009EE1C766CD1F43CF41D60D?sequence=1

World Health Organization. (2020). *WHO Director-General's Remarks at the Media Briefing on 2019-nCoV*. www.who.int/dg/speeches/detail/who-director-general-s-remarks-at-the-media-briefing-on-2019-ncov-on-11-february-2020

Wu, F. (2002). *Yellow: Race in America Beyond Black and White*. Basic Books.

Yang, C., Tsai, J.-Y., & Pan, S. (2020). Discrimination and Well-Being Among Asians/Asian Americans During COVID-19: The Role of Social Media. *Cyberpsychology, Behavior, and Social Networking*. https://doi.org/10.1089/cyber.2020.0394

Zhang, Q. (2010). Asian Americans Beyond the Model Minority Stereotype: The Nerdy and the Left Out. *Journal of International and Intercultural Communication*, *3*(1), 20–37. https://doi.org/10.1080/17513050903428109

9

"BALANCING IT ALL"

The Implications of the COVID-19 Pandemic on Working Mothers in Texas

Nazgol Bagheri and Joshua Yates

Introduction

> *Wars were never gender-neutral, and so was the COVID-19 pandemic.*
>
> Mother of three, teacher, El Paso

In the United States, the pandemic has highlighted not only the racial and class divides but also the gender divide. Unlike usual economic recessions (e.g., the 2007–2009 Great Recession) in which men's employment has been affected more adversely than women's, during the pandemic, women's employment has dropped at a faster rate than men's, due to government-mandated social distancing measures and the high female-to-male ratio in labor markets affected by the lockdown. The numbers are telling (U.S. Bureau of Labor Statistics; National Women's Law Center): women have lost nearly one million more jobs than men during the first nine months of the pandemic (March to November, 2020); while in December, Black, Hispanic, and Asian women made all of women's job losses that month. While nearly eight out of ten say the pandemic is a significant source of stress in their life; women seem particularly afflicted as they are considerably more likely than their male counterparts to deal with job loss, serve as an "essential" worker, and/or care for children out of school as well as the elderly. However, job losses in healthcare were just one reason for women's income (and independence) loss; the closure of daycare centers and schools forced many women to return to the home and to unpaid domestic and care work (Alon et al., 2020, Bateman, & Ross, 2021). In this chapter, we aim to illustrate how the enforced lockdown measures by the federal government and the State of Texas have affected the everyday lives, and mental, physical, and emotional health, of women across the state.

We have particularly investigated the impacts on working mothers who self-identify themselves as immigrants (not women of color). There remains an

DOI: 10.4324/9781003268710-9

urgency to a gendered analysis of the implications and the potential responses to this multidimensional crisis. Most of the research on the COVID-19 implications on women has focused on either semi-rural women working in informal economies in developing countries or highly educated women in leadership positions in developed countries. So far, the results of these studies have been published mostly by the United Nations (UN), the World Health Organization (WHO), the World Bank, and major international news outlets. While both groups of women are important representatives of gendered equality in society and account for a large portion of women worldwide, they do not represent many women's experiences. Crenshaw (1990, p. 1242) reminds us that "although racism and sexism readily intersect in the lives of real people, they seldom do in feminist and antiracist practices." As feminists and antiracists, we[1] believe that our positionalities not only facilitate our research, but also enhance it through incorporating identity factors of women with whom we came to create a collective solidarity during the course of this research, from March 2020 to March 2021. We draw on Lawson's (2007, pp. 3–4) seminal work in which collective solidarity and care ethics "begins from a relational social ontology, understanding our world in terms of the connections that bind us together."

We open the chapter by recognizing the differentiated experiences and afflictions for women and men; we then contextualize our research in the thin but growing literature and data on gendered consequences of the 2020 COVID-19 pandemic. We draw on postcolonial and Marxist feminism works to explore the reductive and normative subjectivities and to examine inter-related structures of racial, gendered, and classed power and privilege. We then turn into the extra burden of intergenerational care work forced on women and recognize the intersectionalities of power that operate, in part, through the very mechanisms of care itself. Studies on care also show that daughters, not sons, are often the ones who care for their elderly parents, even when they leave the home country (see De Silva, 2018 and Pettit 2021). According to the U.S. Bureau of Labor Statistics, even before the pandemic, women—both employed and unemployed—spent an average of one hour per day more than men in the "caring for household member" (see Table 9.1).

The earlier care for others category includes childcare, homemaking services (informal work), and elder care. Hence, the concept of intersectionality is used as a key theoretical resource and a reference point to further develop care ethics. We use this concept to explore the different ways in which gender, race, class, and profession interact to shape the various struggles and experiences of the interviewees (Crenshaw, 1990).

Second, in order to offer a more realistic and intimate picture of the gendered dimensions of the pandemic, we draw on concrete examples of working mothers, striving to "balance it all" during the 2020 COVID-19 pandemic. We rely on semi-guided interviews with Texan women in six cities, including Austin, El Paso, Dallas, Houston, Laredo, and San Antonio (see Figure 9.1).

Their stories demonstrate how valuable expression and reflection have been during the pandemic to make sense of and cope with the turbulence many of them

TABLE 9.1 American Time Use: Average Hours Per Day Spent in Selected Activities by Employment Status and Sex, 2019 Annual Averages (Pre-Pandemic)

	Female Employed	Female Unemployed	Male Employed	Male Unemployed
Personal care, including sleep	9.46	10.19	9	10.04
Household activities	1.69	2.7	1.23	1.72
Purchasing goods and services	0.83	0.94	0.57	0.69
Caring for household members	0.66	0.61	0.40	0.16
Caring for non- household members	0.16	0.25	0.13	0.22
Working and work-related activities	5.69	0.10	6.69	0.22

Source: U.S. Bureau of Labor Statistics (2019). Charts related to the latest "American Time Use Survey" news release | more chart packages. U.S. Bureau of Labor Statistics. Retrieved 2020, from www.bls.gov/charts/american-time-use/activity-by-work.htm.

Note: This table contains the average time spent on selective activities.

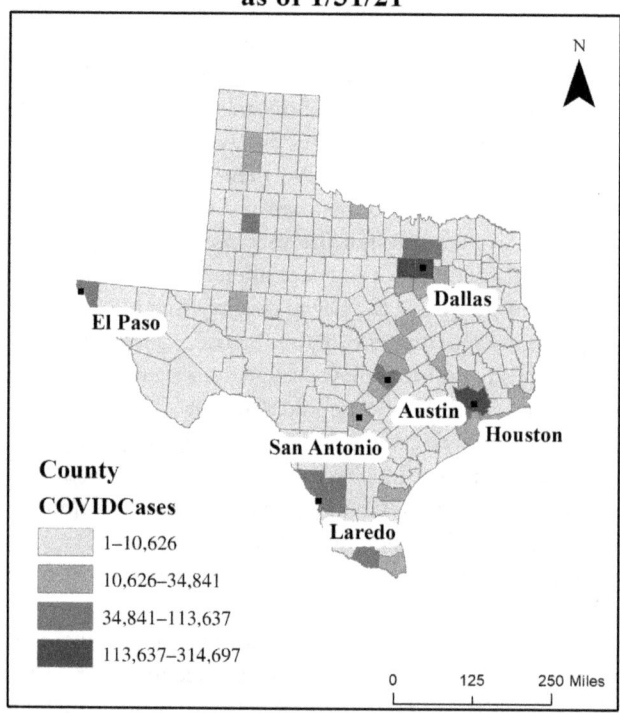

Texas COVID-19 confirmed cases by county as of 1/31/21

FIGURE 9.1 Texas COVID-19 Confirmed Cases by County (map created by the authors) The figure contains confirmed COVID-19 cases in Texas.

Data Source: Texas Department of State Health Services-Texas COVID-19 data portal, https://dshs.texas.gov/coronavirus/).

have experienced. But most importantly, these stories make these invisible women and their care labor and sufferings visible.

That listening and sharing—by scholars and by policymakers alike—gives women themselves a voice and is vital for any responses to these complex and pressing crises that deeply threaten human rights and democracy around the globe. We have conducted online ethnographic interviews with 41 women who self-identified as first- or second-generation immigrants to the United States, who were fully employed before the pandemic, and who are mothers. Ninety-seven women were first invited to participate in this research via a personal email and/or social media invites, using a snowball (chain-referral) sampling. The initial email included a link to an online, closed-question survey, comprised of ten questions that asked women about their self-identification with this study's specifics (e.g., race, immigration, age, motherhood, occupation), their knowledge of the COVID-19 pandemic, and its implications on their lives in relation to women's economic vulnerability and job stability, women's physical health and mental well-being, and finally women's access to various resources.

Next, in order to offer a more realistic and intimate picture of the gendered dimensions of the pandemic, we draw on concrete examples of working mothers, striving to "balance it all" during the 2020 COVID-19 pandemic. We rely on semi-guided interviews with Texan women (see Table 9.2) in six cities: Austin, El Paso, Dallas, Houston, Laredo, and San Antonio.

They were also asked to rank the extent of their anxiety regarding the various dimensions, including income loss, childcare, relationship, and getting sick. During the interviews, they explained further how their work and home lives have changed, how their parenting roles and responsibilities have shifted, and whether they have been supervising remote schooling or caring for sick, isolated, or aging relatives.

Lastly, we argue the COVID-19 pandemic has re-created and will continue to deepen the engrained gendered, racialized, classed, and ableist inequalities via caring labor, its devaluation, and invisibilization. People who are educating our children, providing home healthcare, cleaning our houses, processing our food, caring for our elderly, and nurturing our communities have been called "heroes." We emphasize the urgency of adapting a gender lens in order to create gender-sensitive policy measures and responses to these interlocked crises and a more just and resilient recovery from them. Our ultimate goal is to contribute to the growing methodological and theatrical bodies of work that confront and transform the deeply entrenched interlocking power inequalities and locate the care labor in a complex context of national and international policy and politics.

Women in Crises

On the last day of 2019, WHO was formally informed about a cluster of cases of pneumonia, later discovered to be caused by a novel coronavirus, SARS-CoV-2, in Wuhan City, a central Chinese cultural and economic hub of over ten million people. Almost a month later, WHO declared the outbreak of a worldwide public

TABLE 9.2 Interviewees' Demographic, Geographic, and Socioeconomic Characteristics

	Austin(8)	El Paso(5)	Dallas(6)	Houston(7)	Laredo(5)	San Antonio (10)
Family Arrangement						
Living with her partner	4	2	4	5	3	7
Separated from her partner	4	3	2	2	2	3
Living with elderly parents	2	1	0	0	3	2
Having one or more children less than 5 years old	4	4	5	6	5	7
Having one or more children between 5 and 12 years old	3	1	3	1	5	4
Having one or more children between 13 and 18 years old	2	0	2	1	0	2
Education						
High school diploma or less	3	2	4	4	4	5
Bachelor	3	2	1	2	1	3
Master or higher	2	1	1	1	0	2
Income						
$15,000 or less	0	1	0	0	2	1
$15,100–$50,000	6	3	4	4	3	7
$50,100–$85,000	1	2	1	2	0	1
$85,100 or more	1	0	1	1	0	1
Race						
White American (having originated in Europe, the Middle East, or North Africa)	4	2	2	2	2	5
African American	2	1	2	2	2	2
Asian American	1	2	1	2	1	1
American Indians/Alaska Native	1	0	1	0	0	1
Native Hawaiian/Other Pacific Islanders	0	0	0	0	0	0
People of two or more races	0	0	0	1	0	1

Notes: Data gathered and Organized by the Authors During in-Depth Zoom and Phone Interviews of 41 Texan Working Mothers from March 2020 to March 2021)

This table contains demographics of the interviewees for this study health crisis. At the time of writing, 192 countries are affected by the virus, with 128,377,922 confirmed cases and 2,806,679 global deaths. According to the UN report of April 2020 referred to earlier, the COVID-19 pandemic has negatively and disproportionately affected millions of women's economic lives and productivity at higher rates than for men (UN, 2020a, Bernstein, 2020).

The year 2020 was meant to mark an exciting year for women in the world, and the UN was about to celebrate the 25th anniversary of a ground-breaking moment, the Beijing Platform for Action for Gender Equality. However, the COVID-19 pandemic and its economic fallout put a halt on any further gender equality progress, causing women to lose jobs due to caregiving challenges and sending them back to the "private, domestic sphere" of homes. The pandemic's regressive effect on gender equality did not only expose gender biases but also exacerbated them at the work place and home. In addition to the existing gender inequalities, the increased time women have to spend on caregiving responsibilities has caused an adverse impact on working mothers' productivity. McKinsey Global Institute has estimated that female job loss rates due to COVID-19 are almost double male job loss rates globally, at 5.7% versus 3.1%, respectively. In other words, while women make up only 40% of global employment, they account for the majority of the job losses (~55%). Another report by LeanIn.org, the nonprofit for women in the professional workplace, suggested that the pandemic and accompanying recession have brought a halt to progress toward gender parity in several economies and industries. While there remains an urgent need for more gender-disaggregated data at both global and country levels, similar patterns have been observed in Texas. According to the Texas Workforce Commission (2020), women's job loss remained considerably higher than men in different stages of the pandemic.

There are several reasons explaining such uneven job loss among women and men worldwide: the first reason is the overwhelming percentage of women working in industries that were hit most by the pandemic. In many countries, including the United States, curfews and lockdowns have affected the parts of the economy that were female dominant. The service jobs (e.g., restaurants, bars, entertainment, and hospitality) were vanished; the federal and local government employers (e.g., education and administration sections when women outnumber men) were furloughed or given reduced hours to work from home, due to the decrease of economic activity and the decreased taxes collected by the cities. For example, in the United States, the shutdowns and physical distancing required by federal and local governments have affected certain industries—often low-wage jobs with high-customer interaction—in which women, particularly women of color (Najmabadi, 2020), are disproportionately employed. According to a *New York Times* analysis of census data crossed with the federal government's essential worker guidelines, one in three jobs held by women has been designated as essential. These essential workers work in healthcare, building and cleaning services, social services, public transit, grocery, and delivery and warehouse. Nationwide, women hold the majority of jobs in cleaning services and healthcare and more than 80% of jobs in childcare and community and family services. According to *Texas Tribune*, 62% of essential workers in Texas' top ten cities with the largest populations of essential workers are women, while women account for only 48% of the total workforce in those cities.

The second reason for the uneven job loss is the increased burden of unpaid care for children. Women are once again at the heart of caregiving; mothers are at home and caring for their kids, due to the closing of childcare centers and the shift to remote schooling. Working mothers, much more than fathers, are burdened with overwhelming household responsibilities in addition to their paid jobs. Even before the pandemic, most workplaces penalized women who chose to work from home, work fewer hours, and/or needed more flexibility to meet their family needs. This has been exacerbated during the pandemic and faced many working women with inevitably difficult choices about whether to quit their jobs and stay home with their children (Petersen, 2020, Robertson and Gebeloff, 2020, San Antonio Express-News 2020). Collins et al. (2020) found out that the gender gap in hours worked (at paid jobs) grew during the COVID-19 pandemic. Hard financial and emotional decisions (and involuntary sacrifices) had to be made, mostly by women, and that has resulted in a faster rate of women's employment loss than average, even considering the fact that women and men work in different sectors of the economy.

The third reason, which may have had less effect on women's job loss, is the virus itself and the very real occupational hazard that healthcare workers had to face due to close proximity to patients, lack of personal protective equipment, and other unknown risks during early stages of the pandemic. According to the WHO's sex distribution of healthcare workers data for 2018, women made up over 80% of nursing personnel in the United States. The pandemic has placed a sudden, immense burden on healthcare workers. The frontline healthcare workers have been designated as "essential workers" (also called heroes, "but not treated as truly [such]" according to Mina, mother of two, a registered nurse in Austin). They had no choice except to work close and for prolonged periods with COVID-19 patients, exposing themselves and their household members to the potential risk of infection. One early study suggested that healthcare workers were at increased risk for reporting a positive COVID-19 test. The International Council of Nurses (ICN) has continuously reported on the tragic deaths of nurses who died from the infection, the lack of personal protective equipment among nurses, and the psychological toll on their mental health. The largest healthcare occupation is registered nurses, dominated by female workers worldwide. In the United States, women make 75% of full-time, year-round healthcare workers (ICN, 2020). Women account for over 80% of registered nurses, nurse practitioners, psychiatrists, and home-help aids, while comprising only 30% of the physicians and surgeons. In addition, there is an invisible component to the frontline healthcare heroes, and that is the underpaid, undervalued, and essential workers who look after, clean, assist, cook, and care for patients, nurses, and doctors. They are nursing assistants, phlebotomists, home health aides, housekeepers, medical assistants, cooks, all of whom are mostly women and disproportionately people of color. These women also have been faced with a difficult decision: quitting their jobs and prioritizing their health (while losing the income) or exposing themselves and their families to the virus. Several of these physically overworked and mentally exhausted women that we surveyed had quit their jobs, not because of unpaid care labor at home, but because they feared for their lives and those of their loved ones.

Works in feminist ethics of care and political geography provide an intellectual framework within which one can make sense of the overwhelming outnumbering of women in the care industry. These numbers address what has been studied by feminists across disciplinary boundaries under the label of "the feminization of carework" (see Brennan, 2004; De Silva, 2018; Domosh & Seager, 2001; England, 2005; Gregson & Lowe, 1993; Lawson, 2007; McDowell, 2016; Mullings, 2005; Pratt, 1999; Williams, 2002). As Nakano Glenn (2012) suggests, women have historically been "forced to care," often out of love, responsibility, or both, and yet it is associated with "unpaid" and "unskilled." Care is

> highly emotional and irrational. It is women's work … Yet care is political precisely because it embodies issues typical of politics in a democracy; questions over the allocation of public resources as well as agonist relations wherein equity, justice, obligation and rights are lived.
>
> *Brown, 2003, p. 835*

This feminization of care work has resulted in low wages for caregivers, from in-home to hospice care, from daycare to assisted living centers. These women are often immigrants, and particularly vulnerable to any economic changes—especially because of exclusive labor laws and policies—and that is why these women were first to be furloughed or fired in the COVID-19-induced economic downturn.

The uneven job losses highlights the pre-existing gendered inequalities; they also explain why moms are working (at paid work) dramatically fewer hours than dads during the pandemic. Collins et al. (2020) suggests that between March and April 2020, mothers' work hours fell four to five times as much as those of fathers. Ultimately, all the current studies reveal that gender inequality—at work and home, alike—has worsened during the pandemic.

On the anniversary of the COVID-19 shutdown, an increasing body of scholarly work argues that women's suffering goes well beyond losing their incomes, jobs, independence, or managing the forced, unpaid care work at home; they have also been disproportionally vulnerable in many other dimensions, including physical health, mental well-being, gender violence, and educational opportunities. In fact, from health to the economy, security to social protection, exercising to nutrition, education to access to technology, domestic violence to sexual and reproductive health, the impacts of COVID-19 are exacerbated for women.[2] The first UN report on the subject, *The Impact of COVID-19 on Women*, published in April 2020 recognized four dimensions for the gendered inequality highlighted by the pandemic: (1) compounded economic impacts, (2) health (both physical and mental), (3) unpaid care work, and (4) gender-based violence (UN, 2020b). The report concluded with a strong recommendation to all nations: to "place women and girls—their inclusion, representation, rights, social and economic outcomes, equality and protection" first. We suggest such gendered response is possible through gathering gender data, not only mere statistics of women whose lives and livelihoods have been affected by the pandemic but also the qualitative narratives of their very personal, yet political, stories. In what follows, building from this understanding of women's stories and their importance, we (re)present 41 of those stories, of Texan working mothers who have dealt with the unexpected, sudden implications of the 2020 pandemic.

Texan Working Mothers' Lived Realities

> *It came a day that I could not care anymore, my body just quit; but I had no choice, I had to put on my gown, gloves, and mask and go!*
>
> Amanda, mother of three, registered nurse, Austin

Between March 21 and May 5, 2020, using snowball sampling, we reached out to 97 women through our friends circle, colleague network, and Mommy & Me groups. The initial contact was made either by an email or a social media invite. Women were invited to volunteer to participate in our research by completing a multiple-question online survey. The questions were skewed toward women's self-identification questions (e.g., whether they see themselves as either first- or second-generation immigrants), working status before the pandemic (e.g., type of profession, weekly hours, and income ranges), motherhood (e.g., how many kids they have and the ages of them), basic demographic data (e.g., age, education, and the city where they live), and their knowledge of the COVID-19 pandemic (e.g., how serious do you think the global public health crisis is? how has the pandemic affected your work-life balance? how do you find your information about the pandemic?). Of the 47 responses we received from the initial online survey, 42 met our criteria for the informants—working mothers who self-identified themselves as first- or second-generation immigrants.

Of the initially invited women, 41 women took part in an hour-long semi-guided interview via Zoom video platform. In the early stage of our interviewing, one woman had to drop from her participation in the study due to her COVID-19 severe illness. Participants represent a wide range of race, age, geographical locations, occupations, and family arrangements. The informants comprised 11 women in the 25–34 age group, 19 in the 35–44 age group, and 11 in the 45–54 age group. They represent the urban low- to high-income class of Texan women (annual income ranged from $32,000 to $101,000) but had differing access to resources such as childcare, other family income, internet, personal vehicles, and assistance of domestic partners.

In most cases, the initial Zoom interview was followed by a phone-call interview, if necessary. All were carried out between May 12, 2020, and February 2, 2021. Both Zoom and phone interviews were conducted by the first author in English and were recorded, transcribed, and returned for editing. Only edited transcripts are used for quotation. Using a grounded theory method, we have interpreted and coded the interviews, adapting the feminist approach to content analysis. In this approach, women's responses and stories were considered subjective, partial, contextual in regard to their specific characteristics, and open for further questions. We strived to respect the distance and difference between us—the researchers— and, Texan women, our research population. Considering the care ethics of doing research with vulnerable informants, we were actively responsive to "our own location within the circuits of power and privilege that connect our daily lives to those who are constructed as distant from us" (Lawson 2007, p. 7). Such consideration was used during the Zoom interview and while we were interpreting the collected data to determine whether a follow-up phone conversation was needed. We have categorized and analyzed the collected data through a hybrid technique, producing both numerical descriptions and qualitative narratives.

Without exception, all our conversation began with discussing women's knowledge of COVID-19 pandemic. On both the initial survey and the Zoom interview, women were asked to choose/explain to what extent the pandemic has affected their daily life, what kind of negative changes the pandemic and the governmental lockdown measures have brought into their lives, and if they saw these changes as gendered and whether they felt that life under new circumstances was worse for women than for men. We then discussed the following without any certain order: the pandemic implications for women's economic vulnerability and job stability; women's physical health and mental well-being; and women's access to various resources, including medical, reproductive health, and job training and search opportunities. However, women's concerns went beyond these initial categories; they brought up various personal and societal concerns, from ideological questioning of self (e.g., life satisfaction, career goals) to more intimate issues of relationship/marriage or vaccine safety. Building from these insights and using women's quotes (identified by pseudonyms), we engage in thinking through the spatial extensiveness of gendered care work during crises and re-considering the micro- and macro-level analyses of the relationship between "essential workers" and gender on a global scale.

Almost all women (40 out of 41) stated that they believed that they were affected differently than men by the pandemic; in Amanda's words:

> Men are infected worse and more, sure, but who takes care of those men? We do! I take care of my elderly dad who lives with us at home, then I go to work and take care of others' fathers, husbands, and sons ....of course, it makes a difference to be a woman during this pandemic!

Amanda is a mother of a toddler and five-year-old twins. She is a registered nurse, she self-identified herself as a second-generation Venezuelan immigrant. She came to Austin because of her husband's job but found a "rewarding job" at a local hospital. Her mother passed away a few years ago, and since then, her father lives with them. Amanda is among some 800 licensed registered nurse practitioners in

Travis County who had to work over 60 hours per week; she has experienced the early wave of burning out as the pandemic hit Texas back in July 2020 (according to the *New York Times*, some 40% of the American workforce was working from home). While her essential care work is seen as

> act ITALICS? of love … in one hand, nurses and doctor assistants' work is priceless and on the other hand, it doesn't have a monetary value. The incentive is expected to not be higher pay; at least not for female dominate middle-income female-dominant health care workers. That leave (sic) you both valued and devalued at the same time!

The confusion, anxiety, stress, and loneliness Amanda shared were not unique, and they were not always related to profession. National research has shown that during the early months of the pandemic, almost one in three women in the American workforce had school- or daycare-aged children and struggled to balance everything at home with school closures.

> *I am not sure if I will have a job tomorrow or next week. This keeps me awake at night, I feel like a failure as a mother to my kids! You know what if I cannot even provide food for them?*
>
> Rosa, Mother of two, Grocery stocker, El Paso

Rosa's job is categorized as "essential." She expressed, nevertheless, the mixed feelings of being deemed an essential worker and not having any work security and benefits after the pandemic is over. She mostly talks about her motherhood responsibilities; her husband went back to Mexico but was not able to get back to the United States. She is a single mother who not only provides the income for her family of three but also is responsible for her daughter's remote schooling. During the pandemic, it has become even more apparent that the existing school and childcare system do not meet the needs of working mothers. According to the Brooking Institution, in the United States, over 50% of women aged between 18 and 64 work, 25% of those women are mothers with at least one kid at home. Rosa felt "alone" and "frustrated" when she found out about the school closures; she had to teach herself to teach second-grade math in less than a week. Rosa's notion of "failing as a mother" is what many mothers do ponder during the course of raising a child. During crises, and when a mother is dealing with personal mental health problems, including the very real chance of losing her household's sole source of income, she often blames herself.

While our interviewees perceived, experienced, and navigated the extra stress caused by the COVID-19 pandemic—either related to fear of losing job, getting sick, domestic violence at home, or the extra shift at work—we want to recognize that there was a difference among women's dealing with the stress. Women with higher education (and therefore, higher incomes) and a present partner were more inclined to take breaks for themselves, possibly taking a nap or going for a walk. During the course of our conversation with such a diverse group of mothers, it became apparent that recognition of these in-group privileges and limitations was necessary. As Crenshaw (1990, p.1242) reminds us "the problem with identity politics is not that it fails to transcend difference, as some critics charge, but rather the opposite—that it frequently conflates or ignores intragroup differences." We observed the in-group differences in various dimensions of women's lives. For example, Connie (mother of three and a middle school teacher) and Shirin (mother of two, dish washer, and immigrant to Laredo from Honduras) expressed their anger, frustration, and disappointment respectfully:

> *I do not know what they mean by "we are in this together?" They simply cannot be serious. I cook, cleans (sic), washes (sic) the sheets, make sure my kids sign up on the computer and work. My husband still work (sic) from 9-5, like not much has changed. We are not in this together!*
>
> *I came to this country to have my independence and give a better future to my kids; right now, I am unable to do either, I was fired from the restaurant I worked at, trying to complete job applications online while helping my kids with their online classes. This seems impossible.*

The pandemic did not affect us all equally. All pre-existing inequalities have been made worse by COVID-19. Some, like Connie, had to learn to discuss gender equality issues with their partners and ask them to accept more responsibilities around the house. Connie and I re-connected after several weeks, she reported she was still striving to change their gendered roles at home, while educating her students about a shift in gender division of labor at society (Glynn, 2018, Madgavkar et al. 2020). Unfortunately, for Shirin, life proved to be more difficult; her husband lost income due to being infected by the virus, and it turned out to be literally impossible for her to find an online job while home schooling her kids. She is currently working in an informal, underpaid setting, making handmade, traditional Honduras dolls for a boutique store in New York City.

Unlike Connie and Shirin, Mariam, a software engineer at a high-profile company in Austin who gave birth to her baby while the pandemic was unfolding in Texas, expressed gratitude for her extra time at home: not all care work is dreadful; "certainly raising my baby and playing with my twins is joyful." Mariam admitted, however, that she might be enjoying motherhood as she decided to quit her job and left the work-related stress to her husband.

> *This is not a voluntary leave of absence. My husband and I had a very difficult decision to make, since we both have been career-oriented. I feel I moved years back when women were still expected to stay home and raise children, but with our twins are at home 24/7, and now we have a new baby! We just cannot manage it all. I cannot do it all! So I was the one who had to sacrifice.*

Mariam acknowledged her privilege: having an access to multiple available choices. She self-identified herself as a second-generation immigrant from Iran; her parents left Iran in the late 1980s and she was born here, in Dallas. Because of the need for more software engineers in Texas due to the recent technological move from California to the state, Mariam felt safe leaving her job and picking it up again after a year or two. Not all women had "the privilege" of picking their jobs after the pandemic.

> It felt like a slap in our faces—the day care manager told us we had to either quit and collect unemployment or work extra shifts to meet the new increased need of childcare by parents and the social-distancing requirements by the state. It felt like I was given no choice at all.

Nonetheless, Ameneh, a young mother and a recent refugee from Syria, could not apply for any state or federal unemployment benefits as she was still awaiting her legal residency paperwork and, perhaps, would be denied the full benefits of citizenship. She and her husband both worked full-time before the pandemic, but her husband lost his job at a nearby restaurant. In the middle of the pandemic, when the daycare centers were "safe" to re-open, she worked over 60 hours, sometimes skipping the weekend, to make up her family's lost income from the center's temporary closure. The daycare center extended its one shift from 7:00 a.m. to 5:00 p.m. to three shorter shifts, running from 6:30 a.m. to 7:30 p.m. to offer all its clients (other mothers) a time without their kids, while following the state-regulated numbers of kids per class. Some women worked part time or had a family member on whom they could rely to provide supervision for their young and school-aged children. But the majority relied on childcare and schools to keep their children safe while they worked. After the sudden mass closure of daycare centers, schools, and afterschool programs across the country, working mothers found themselves at the center of care giving (Savat and Collins, 2020, Zamarro, 2020). An early study on gender differences of the pandemic impacts found that women reported being the only one in the household providing childcare almost three times as often as men reported that. As an essential worker at one of the few open daycare centers in El Paso, Ameneh is sure of one thing:

> I am exhausted, physically, I come home and fall asleep; my only reward now is to think of the days that we have been vaccinated and I can stay home on weekend and play with my own kids too! Then we all have choices.

Even higher-educated women who did not work in the service industry were challenged with their career and family planning choices.

> I finally got a job in academia—after five years of being on contract and moving my kids from one city to another. With my kids and no help at home, I cannot focus, read, nor write, but I also cannot afford losing a tenure-track job!

Tina, a 39-year-old assistant professor, shared her hesitation to start a family with her long-term partner. She felt she was fighting against two clocks, professional and biological. According to a recent study done by the *Chronicle of the Higher Education*, mother professors have lost, on average, about an hour of research time per day— that is, in addition to what childless scholars have lost due to the pandemic's social and economic impacts. Tina is among those women who were disproportionally more affected than her husband was—who is also a professor—competing demands from her students, parenting, homeschooling, and other caring duties. One university went so far (Burke 2020), trying to forbid faculties from parenting while working at home. Tina's response was:

> *the rules are often written by male administration who are way above regular professor's tax bracket!*

We listened to several other women who, unlike Tina, did not even have the choice to quit their paid jobs. According to the Brookings Institution, most mothers were either breadwinners earning the majority of their family's income or co-breadwinners earning less than half but at least one-quarter of their families' income. Paulina's situation is one among several Black mothers and heads of the household who could not simply quit and care for their kids. These rates are even higher for non-White mothers. Paulina is a single mother of two high school kids; they live in a 700-square foot apartment in East Austin. She reluctantly confessed:

> *There are days I wished my sons were gone—gone to college, or camping, or I could quit my job but I am the only income source for my home, I want my boys to focus on their school—I am a janitor, it is hard physical work, and now people expect even more, you have to sanitize everything … I keep look forward to that quiet rest day at home!*

In our follow-up conversation, Tina discussed how both she and her husband were challenged by the sudden digital neoliberalization of academia, the sudden move to "online learning," where only her husband—and not herself—was able to attend an online workshop on converting his courses to online modality. "*For now, I think we will focus on the tenure clock*," Tina expressed in tears, "*I worked so hard for so many years; we … I may have to let go of having kids.*"

As several interviewees mentioned, specific services such as childcare (or lack thereof) played an important role in the gender-equality gap in the labor force. According to a survey of some 2,500 working parents conducted by Northeastern University from May 10 to June 22, 2020, almost 15% of American parents had to quit a job or reduce their working hours due to a lack of childcare (Modestino, 2020). As *The Washington Post* suggests, "the pandemic may set women back by a whole generation;" more women are pushed to leave their paid work, and building inclusive and balanced economies and societies face more barriers.

We would like to end this section with Lucy's story. Lucy is a mother of two, her first child is disabled; she used to care for him for years while working as a counselor at a nursing home in Houston. Not only from her own lived experiences but also from her own work with elderly dealing with anxiety, memory loss, and isolation, Lucy is familiar with a sense of precarity. But she was "caught off guard" by the pandemic and its complex implications for her personal and professional lives.

> *I am not sure who cares for me? I know I care for my kids, my husband, my patient at the work, I care for my family, neighbors, colleagues, and my friends. I have to use the mask they have given me several times before they give me a new one, I have to stay in a room, separated from my family to avoid infecting them, I have to wash and sanitize my already cracked, dried hands several times a day .... yes, I am not sure who cares for me?*

"Care as a political concept requires that we recognize how care—especially the question, who cares for whom?—marks relations of power in our society and marks the intersections of gender, race, and class with care-giving" (Tronto, 1993, pp. 168–169). In this sense and for Lucy, care becomes an expansive category, crossing the several boundaries between the economic and the noneconomic, the public and the private, the valued and the undervalued, and the personal and the political. The intersectional and intergenerational vulnerabilities experienced during the COVID-19 pandemic by these Texan working mothers generate a messy, contested, and yet fluid network of inter-relations, which affect various axis of difference including sex, gender, age, race, class, education, disability, marital status, income, and motherhood. Lucy re-connected with us after a few months when the infection rate in Texas started to decline, bringing a feeling of hope to her life, personal and professional alike.

Epilogue

The results highlight—despite the wide execution of work-from-home and tele-commuting flexibility policies and governmental assistance funds and programs—the disproportional emotional, mental, social, and professional challenges for working mothers. We argue how the lack of gender lens puts women, especially minority women who in this study are already vulnerable, at more risk. While the long-term consequences of these global, complex health and economic crises are yet to be explored, we contend that it is only through a gendered lens and deep examination of the pandemic's disproportional effects on women's lives that we can understand the changes, policies, and programs required to cultivate more just and inclusive communities. Among these considerations are understanding the power by gathering disaggregated, intersectional data; recognizing the essentiality of care work by supporting funding and training for early learning and childcare; and finally by ensuring women and minorities' voices and stories are heard during post-pandemic decision-making and planning.

Notes

1 The first author is a first generation immigrant to the U.S., feminist professor, and mother; the second author is a graduate student in Geography & Environmental Sustainability, is born and raised in United States, and he aims to engage in feminist participatory and community research.
2 The exception is that the rates of infection and death among women have been less; however, the limited studies reported that the COVID-19 vaccine side effects are more severe for women, perhaps due to their stronger immune response.

Acknowledgments: We are indebted to several people who have pushed this project along. First, we wish to thank the women who generously participated in this study. Nazgol wishes to thank her friend and mentor, Dr. Steven L. Driever, for his beneficial comments. We thank Steve and Darya Cochrane as well as Theresa and Barry Yates for their continuous love and support, especially during the early hard months of the pandemic. Special thanks go to Dr. James Vaughan for his resilience for life, and against the coronavirus itself, and the inspiration he seeded in our hearts.

References

Alon, T., Doepke, M., Olmstead-Rumsey, J., & Tertilt, M. (2020). The Impact of COVID-19 on Gender Equality. NBER.

Bateman, N., & Ross, M. (2021, April 5). Why Has COVID-19 Been Especially Harmful for Working Women? Retrieved from www.brookings.edu/essay/why-has-covid-19-been-especially-harmful-for-working-women/

Bernstein, A. (2020). COVID-19 Dealt a Blow to Working Women. Can We Emerge Stronger? Retrieved from www.nytimes.com/2020/12/07/opinion/covid-women-work-careers.html

Brennan, D. (2004). Women Work, Men Sponge, and Everyone Gossips: Macho Men and Stigmatized/ing Women in a Sex Tourist Town. *Anthropological Quarterly, 77*(4), 705–733.

Brown, M. (2003). Hospice and the Spatial Paradoxes of Terminal Care. *Environment and Planning A: Economy and Space, 35*(5), 833–851.

Burke, L. (2020). Florida State BARS Parenting During Remote Work. Retrieved from www.insidehighered.com/quicktakes/2020/06/30/florida-state-bars-parenting-during-remote-work

Collins, Landivar, L. C., Ruppanner, L., & Scarborough, W. J. (2021). COVID-19 and the gender gap in work hours. Gender, Work, and Organization, 28(S1), 101–112. https://doi.org/10.1111/gwao.12506

Crenshaw, K. (1990). Mapping the Margins: Intersectionality, Identity Politics, and Violence against Women of Color. *Stanford Law Review, 43*(6), 1241–1299.

De Silva, M. (2018). Making the Emotional Connection: Transnational Eldercare Circulation within Sri Lankan-Australian Transnational Families. *Gender, Place & Culture, 25*(1), 88–103.

Domosh, M., & Seager, J. (2001). Putting Women in Place: Feminist Geographers Make Sense of the World. New York: Guilford Press.

England, K. (2005). *Who Will Mind the Baby? Geographies of Childcare and Working Mothers.* New York: Routledge.

Glenn, E. N. (2012). *Forced to Care: Coercion and Caregiving in America*. Cambridge: Harvard University Press.

Glynn, S. J. (2018). An Unequal Division of Labor. Retrieved from www.americanprogress. org/issues/women/reports/2018/05/18/450972/unequal-division-labor/

Gregson, N., & Lowe, M. (1993). Renegotiating the Domestic Division of Labor? A Study of Dual Career Households in North East and South East England. Retrieved from https:// journals.sagepub.com/doi/10.1111/j.1467-954X.1993.tb00074.x

International Council of Nurses (ICN). (2020). ICN COVID-19 Update: Occupational Risks to Nurses Must Be Minimized to Enable Them to Continue Their Vital Work. Retrieved from www.icn.ch/news/icn-covid-19-update-occupational-risks-nurses-must-be-minimised-enable-them-continue-their

Lawson, V. (2007). Geographies of Care and Responsibility. *Annals of the Association of American Geographers, 97*(1), 1–1.

Madgavkar, A., White, O., Krishnan, M., Mahajan, D., & Azcue, X. (2020). COVID-19 and Gender Equality: Countering the Regressive Effects. Retrieved from www. mckinsey.com/featured-insights/future-of-work/covid-19-and-gender-equality-countering-the-regressive-effects

McDowell, L. (2016). Reflections on Feminist Economic Geography: Talking to Ourselves? *Environment and Planning A: Economy and Space, 48*(10), 2093–2099.

Modestino, A. S. (2020). Coronavirus child-care crisis will set women back a generation. Washington Post. Retrieved from https://www.washingtonpost.com/us-policy/2020/07/29/childcare-remote-learning-women-employment/

Mullings, B. (2005). Women Rule? Globalization and the Feminization of Managerial and Professional Workspaces in the Caribbean. *Gender, Place & Culture, 12*(1), 1–27.

Najmabadi, S. (2020). Texas' Front-Line Workers in the Pandemic Are Predominantly Women and People of Color, Analysis Finds. Retrieved from www.texastribune.org/2020/05/01/texas-coronavirus-frontline-workers/

Petersen, A. (2020). "Other Countries Have Social Safety Nets. The U.S. Has Women." Retrieved from https://annehelen.substack.com/p/other-countries-have-social-safety

Pettit, E. (2021). Covid-19 Has Robbed Faculty Parents of Time for Research. Especially Mothers. Retrieved from www.chronicle.com/article/covid-19-has-robbed-faculty-parents-of-time-for-research-especially-mothers?utm_source=Iterable&utm_medium=email&utm_campaign=campaign_1936274_nl_Academe-Today_date_20210126&cid=at&source=ams&sourceId=5077842

Pratt, G. (1999). From Registered Nurse to Registered Nanny: Discursive Geographies of Filipina Domestic Workers in Vancouver, B.C. *Economic Geography, 75*(3), 215–236.

Robertson, C., & Gebeloff, R. (2020). How Millions of Women Became the Most Essential Workers in America. Retrieved from www.nytimes.com/2020/04/18/us/coronavirus-women-essential-workers.html

SAExpress-News Editorial Board. (2020). Editorial: In Pandemic, Women Take the Hardest Hit. Retrieved from www.expressnews.com/opinion/editorials/article/Editorial-In-pandemic-women-take-the-hardest-hit-15676271.php

Savat, S., & Collins, C. (2020). Mothers' Paid Work Suffers During Pandemic, Study Finds. Washington University in St. Louis. Retrieved from https://source.wustl.edu/2020/07/mothers-paid-work-suffers-during-pandemic-study-finds/

Texas Workforce Commission's Labor Market & Career Information (2020). Texas Workforce Report 2019 to 2020, https://lmci.state.tx.us/shared/PDFs/Workforce_Report.pdf.

Tronto, J. (1993). Moral Boundaries. A Political Argument for an Ethic of Care. New York and London: Routledge.

United Nations. (2020a). Put Women and Girls at Center of COVID-19 Recovery: UN Secretary-General. *UN News*. Retrieved from https://news.un.org/en/story/2020/04/1061452

United Nations. (2020b). Policy Brief: The Impact of COVID-19 on Women. Retrieved from www.un.org/sexualviolenceinconflict/wp-content/uploads/2020/06/report/policy-brief-the-impact-of-covid-19-on-women/policy-brief-the-impact-of-covid-19-on-women-en-1.pdf

Williams, A. (2002). Changing Geographies of Care: Employing the Concept of Therapeutic Landscapes as a Framework in Examining Home Space. *Social Science & Medicine, 55*(1), 141–154.

Zamarro, G. (2020). Gender Differences in the Economic and Social Impact of the COVID-19 Pandemic. Retrieved from www.wiareport.com/2020/07/gender-differences-in-the-economic-and-social-impact-of-the-covid-19-pandemic/

10

ESSENTIAL, CONTINGENT, INFORMAL, AND INFECTED

Work and Ethnicity During COVID-19[1]

Amy Schoenecker and Elizabeth Alejo

Introduction

As COVID-19 spread throughout the United States in early 2020, a startling trend emerged: the virus was disproportionately affecting non-White communities. The Centers for Disease Control and Prevention (CDC) (2020b) indicated that cases, hospitalizations, and death rates were higher for communities of color. For example, in June 2020, 33.8% of COVID-19 cases were found in the Latinx community, while they represent only 18% of the population (Tai et al., 2020).[2] Why were communities of color being overly exposed to the virus?

Several media outlets responded to this question by explaining that Black and Latinx workers were excessively represented in industries, like meatpacking, which were COVID-19 hotspots. By early December 2020, there were over 44,500 cases and at least 232 worker deaths in meatpacking plants (Chadde & Ag, 2020). Other explanations were a lack of healthcare (CDC, 2020a; Clark et al., 2020; Tai et al., 2020), and that Black and Latinx people worked in "essential" jobs, jobs deemed necessary to the economy, which cannot be done from home (CDC, 2020a; Thorbecke, 2020). Despite truth to these explanations, they are incomplete answers.

This chapter addresses why Latinx communities were more susceptible to COVID-19 by focusing on one neighborhood in Chicago. Early on, Little Village, a Mexican American immigrant neighborhood, became the epicenter of disease spread in the city (Hickey, 2020; Zamudio, 2020). By May 2020, the zip code associated with Little Village had the most confirmed cases of any zip code in the state (Hickey, 2020). By December 2020, the zip code was no longer number one, but still had a stunning 8,714 cases (Illinois Department of Public Health, 2020) out of 85,979 residents (City of Chicago, 2020a). We argue that Little Village residents overwhelmingly work in "essential," informal,[3] and contingent employment, which helps explain their overrepresentation in COVID contraction. Each type of work is

DOI: 10.4324/9781003268710-10

low-paying, flexible, and often without benefits like healthcare and sick leave. The segmented labor force in the United States means that Black and Latinx workers are overrepresented in such positions. This segmentation, coupled with the labor trends of flexibilization, informalization, and contingency of labor, is critical to understanding why certain communities were overly exposed to COVID-19. Moreover, essential, contingent, and informal work interact and overlap with one another in ways that heightened the risk for Little Village residents. Finally, we reconceptualize the term "essential" beyond the market-oriented definition that casts certain jobs as vital to the economy. We propose a worker-oriented perspective, finding that essential means vital for workers' livelihood.

We begin by describing the data used, followed by a discussion of the Latinx population in Chicago. Next, we detail low-wage work done in the United States. After this, we present findings on how Latinx and especially Little Village residents are concentrated as essential, contingent, and informal workers. We end the chapter by comparing Little Village with another neighborhood, highlighting the interplay of the three work categories and discussing the potential paths forward.

The Spatiality of Labor

The context of a hyper-segregated city like Chicago means that White, Black, and Latinx populations[4] reside in separate parts of the city, not readily captured by the city's administrative (ward) boundaries. Thus, we utilize data from myriad levels, including ward, community area, and county, among others. Data that put Little Village as the hardest hit neighborhood rely on zip code. However, the zip code associated with these figures is 60623, encompassing multiple wards (22nd, 24th, and 12th), racial and ethnic groups (Black residents live North in the zip code, Latinx residents South), neighborhoods (Lawndale and Little Village), and community areas (North and South Lawndale). Therefore, associating 60623 with *only* Little Village may be misleading (see Figure 10.1). Given the segregation patterns of Chicago, and the limited scope of this project, we focus on the Latinx population mostly residing in the Little Village neighborhood, rather than the 60623 zip code.

Little Village is not a neighborhood with specified boundaries on which data are easily available. However, Chicago formally recognizes community areas, releasing demographic data on them. Thus, we primarily use data on the community area of South Lawndale, which has virtually identical boundaries with Little Village. The terms/names will be used interchangeably. South Lawndale is comprised of much of the 22nd and 12th wards.

To understand the work patterns of Little Village residents, we matched U.S. census tracts to the boundaries of South Lawndale and gathered industry data for these tracts.[5] We compared these industries with the executive order by Illinois Governor J. B. Pritzker regarding essential work during the March 2020 shutdown. While a precise match is impossible, the data give a good indication of which industries Little Village residents do and do not work in. Additionally, we map known hotspots and essential industries in and immediately surrounding the

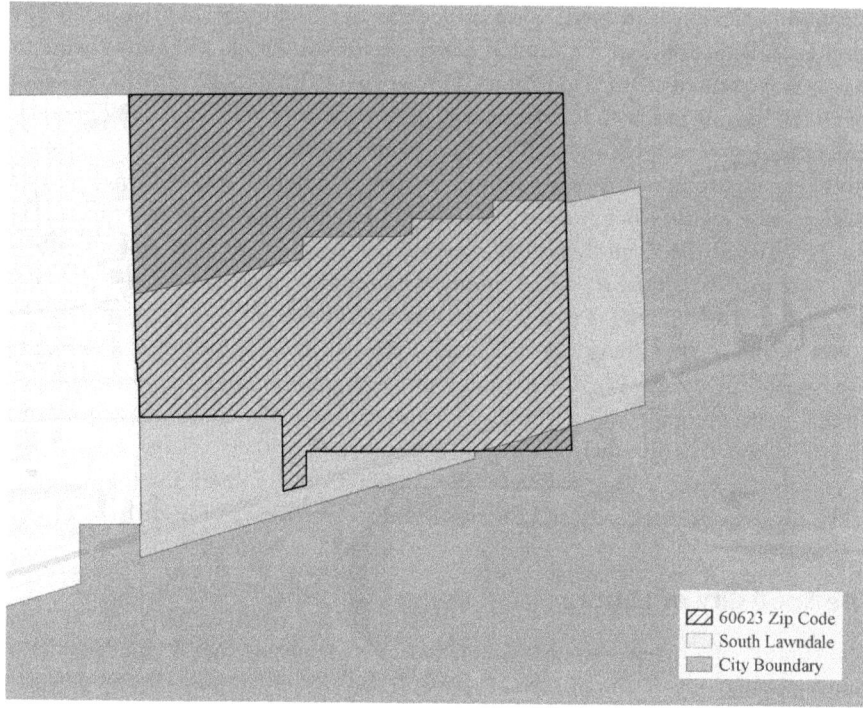

FIGURE 10.1 Zip Code and Community Area Overlay

neighborhood. For the contingent workforce, we examine the temp industry in Chicago and Cook County and provide estimates of the contingent workforce using recent surveys by Chicago Workers' Collaborative and Temp Workers Justice. We also created a map of temp agencies using data from the Illinois Department of Labor, the city of Chicago, and Google Maps.

Finally, to showcase the spatiality of the visible informal economy, we employ original spatial data collected in the spring/summer of 2019 on street vending in Little Village. We canvassed the neighborhood for early morning and afternoon vendors, seven days a week to distinguish vendors who sell daily, or on the weekend, from those who vend only sporadically.[6] We found 280 street vendors and 15 itinerant vendors in and around Little Village. In addition, we found 35 daily rummage sales, and pop-up food stands. Data points with at least two observations were mapped and are presented as a heat map to protect exact vending locations.

Placing the Latinx Population

Historically, Latinx migration into the United States has been tied to labor demands (DeGenova, 1998; Tienda & Sanchez, 2013). Through the early 20th century Mexican laborers were recruited by agricultural and later manufacturing industries

TABLE 10.1 Select Demographic Data

Community Area	Per Capita Income	% Latinx	% of Households Below Poverty[1]	Population	% Without Health Insurance
South Lawndale	$10,402[a]	86.6%[b]	30.7%[a]	72,157[b]	29.2%[d]
Chicago	$28,202[a]	28.8%[c]	19.7%[a]	2,695,652[c]	9.8%[d]

Sources: a. City of Chicago, 2014; b. U.S. Census Bureau, 2019a; c. U.S. Census Bureau, 2019b; d. Chicago Health Atlas, 2019.

Note: This table gives select demographic data comparing residents of South Lawndale with residents of Chicago, demonstrating that South Lawndale residents are poorer, have a greater percentage of their population without health insurance, and have higher concentration of Latinx residents than Chicago residents overall.

(Reisler, 1976). The Bracero Program (1942–1964) recognized immigrants as a key source to satisfy labor shortages and demands for inexpensive labor. Promoting short-term labor contracts, the Program was neither a visa nor a path to citizenship. Though many early Latinx migrants entering the United States went to the Southwest, many followed railway jobs to Midwestern cities like Chicago (Arredondo, 2008; Delgadillo & Weaver, 2017; Reisler, 1976).

Early Mexican immigrants to Chicago settled near the city's steel plants, meatpacking industry, and railway yards. By 1945, they had mostly settled into the Near West Side, Back of the Yards, and South Chicago neighborhoods (Betancur, 1996; Nuevo-Kerr, 1984). Eventually, urban renewal pushed them south into Little Village. Today, Little Village is 86.6% Latinx (Table 10.1) and 80% Mexican origin (U.S. Census Bureau, 2019a). Sometimes referred to as "Mexico of the Midwest" (Gamboa & Armas, 2017; Keating, 2004), the heart of Little Village is 26th street, only second in income revenue to the city's downtown shopping district, the Magnificent Mile (Yi, 2019). Despite this, Little Village residents are largely poor. According to City of Chicago data (2008–2012), South Lawndale's per capita income is $10,402, and 30.7% of households live below poverty (Table 10.1). Additionally, South Lawndale shows the highest percentage of people among the city's 77 community areas without health insurance: 29.2% (Chicago Health Atlas, 2019).

Understanding Low Wage Work in the United States

To understand why Latinx communities saw high COVID case counts, we analyze the labor of Little Village residents as essential, contingent, and informal. With literature on essential work limited to times of war and other pandemics, we focus here on the latter two types of work: contingent and informal. Additionally, we discuss the segmentation of communities of color in low-wage jobs.

Contingent, temporary, or nonstandard work, is often described in distinction to what it is not: full-time, fixed-schedule, single-employer (Hatton, 2011). In their conceptualization of nonstandard work, Kalleberg et al. (2000) include part-time employment, day labor, on-call, temp work, contract, and self-employment. Here, we focus on one type of contingent work—temp agencies. Hatton (2011) identifies temp agencies by their "triangular employment relationship" (p. 11), where they serve as a legal employer, contracting out their workers. This complicates the employer-employee relationship, impeding the ability to form unions and demand better wages and working conditions (Wills, 2009). By the early 20th century, temp agencies were working with 90% of employers, altering the work landscape by contributing to a general downward pressure on wages and decreased employment security (Hatton, 2011). Temp work in the form of the archetypal Kelly girl was initially confined to clerical work (Hatton, 2011), but many manufacturing companies in the United States rely on temp agencies to keep domestic labor costs low (Peck & Theodore, 2001).

Like contingent work, informal workers often have a vulnerable work status. The term "informal economy" was coined in the 1970s by Keith Hart (1973). Domestic work, home-based work, street vending, and waste picking are some of the oldest and largest informal industries (International Labour Organization, 2013). Informal and contingent work have many similarities, including lack of sick and vacation time, ambiguous employer-employee relationship, and a flexible work status. Informal work was initially discussed in the context of developing countries; however, subsequent research has shown it to be of continued importance in developed countries (see Koch, 2015; Leonard, 1998; Portes et al., 1989; Portes & Sassen-Koob, 1987). Labor relationships in the informal economy vary. Some are entrepreneurs, some contract their labor out, while others have informal wage employment, including domestic or industrial outwork (Chen, 2012). The line between contingent and informal work is blurry. For example, day laborers can be considered both contingent and informal.

Communities of color are overwhelmingly represented in low-paying jobs. Kalleberg et al. (2000) demonstrate that White men are the least likely to have bad jobs compared to women and men of color. Echoing the findings of Glenn (1992), Duffy (2007) points out that women of color have always been the ones doing the "dirty work" of reproductive labor, like cooking and cleaning, but increasingly Hispanic men are as well. Luthra and Waldinger (2010) find that recently arrived Mexican migrants cluster in nonstandard employment at rates higher than White workers. Additionally, second- and third-generation Mexican Americans often take jobs that are standard, but not sufficient, lacking healthcare and retirement benefits (Luthra & Waldinger, 2010).

What accounts for the lumping of communities of color into the lowest and worst-paid positions? Kirschenman and Neckerman (1991) found that employers often used racial and ethnic characterizations when making hiring decisions. Changhwan and Tamborini (2006) argue that race is not a significant factor in hiring for technique-based positions but is a factor when hiring for social-skills-oriented work. Ndobo et al. (2018) compare native-born with immigrant applicants, finding the former were preferred for more prestigious positions, while the latter tended to be chosen for lower-skilled positions. Finally, citizenship matters. Bauder (2008) describes citizenship status as "a strategically produced form of capital" (p. 315). Without it, migrant workers are more vulnerable, often channeled into the secondary labor market or informal economy.

The above paragraphs demonstrate that many vulnerabilities are associated with contingent and informal work and discuss how and why communities of color are overrepresented in low-paying positions. Next, we present findings on the labor characteristics of Little Village as essential, contingent, and informal.

Essential, Contingent, Informal, and Infected

Essential Workers

In this section, we discuss essential work in Little Village in two ways. First, we use census industry data to show that many Little Village residents work in industries likely considered essential by Illinois Governor Pritzker's initial executive order. We also highlight recent surveys by the U.S. Bureau of Labor Statistics (BLS) to determine the possibility of certain employees being able to work from home. Second, we employ spatial data on known COVID hotspots and essential industries surrounding Little Village to suggest that the proximity to these industries and hotspots may have played a role in exposure to the disease.

On March 21, 2020, Illinois Governor Pritzker issued an executive order directing everyone but essential workers to stay home. The order outlined which businesses could remain open, including grocery stores, food and beverage manufacturing and production, and manufacturing and supply chains providing critical goods, among others (Pritzker, 2020).

Census data provide insight into the types of jobs Little Village residents fill. While it is impossible to determine the exact numbers of people who worked outside the home during the pandemic, we roughly match the industries that residents work in with the industries kept open during the early stages of the pandemic and according to Pritzker's executive order. A total of 25,414 Little Village residents are formally employed (U.S. Census Bureau, 2019c). Figure 10.2 shows the largest concentration of Little Village residents are in manufacturing (21% or 5,375 people).[7] Governor Pritzker's executive order allowed food and beverage manufacturing and manufacturing of items related to supply chains to remain open. Next, coming in between 10% and 13% of workers are Arts and Entertainment (13%, 3,299 people), Education and Health (11.7%, 2,972 people), Professional (13.7%, 3,484 people), and Retail Trade (10.5%, 2,675 people). Just under 10% (or 2,388) of residents work in construction.

A further breakdown of these industries shows that Little Village residents are clustered in the lowest-paid categories, in line with the discussion of low-wage labor above (see Figures 10.3–10.5). For example, in the Professional, Scientific, Management, and Administrative and Waste Management Services category (Figure 10.3), 663 of the 3,484 (19%) of those employed in this category worked in

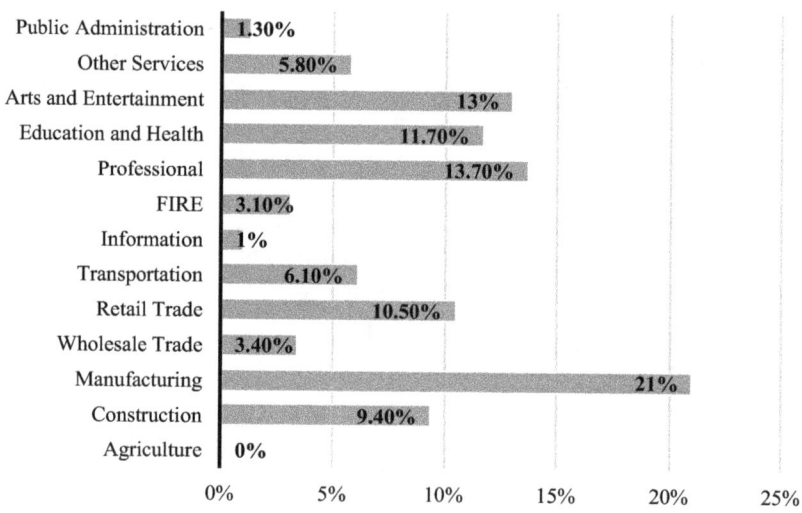

FIGURE 10.2 Percent of Little Village Workers by Industry

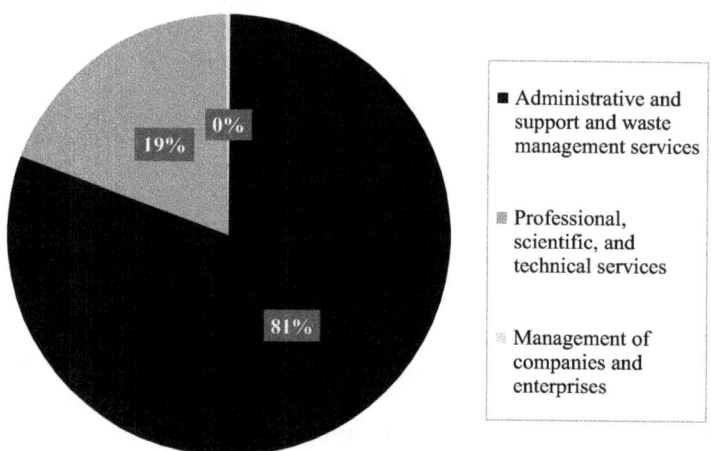

FIGURE 10.3 Professional, Scientific, Management, and Administrative and Waste Management

professional, scientific, and technical services, while only 11 (>1%) worked in the management of companies and enterprises. Most in this category (2,810 people, or 81%) are employed as administrative and support staff for waste management services. Governor Pritzker's executive order classified solid waste and recycling collection as essential infrastructure to remain open.

Figure 10.4 breaks down the Education and Health industry into two categories, showing that 62% of residents (1,832 people) in this industry were working in healthcare and social assistance; healthcare and public health operations were

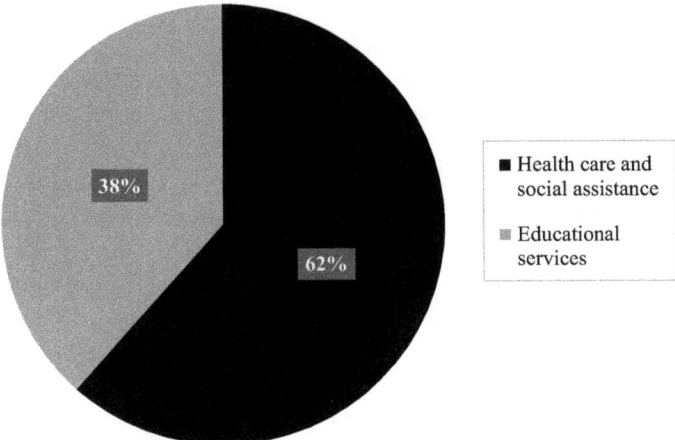

FIGURE 10.4 Educational Services, and Healthcare and Social Assistance

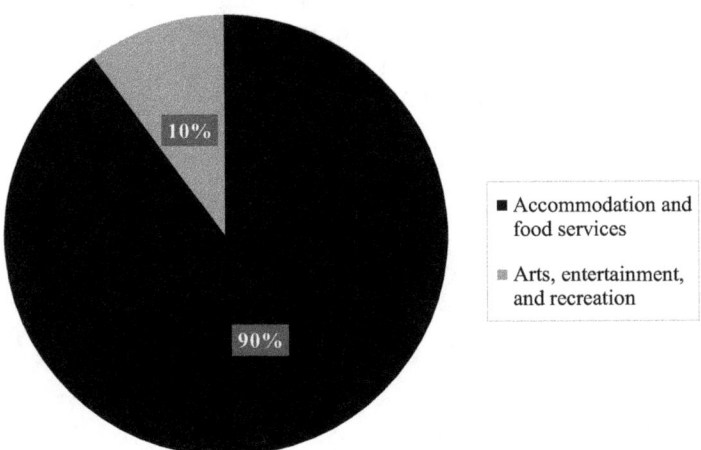

FIGURE 10.5 Arts, Entertainment, and Recreation, and Accommodation and Food Services

also ordered open by the executive order. Figure 10.5 shows that in the Arts and Entertainment industry, 90% or 2,967 of the 3,299 employed in this industry were in accommodation and food services. Many of these businesses remained partially open during the initial stages and are covered under the 12th category in the executive order. Again, these figures cannot tell us who were working from home or not, but they capture the extent to which Little Village workers are clustered into industries considered "essential." Additionally, the data show the segmentation of Little Village workers into the likeliest lowest-paying positions in each industry.

Also telling is the industries that Little Village residents are *not* working in, including the information or FIRE industries (finance, insurance, and real estate) (see Figure 10.2). Their numbers represent 1% and 3.1% of formal sector workers in Little Village, respectively. Professional services are mentioned in the executive order, but many of these jobs can be done from home. For example, a recent BLS survey indicates 81% of those in the financial activities industry and 80% in information industries reported being able to work from home during the pandemic (Dey et al., 2020). This is compared with only 41% in manufacturing, 21% in construction, and 20% in leisure and hospitality (Dey et al., 2020), many of the industries Little Village residents work in. Disaggregating by race and ethnicity, the report also estimates who can/cannot work from home. Using data from two previous surveys (the American Time Use Survey, or ATUS, and the National Longitudinal Survey of Youth, 1979, or NLSY79), the report shows distinct differences in telecommuting. According to the ATUS survey, Hispanic workers show some of the lowest levels of being able to work from home at 29%, compared with 39.5% of Black and 49% of White workers. The NLSY79 survey shows that 39% of Hispanic workers can telework, while 47% of White workers can (Dey et al., 2020).[8] Combining the industry and race/ethnic makeup of who can and cannot telecommute, it is likely that many Little Village residents were working in-person during Chicago's initial shutdown. We turn next to known hotspots and essential industries around Little Village.

As early as March 2020, the Cook County Department of Corrections (see Figure 10.6) noted positive COVID cases, reaching 350 inmates and staff within two weeks (Williams & Ivory, 2020). It quickly became the largest hotspot in the United States. According to tracking by the New York Times (2020), the top 41

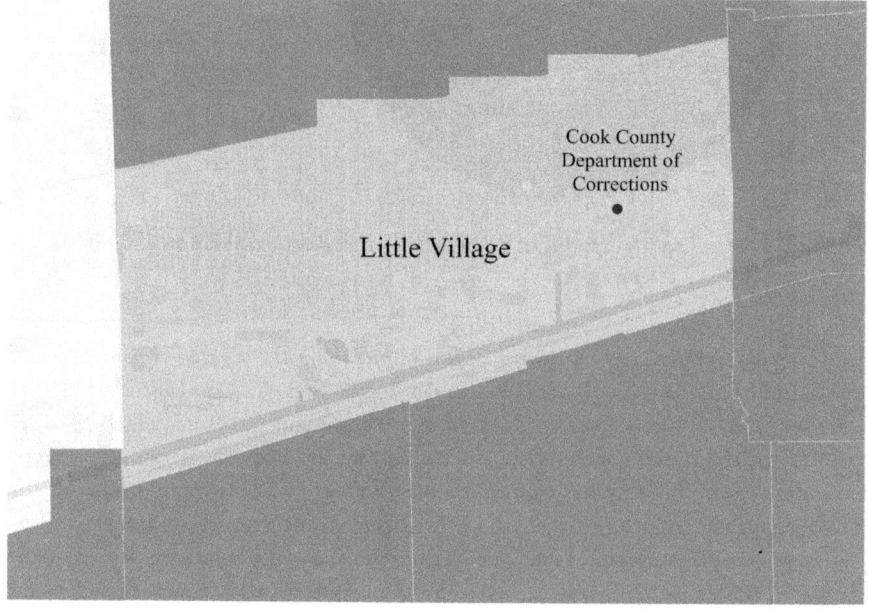

FIGURE 10.6 Cook County Department of Corrections

places for outbreaks in Illinois were prisons, correctional, and juvenile centers. Cook County Department of Corrections led the way with 2,106 cases (New York Times, 2020).

A contentious industry that remained open early on was meatpacking. The number of COVID cases in these plants soared as then-President Trump signed an executive order mandating they stay open with only a good faith effort needed in following safety protocols (Grabell et al., 2020). In Illinois, there were at least 1,029 cases tied to 26 plants, including 21 cases from Rose Packing on Chicago's South West side (~3 miles south west of Little Village). Figure 10.7 indicates the meatpacking and food plants (including produce wholesalers) in and around Little Village. Each dot represents a distinct site; a total of 45 sites were found. In addition to food production and distribution plants and the Cook County Department of Corrections, Little Village is uniquely surrounded by additional essential industries, including transportation, distribution, and logistics (Figure 10.8), and construction and other "essential" services like waste management, recycling, and utility companies (Figure 10.9).[9]

Given the industries Little Village residents worked in, the industries kept open during the pandemic, and the high concentration of "essential" industries (some of which were known COVID hotspots) in and surrounding Little Village, it is not surprising that cases soared here early in the pandemic. Next, we explore contingency in Chicago.

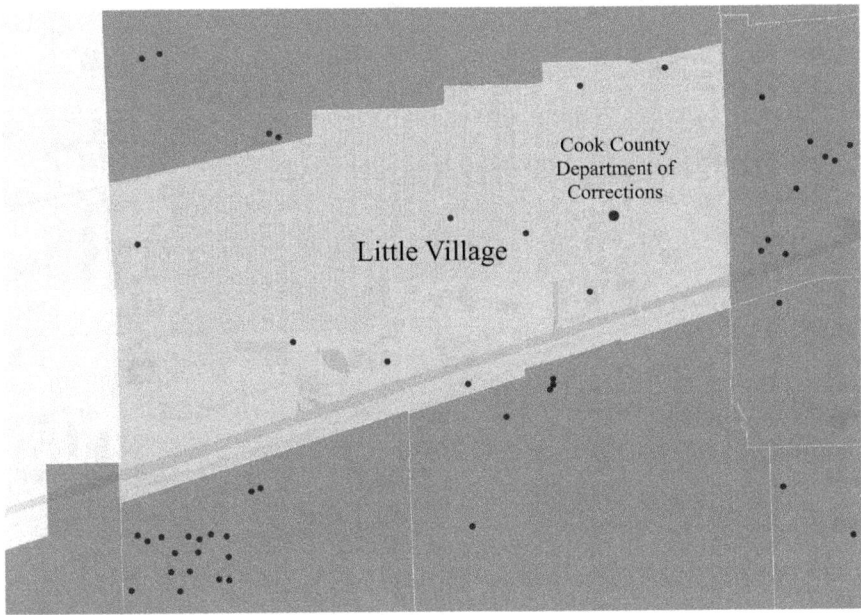

FIGURE 10.7 Meatpacking and Food Production

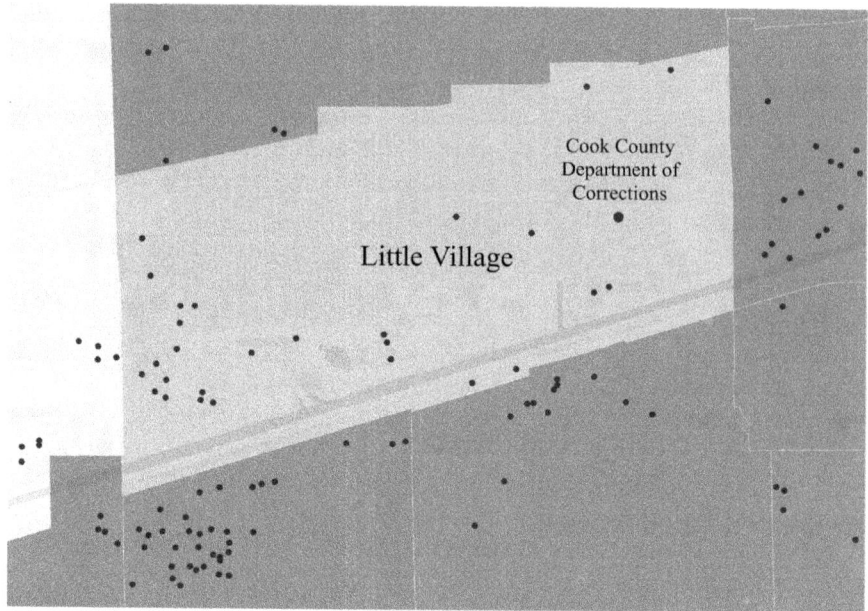

FIGURE 10.8 Transportation and Logistics

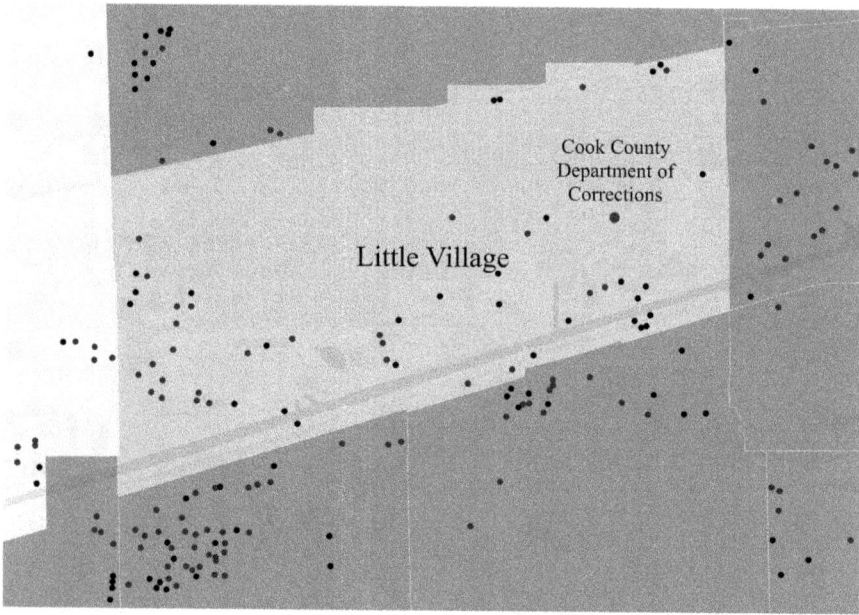

FIGURE 10.9 Essential Construction and Services

Contingent Workers

Contingent workers are distributed across sectors, tend to earn less than their non-contingent counterparts, and are less likely to have health insurance (BLS, 2018). The latter point is echoed in a report by Temp Workers Justice and the Chicago Workers' Collaborative who surveyed temp workers in Illinois during the pandemic: three out of every four temp workers reported not having health insurance (Hernandez, 2020). They also found that around 80% of respondents were unable to get paid sick leave. Respondents said they were unable to follow social distancing guidelines while working and were not provided necessary personal protective equipment (Hernandez, 2020). Some noted having to bring their own toilet paper, soap, goggles, disinfectants, and hand sanitizer to work, even facing retaliation for doing so (Hernandez, 2020).

In 2019, ProPublica audited temp agencies in Illinois, finding about 42% of temp workers, of a total of 675,000, are Latinx (Sanchez, 2020). Overall, the Latinx community is 17.5% of Illinois' population (U.S. Census Bureau, 2019d), indicating an overrepresentation in this workforce. Another report by Temp Worker Justice found that Black and Latinx workers are overrepresented in blue-collar temp assignments specifically (DeSario & White, 2020). Their data show that in Cook County, approximately 211,500 temp assignments were generated in 2019. Of these, 40.2% were filled by Black workers and 47.5% by Latinx workers. These figures count assignments rather than individual workers meaning that an individual might be counted multiple times if they received multiple temp assignments. While these figures render a fuzzy estimate of the temp workforce, they align with research by Peck and Theodore (2001), who demonstrate that Black and Latinx workers are overrepresented in contingent work in Chicago.

To better understand temp agencies in Chicago, we pulled business licensing records from the city of Chicago and the Illinois Department of Labor, finding 143 licensed and currently active temp agencies.[10] Given that these agencies pop up and disappear quickly, we also included a Google Map search to find additional agencies. Upon confirmation that they still operated, we found an additional 50 agencies, taking our total to 194. Figure 10.10 shows the locations of these temp agencies, with the majority race or ethnicity by community area included.[11] The densest cluster of agencies is in the central business district, often filling white-collar positions. Following this, agencies are predominately located in Latinx communities; very few are in predominately Black neighborhoods. Figure 10.11 shows the temp agencies in and around Little Village, many of which fill manufacturing and blue-collar openings. Further entrenching racialized selection of workers, elaborate busing systems known as "raiteros" have emerged to transport workers from Little Village and other Latinx neighborhoods to suburban factories, including in Cicero (Grabell, 2013). Some of these suburban locations (in proximity to Little Village) have been included in Figure 10.11.

The findings on temp workers demonstrate that Black and Latinx workers are overly represented in this industry, and that many of the assignments were in places

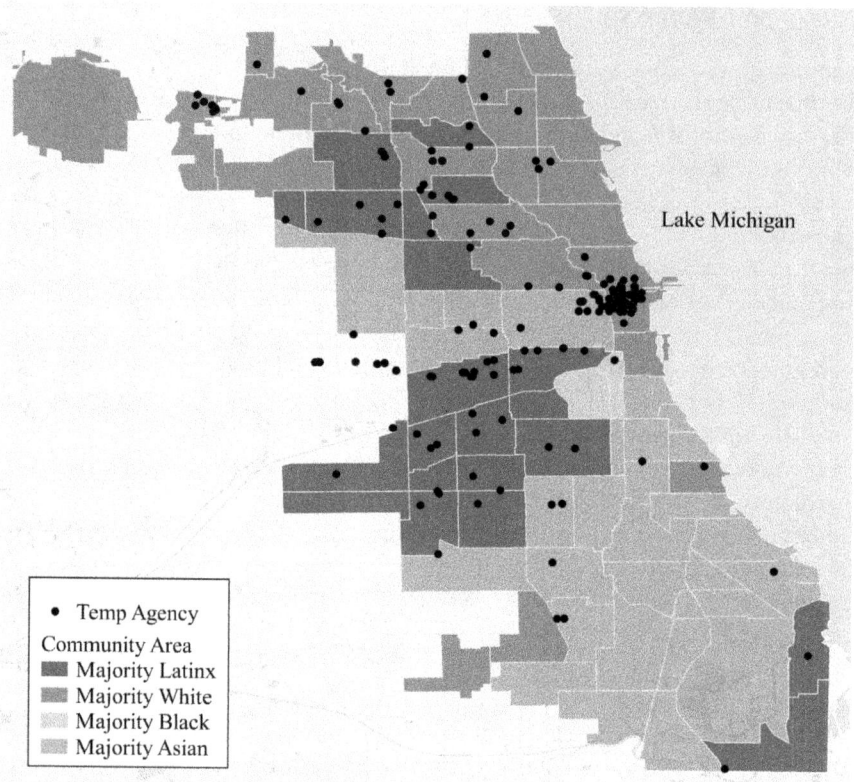

FIGURE 10.10 Temp Agency Locations by Race/Ethnicity of Community Area

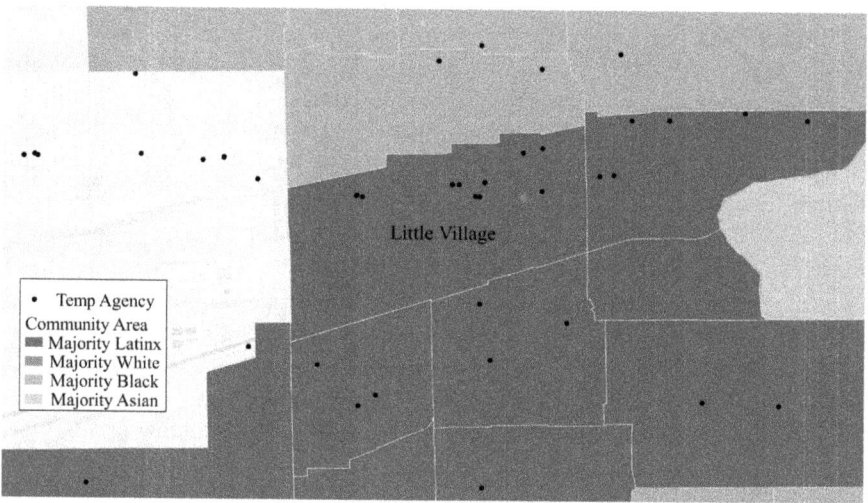

FIGURE 10.11 Temp Agency Locations in the Little Village Area

not aligned with COVID safety protocols. Moreover, the surveys demonstrate that many temp workers were afraid to take sick leave for fear of losing their jobs. Finally, the maps of temp agencies, coupled with the "rateiros," show how Latinx, including Little Village residents, are targeted for this type of work.

Informal Workers

The most visible type of informal work in Chicago is street vending. Common types of vending include itinerant vendors (e.g., dessert vendors) and stationary vendors who return daily to the same spot.[12] Illinois Policy estimates Chicago street vendors at 1,500–2,000 (Berg, 2016). Prior to 2015, it was illegal to sell precooked, made-on-the spot food or drinks. This was restrictive for many Little Village vendors who sell traditional Mexican treats, such as *elotes* (corn with butter, mayonnaise, and other flavorings), *tamales*, and *atole* (masa-based warm drink). Policy changes in 2015 allowed vendors to sell prepacked food if cooked in a licensed industrial or shared kitchen. Thus far, only 18 licenses have been granted for this new category (City of Chicago, 2021),[13] suggesting that cooking in a licensed industrial or shared kitchen is prohibitive for many vendors. Chicago vendors are overwhelmingly represented in Latinx communities, with the largest concentration in Little Village (Lucci & Gowins, 2015). In 2015, Illinois Policy interviewed 197 vendors in Chicago, finding that 100% were Hispanic, and most were Mexican (Lucci & Gowins, 2015).[14] Vendors work at busy intersections and areas with high levels of foot traffic, including near schools and churches.

In the summer of 2019, we conducted a canvass of the visible workforce in Little Village. The workforce includes informal entrepreneurs like street vendors who operate in public spaces, daily rummage sales or trinket vendors operating out of their front yards or on busy street corners, and *cocinas economicas*, small, backyard pop-up food stands. Figure 10.12 shows the concentration of the visible informal workforce. South Lawndale is lightened in color compared with surrounding community areas. Darker clusters on the map below represent larger concentrations of street vendors, while lighter clusters represent ~1–3 vendors.

Lucci and Gowins (2015) found that the average Chicago vendor earns $328 weekly (or $15,744 annually) and that most (95%) support at least one dependent on this income. Reports indicate that many vendors continued to operate during the pandemic (Nakayama, 2020), given the low incomes and associated economic vulnerability of such work. Additionally, since vendors interact face-to-face with their clientele, they may have been at heightened risk during the early days of the pandemic, before widespread mask usage was in effect.

Comparing Little Village and Norwood Park

While we focus on Little Village, it is helpful to compare with another neighborhood. Keeping in mind the segmentation of labor by race and ethnicity, we compare Little Village to a majority White neighborhood. To determine a comparative

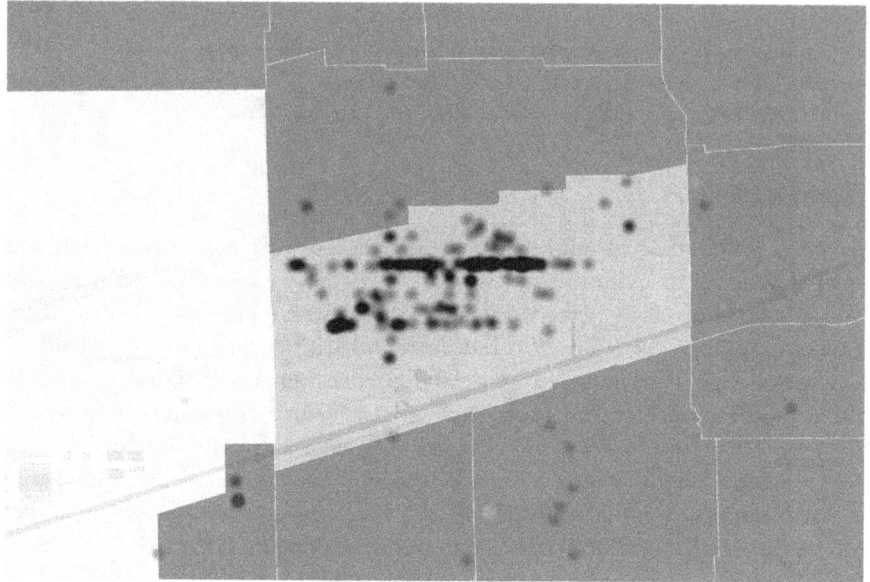

FIGURE 10.12 Heat Map of Vendors

neighborhood, we used census data and matched census tracts to the city's 77 community areas, then organized these areas by race and ethnicity (based on an average percentage of the racial/ethnic makeup of the census tracts in each community area). To roughly match the size, income, and percentage racial/ethnic concentration of Little Village, we compare it to Norwood Park.[15]

Norwood Park has a per capita income of $32,875 compared to South Lawndale's $10,402 (City of Chicago, 2014), a hardship index[16] of 21, compared to South Lawndale's 96 (a higher number indicates more hardship), and a 9% unemployment rate compared to South Lawndale's 15.8% (City of Chicago, 2014). Community areas at the highest end saw unemployment numbers between 33% and 36%, suggesting that low-paying (or infrequent) work may be more of an issue in Little Village than unemployment. This comports with the concentration of Latinx and Little Village residents in low-wage and contingent positions. Finally, 29.2% of Little Village residents are without health insurance as compared to 5.5% of Norwood Park residents (see Table 10.2).

Figures 10.13 and 10.14 compare the essential industries in and around Norwood Park and Little Village,[17] including food product plants, transportation, construction, and utilities (each dot represents a single business). There are no jails or prisons in or around Norwood Park, and it has one meat processing plant. The maps demonstrate the unique density of these industries in and around Little Village and the dearth of these industries in and around Norwood Park. Only one temp agency was found in Norwood Park, with a few others in the surrounding community areas (Figure 10.14). Finally, while we have never canvassed Norwood Park for street

TABLE 10.2 Select Comparative Demographic Indicators

Community Area	% Latinx	% White	Per Capita Income	Hardship Index	Unemployment Rate	% Without Health Insurance
South Lawndale	86.6%[a]	3.9%[a]	$10,402[b]	96[b]	15.8%[b]	29.2%[c]
Norwood Park	13.9%[a]	78.9%[a]	$32,875[b]	21[b]	9%[b]	5.5%[c]

Sources: a. U.S. Census Bureau, 2019a; b. City of Chicago, 2014; c. Chicago Health Atlas, 2019.

Note: This table is a comparison of select demographic data of the two community areas, South Lawndale and Norwood Park, showing that South Lawndale residents are overwhelming Latinx, are poorer, have a higher unemployment rate, and have higher percentage of their population without health insurance compared to Norwood Park residents.

vendors, the report from Illinois Policy did not report any vendors in this area. Additionally, their report found 100% of vendors were Hispanic, and Norwood Park is mostly White. Thus, it is unlikely there are street vendors who operate here.

This comparison highlights the unique combination of employment and labor-related factors, which put Little Village and, in many cases, other Latinx communities at heightened risk for COVID-19 exposure. The comparison also demonstrates the stark differences between a majority White and majority Latinx neighborhood when it comes to critical factors such as labor and poverty.

Discussion

The instability that low and infrequent wages produce likely contributed to Little Village residents feeling that it was essential to work throughout the pandemic. This is mentioned by street vendors as indicated above, and by temp workers surveyed by the Chicago Workers' Collaborative. A quarter of respondents believed they would lose their jobs if they had to quarantine, while 33% were unsure if they could keep their jobs after quarantining (Hernandez, 2020). One worker reported being fired after missing work due to contracting COVID, despite a doctor's note, and their status as a "permatemp" (temping at the same job for five years). Another worker reported that a group of six from the same company got sick, and all six were fired (Hernandez, 2020).

On their own, each type of work—essential, contingent, and informal—presented heightened exposure to COVID. However, more important than understanding each on their own is to understand how they are interconnected. First, street vendors continued to operate throughout the pandemic, selling hot and cooked food. Early morning *tamale* and *atole* vendors serving people on their way to work is the norm, as is hot and cooked food stands clustered on 31st and 26th streets, near foot traffic, and around essential industries. Vendors also work mere blocks from the Cook County Department of Corrections. If many residents of Little Village were "essential" and continued their normal consumption habits of

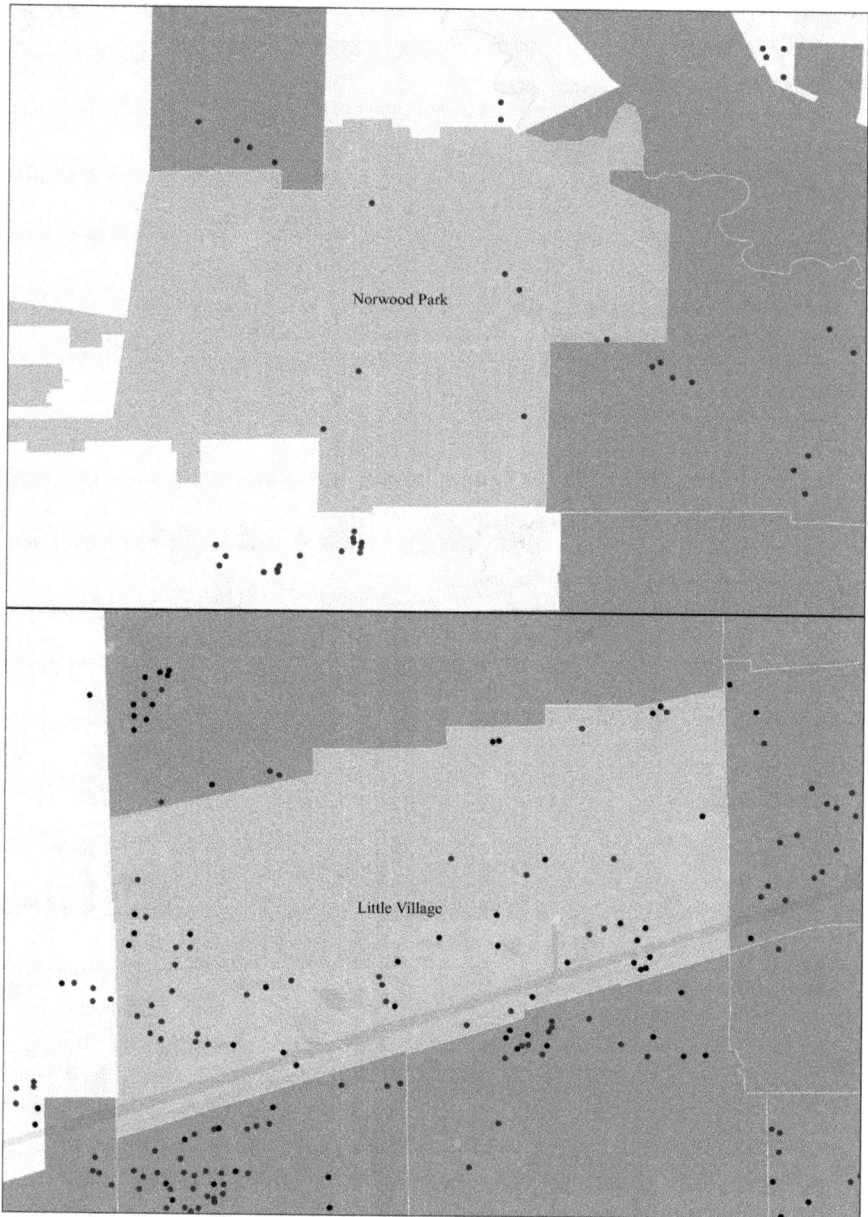

FIGURE 10.13 Essential Industries Comparison

buying from local vendors, especially early during the pandemic, it is no surprise that there was greater incidence of spread here.

Second, the area just south of Little Village is home to numerous produce wholesalers (see Figure 10.7), where many street vendors get their products in

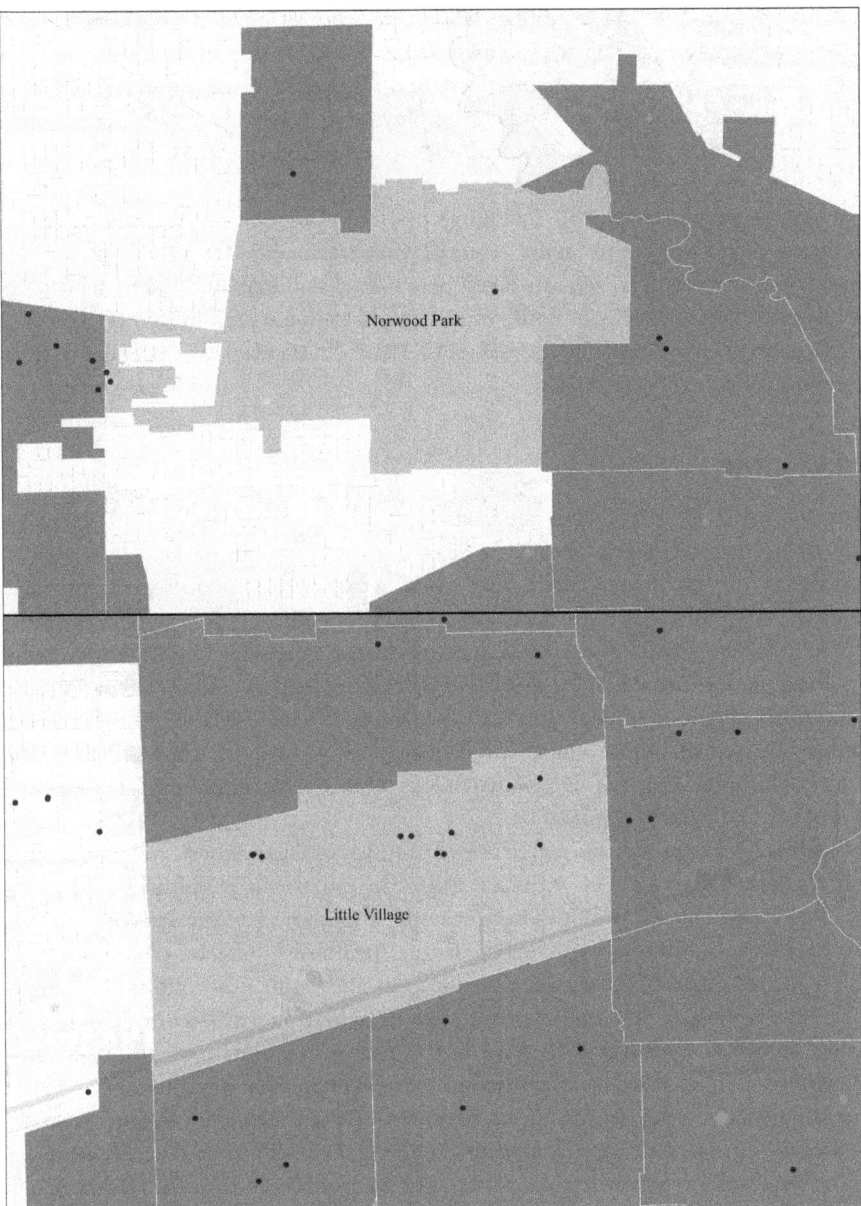

FIGURE 10.14 Temp Agency Comparison

the morning before selling to the public (Berg, n.d.). As food plants were kept open during the pandemic, and vendors continued to work, the proximity and co-dependence of these industries could have been another factor leading to increased chance for virus spread.

Third, some vendors combine vulnerable employment types. One vendor interviewed by Illinois Policy explained that she sold tamales in the morning, then began her factory job at 1:00 p.m. (Berg, n.d.). The low wages produced by these jobs necessitates multiple methods of employment. Unfortunately, working multiple jobs also provided more opportunities for community spread of COVID.

Fourth, and finally, as the above research on contingent labor suggests, many manufacturing plants rely on a contingent labor force. Given that many manufacturing plants were considered essential, mandated open by either the state or federal executive orders, workers faced heightened vulnerability due to their temporary and replaceable work status and the need to maintain a livelihood. In other words, going to work, despite the risk of COVID contraction, was essential to their livelihood.

Conclusions

While many early reports on the racial and ethnic disparities of COVID cases pointed to essential work or lack of healthcare as contributing factors, we argue that this is too simplistic. Many Latinx workers participate in contingent, informal, and low-wage jobs that reduce access to critical benefits, while leaving them little choice but to continue working in jobs essential to their livelihood. Additionally, healthcare in the United States is tied to employment, making employment type and status more salient of an explanation than a simplistic focus on lack of healthcare. In Little Village, several other spatial and economic issues worsened the situation. The neighborhood is bordered by industrial areas with companies considered essential by both state and federal guidelines.

COVID-19 exposed the inequalities at the root of the American labor, health, and residential systems. The virus has made the American public painfully aware of a system which not only ties healthcare to a job but also to a system in which the lowest-paid and most vulnerable work is primarily done by communities of color. Because these jobs exist across industries and result from multiple factors—including labor law and enforcement, and immigration law—a single policy or policy approach is ill-suited to remedy the problems pointed to in this chapter. A combination of social welfare provisions, that include undocumented workers, increased transparency in the hiring practices of temp agencies, free or low-cost healthcare options that are not tied to employment, and a path to citizenship for undocumented groups would be tough, but critical places to begin. Additionally, xenophobia and racism, which are much harder problems to tackle, need to be addressed. When discussing the rollout of vaccines for his state, Nebraska Governor, Pete Ricketts, claimed that undocumented workers at meatpacking plants cannot get the COVID vaccine (Armus, 2021). While health officials later contradicted this statement, it follows a history in the United States of treating Latinx workers as disposable labor.

Notes

1 We have no known conflict of interest to disclose.
2 We prefer to use the term "Latinx." When citing other studies or sources, we use the terminology used therein, including Hispanic or Latino.
3 The informal economy includes "economic activities that are not covered or poorly covered by formal arrangements—be it in law or in practice" (International Labour Organization, 2002).
4 Chicago is 33% White, 30% Black, and 29% Hispanic or Latino (U.S. Census Bureau, 2019b).
5 Census tracts: 3005-09, 3011-12, 3016, 3017.01 3017.02, 3018.01, 3018.02, 3018.03, 8305, 8407-08, 8417, 8435.
6 Our canvassing decisions were premised on our previous street vending research in Little Village, including two years of participant observation of the vending union, *Asociación de Vendedores Ambulantes*, and interviews with vendors, organizers, and aldermen.
7 Industry names are shortened to fit the table. Full names are: Other services, except public administration; Arts, entertainment, and recreation, and accommodation and food services; Educational services, and health care and social assistance; Professional, scientific, management, and administrative and waste management services; Transportation and warehousing, and utilities; Agriculture, forestry, fishing and hunting, and mining. Those not listed here are otherwise listed by their full name above.
8 The surveys asked slightly different questions, accounting for distinctions in the findings.
9 Gray indicates different community areas, with Little Village emphasized. White space is the city of Cicero. Examples of construction businesses included in Map 5 are steel and concrete manufacturers.
10 We omitted businesses we could not confirm were still operational. Additionally, we did not include freelance and project-based work for industries like legal, marketing, and creative content. These latter agencies were 23 in total.
11 This map is inspired by a map of temp agencies and racial/ethnic makeup of neighborhoods from Peck and Theodore's (2001) critical research on the subject.
12 Current licensing data indicate 208 frozen dessert licenses.
13 License Code 4406, Business Activity ID 966. There are at most 10 companies represented among these 18 licenses, as one license is needed per cart/bike.
14 There are also a small number of Asian vendors in Armour Square, and snow cone vending is popular in some Black neighborhoods in the summer.
15 Norwood Park has the third largest concentration of White population. Mount Greenwood and Edison Park have larger White populations, but they are much smaller in population, and wealthier.
16 The hardship index comprises six socioeconomic measures: % of housing crowded, % households below poverty, % aged 16+ unemployed, % aged 25+ without high school diploma, % aged under 18 or over 64, per capita income (City of Chicago, 2014).
17 The scale was kept constant in QGIS (1:15,000) when mapping to ensure that a similar amount of space was compared.

References

Armus, T. (2021, January 6). Nebraska Governor Says Citizens, Legal Residents Will Get Vaccine Priority Over Undocumented Immigrants. *The Washington Post*. Retrieved from www.washingtonpost.com/nation/2021/01/06/nebraska-covid-vaccine-immigrants-meatpacking/

Arredondo, G. F. (2008). *Mexican Chicago: Race, Identity and nation, 1916-1939*. University of Illinois Press.

Bauder, H. (2008). Citizenship as Capital: The Distinction of Migrant Labor. *Alternatives, 33*(3), 315–333. https://doi.org/10.1177%2F030437540803300303

Berg A. (2016, September 15). *Legal Food Carts Roll Into Chicago, but Roadblocks Abound*. Illinois Policy Institute. Retrieved from www.illinoispolicy.org/legal-food-carts-roll-into-chicago-but-roadblocks-abound/

Berg, A. (n.d.). *Tamales y Temor: The World of Chicago's Shadow Chefs*. Illinois Policy Institute. Retrieved from www.illinoispolicy.org/reports/tamales-y-temor-the-world-of-chicagos-shadow-chefs/

Betancur, J. J. (1996). The Settlement Experience of Latinos in Chicago: Segregation, Speculation, and the Ecology Model. *Social Forces, 74*(4), 1299–1324. https://doi.org/10.1093/sf/74.4.1299

Centers for Disease Control and Prevention. (2020a, July 24). *Health Equity Considerations and Racial and Ethnic Minority Groups*. Retrieved from www.cdc.gov/coronavirus/2019-ncov/community/health-equity/race-ethnicity.html?CDC_AA_refVal=https%3A%2F%2Fwww.cdc.gov%2Fcoronavirus%2F2019-ncov%2Fneed-extra-precautions%2Fracial-ethnic-minorities.html

Centers for Disease Control and Prevention. (2020b, November 30). *COVID-19 Hospitalization and Death by Race/Ethnicity*. Retrieved December 19, 2020, from www.cdc.gov/coronavirus/2019-ncov/covid-data/investigations-discovery/hospitalization-death-by-race-ethnicity.html#footnote01

Chadde, S., & Ag, G. (2020, April 16). *Tracking COVID-19's Impact on Meatpacking Workers and Industry*. Midwest Center for Investigative Reporting. Retrieved December 20, 2020, from https://investigatemidwest.org/2020/04/16/tracking-covid-19s-impact-on-meatpacking-workers-and-industry/

Changhwan, K., & Tamborini, C. R. (2006). The Continuing Significance of Race in the Occupational Attainment of Whites and Blacks: A Segmented Labor Market Analysis. *Sociological Inquiry, 76*(1), 23–51. https://doi.org/10.1111/j.1475-682X.2006.00143.x

Chen, M. A. (2012). The Informal Economy: Definitions, Theories and Policies. *WIEGO Working Paper No. 1*, 1–26. Retrieved from www.wiego.org/sites/default/files/migrated/publications/files/Chen_WIEGO_WP1.pdf

Chicago Health Atlas. (2019). *No Health Insurance*. Chicago Department of Public Health. Retrieved from www.chicagohealthatlas.org/indicators/no-health-insurance

City of Chicago. (2014). *Census Data-Selected Socioeconomic Indicators in Chicago, 2008-2012* [Data set]. Chicago Data Portal. Retrieved from https://data.cityofchicago.org/Health-Human-Services/Census-Data-Selected-socioeconomic-indicators-in-C/kn9c-c2s2

City of Chicago. (2017). *Boundaries – City* [Data set]. Chicago Data Portal. Retrieved August 3, 2020, from https://data.cityofchicago.org/Facilities-Geographic-Boundaries/Boundaries-City/ewy2-6yfk

City of Chicago. (2018). *Boundaries-Community Areas (current)* [Data set]. Chicago Data Portal. Retrieved August 3, 2020, from https://data.cityofchicago.org/Facilities-Geographic-Boundaries/Boundaries-Community-Areas-current-/cauq-8yn6

City of Chicago. (2020a). *Chicago Population Counts* [Data set]. Chicago Data Portal. Retrieved December 17, 2020, from https://data.cityofchicago.org/Health-Human-Services/Chicago-Population-Counts/85cm-7uqa

City of Chicago. (2020b). *Boundaries-Zip Codes* [Data set]. Chicago Data Portal. Retrieved January 11, 2021, from https://data.cityofchicago.org/Facilities-Geographic-Boundaries/Boundaries-ZIP-Codes/gdcf-axmw

City of Chicago. (2021). *Business Licenses-Current Active* [Data set]. Chicago Data Portal. Retrieved January 11, 2021, from https://data.cityofchicago.org/Community-Economic-Development/Business-Licenses-Current-Active/uupf-x98q

Clark, E., Fredricks, K., Woc-Colburn, L., Bottazzi, M. E., & Weatherhead, J. (2020). Disproportionate Impact of the COVID-19 Pandemic on Immigrant Communities in the United States. *PLOS Neglected Tropical Diseases, 14*(7). doi:10.1371/journal.pntd.0008484. www.ncbi.nlm.nih.gov/pmc/articles/PMC7357736/

DeGenova, N. (1998). Race, Space, and the Reinvention of Latin America in Mexican Chicago. *Latin American Perspectives, 25*(5), 87–116. https://doi.org/10.1177%2F0094582X9802500506

Delgadillo, T., & Weaver, J. (2017). Work Coalition, and Advocacy: Latinas Leading in the Midwest. In O. O. Valerio-Jimenez, S. Vaquera-Vasquez, & C. F. Fox (Eds.), *Latina/o Midwest Reader* (pp. 236–251). University of Illinois Press.

DeSario, D., & White, J. (2020). *Race to the bottom: The Demographics of Blue-Collar Temporary Staffing.* Temp Worker Justice & Temp Worker Union Alliance Project. Retrieved from www.tempworkerjustice.org/post/race-to-the

Dey, M., Frazis, H., Loewenstein, M. A., & Hugette, S. (2020, June). *Ability to Work from Home: Evidence from Two Surveys and Implications for the Labor Market in the COVID-19 Pandemic.* Monthly Labor Review, U.S. Bureau of Labor Statistics. Retrieved from https://doi.org/10.21916/mlr.2020.14. www.bls.gov/opub/mlr/2020/article/ability-to-work-from-home.htm

Duffy, M. (2007). Doing the Dirty Work: Gender, Race, and Reproductive Labor in Historical Perspective. *Gender & Society, 21*(3), 313–336. https://doi.org/10.1177%2F0891243207300764

Gamboa, S., & Armas, M. (2017, April 9). Chicago's 'Mexico of the Midwest' Fights Fallout from Fear of Trump. *NBC News.* Retrieved from www.nbcnews.com/news/latino/chicago-s-mexico-midwest-fights-fallout-fear-trump-n740411

Glenn, E. N. (1992). From Servitude to Service Work: Historical Continuities in the Racial Division of Paid Reproductive Labor. *Signs: Journal of Women in Culture and Society, 18*(1), 1–43. Retrieved from www.journals.uchicago.edu/doi/abs/10.1086/494777

Grabell, M. (2013, April 29). Taken for a Ride: Temp Agencies and 'Raiteros' in Immigrant Chicago. *ProPublica.* Retrieved from www.propublica.org/article/taken-for-a-ride-temp-agencies-and-raiteros-in-immigrant-chicago

Grabell, M., Perlman, C., & Yeung, B. (2020, June 12). Emails Reveal Chaos as Meatpacking Companies Fought Health Agencies Over COVID-19 Outbreaks in Their Plants. *ProPublica.* Retrieved from www.propublica.org/article/emails-reveal-chaos-as-meatpacking-companies-fought-health-agencies-over-covid-19-outbreaks-in-their-plants

Hart, K. (1973). Informal Income Opportunities and Urban Employment in Ghana. *The Journal of Modern African Studies, 11*(1), 61–89. Retrieved from www.jstor.org/stable/159873

Hatton, E. (2011). *The Temp Economy: From Kelly Girls to Permatemps in Postwar America.* Temple University Press.

Hernandez, E. (2020). *We Do Not Have the Luxury to Work From Home: The Impact of COVID-19 on Illinois' Essential Temp Workforce.* Chicago Workers Collaborative. Retrieved from www.chicagoworkerscollaborative.org/coronavirus-survey

Hickey, M. (2020, May 5). With Chicago's Little Village Hardest Hit by COVID-19, Residents Are Urged to Stay Home. *CBS Chicago.* Retrieved from https://chicago.cbslocal.com/2020/05/05/with-chicagos-little-village-hardest-hit-by-covid-19-residents-are-urged-to-stay-home/

Illinois Department of Public Health. (2020, December 22). *COVID-19 Statistics.* Retrieved December 22, 2020, from www.dph.illinois.gov/covid19/covid19-statistics

International Labour Organization. (2002). *Decent Work and the Informal Economy.* International Labour Conference, 90th Session, Report VI. Retrieved from www.ilo.org/public/english/standards/relm/ilc/ilc90/pdf/rep-vi.pdf

International Labour Organization. (2013). *Women and Men in the Informal Economy: A Statistical Picture* (2nd ed.). International Labour Office. Retrieved from www.ilo.org/stat/Publications/WCMS_234413/lang--en/index.htm

Kalleberg, A. L., Reskin, B. F., & Hudson, K. (2000). Bad Jobs in America: Standard and Nonstandard Employment Relations and Job Quality in the United States. *American Sociological Review, 65*(2), 256–278. https://doi.org/10.2307/2657440

Keating, A. D. (2004). *Chicago Neighborhood and Suburbs: A Historical Guide.* University of Chicago Press.

Kirschenman, J., & Neckerman, K. M. (1991). 'We'd Love to Hire Them, But …': The Meaning of Race for Employers. In C. Jencks & P. E. Peterson (Eds.), *The Urban Underclass* (pp. 203–232). The Brookings Institute.

Koch, R. (2015). Licensing, Popular Practices and Public Spaces: An Inquiry Via the Geographies of Street food Vending. *International Journal of Urban and Regional Research, 39*(6), 1231–1250. doi:10.1111/1468-2427.12316

Leonard, M. (1998). *Invisible Work, Invisible Workers: The Informal Economy in Europe and the U.S.* Springer.

Lucci, M., & Gowins, H. (2015, August). *Chicago's Food-Cart Band Costs Revenue, Jobs.* Illinois Policy Institute, Special Report. Retrieved from www.illinoispolicy.org/reports/chicagos-food-cart-ban-costs-revenue-jobs/

Luthra, R. R., & Waldinger, R. (2010). Into the Mainstream? Labor Market Outcomes of Mexican-Origin Workers. *International Migration Review, 44*(4), 830–868. https://doi.org/10.1111%2Fj.1747-7379.2010.00827.

Nakayama, Y. (2020, March 23). "We're Pushed to the Side": Street Vendor Says They've Been Forgotten amid COVID-19 Pandemic. *ABC News.* Retrieved from https://abc7chicago.com/community-events/little-village-street-vendors-still-working-amid-pandemic/6043049/

Ndobo, A., Faure, A., Boisselier, J., & Giannaki, S. (2018). The Ethno-Racial Segmentation Jobs: The Impacts of the Occupational Stereotypes on Hiring Decisions. *The Journal of Social Psychology, 158*(6), 663–679. https://doi.org/10.1080/00224545.2017.1389685

New York Times. (2020, December 20). Illinois Coronavirus Map and Case Count. Retrieved December 20, 2020, from www.nytimes.com/interactive/2020/us/illinois-coronavirus-cases.html

Nuevo-Kerr, L.A. (1984). Mexican Chicago: Chicano Assimilation Aborted, 1939-1954. In M. G. Holli & P. A. Jones (Eds.), *Ethnic Chicago* (pp. 269–298). William B. Eerdmans.

Peck J., & Theodore, N. (2001). Contingent Chicago: Restructuring the Spaces of Temporary Labor. *International Journal of Urban and Regional Research, 25*(3), 471–496. https://doi.org/10.1111/1468-2427.00325

Portes, A., Castells, M., & Benton, L. A. (Eds.). (1989). *The Informal Economy: Studies in Advanced and Less Developed Countries.* The Johns Hopkins University Press.

Portes, A., & Sassen-Koob, S. (1987). Making It Underground: Comparative Material on the Informal Sector in Western Market Economies. *The American Journal of Sociology, 93*(1), 30–61. Retrieved from www.journals.uchicago.edu/doi/abs/10.1086/228705

Pritzker, J. B. (2020, March 20). *Executive Order in Response to COVID-19 (COVID-19 Executive Order no. 8).* Illinois.gov. Retrieved from www2.illinois.gov/pages/executive-orders/executiveorder2020-10.aspx

Reisler, M. (1976). *By the Sweat of Their Brow: Mexican Immigrant Labor in the United States, 1900–1940*. Greenwood Press.

Sanchez, M. (2020, April 28). What Happens When the Workers Who Make Hand Soap Get COVID-19? They Protest. *ProPublica*. Retrieved from www.propublica.org/article/what-happens-when-the-workers-who-make-hand-soap-get-covid-19-they-protest

Tai, D. B. G., Shah, A., Doubeni, C. A., Sia, I. G., & Wieland, M. L. (2020). The Disproportionate Impact of COVID-19 on Racial and Ethnic Minorities in the United States. *Clinical Infectious Diseases, 72*(4), 703–706. https://doi.org/10.1093/cid/ciaa815. https://academic.oup.com/cid/advance-article/doi/10.1093/cid/ciaa815/5860249

Thorbecke, C. (2020, May 22). "Heroes or Hostages?": Communities of Color Bear the Burden of Essential Work in Coronavirus Crisis. *ABC News*. Retrieved from https://abcnews.go.com/Business/heroes-hostages-communities-color-bear-burden-essential-work/story?id=70662472

Tienda M., & Sanchez, S. (2013). Latin American Immigration to the United States. *Daedalus, 142*(3), 48–64. https://doi:10.1162/DAED_a_00218

U.S. Bureau of Labor Statistics. (2018, July). *Contingent and Alternative Arrangements—May 2017*. USDL-18-0942. Retrieved from www.bls.gov/news.release/pdf/conemp.pdf.

U.S. Census Bureau. (2019a). *ACS Demographic and Housing Estimates, American Community Survey 5-Year Estimates* [Data set]. Retrieved from https://data.census.gov/cedsci/table?g=0500000US17031.140000&tid=ACSDP5Y2019.DP05&hidePreview=false

U.S. Census Bureau. (2019b). *Quick Facts: Chicago City, Illinois*. Retrieved from www.census.gov/quickfacts/chicagocityillinois

U.S. Census Bureau. (2019c). *Industry by Sex for the Civilian Employed Population 16 Years and Over, American Community Survey 5-Year Estimates* [Data set]. Retrieved from https://data.census.gov/cedsci/table?g=1400000US17031300500,17031300600,17031300700,17031300800,17031300900,17031301100,17031301200,17031301600,17031301701,17031301702,17031301801,17031301802,17031301803,17031830500,17031840700,17031840800,17031841700,17031843500&tid=ACSST5Y2019.S2403&hidePreview=false

U.S. Census Bureau. (2019d). *Quick Facts: Illinois*. Retrieved from www.census.gov/quickfacts/IL

Williams, T., & Ivory, D. (2020, April 8). Chicago's Jail Is Top U.S. Hot Spot as Virus Spreads Behind Bars. *The New York Times*. Retrieved April 23, 2020, from www.nytimes.com/2020/04/08/us/coronavirus-cook-county-jail-chicago.html

Wills, J. (2009). Subcontracted Employment and Its Challenge to Labor. *Labor Studies Journal, 34*(4), 441–460. https://doi.org/10.1177%2F0160449X08324740

Yi, J. S. (2019, March 25). The Grid: Little Village's 'Second Magnificent Mile' Captures Heart of Mexico. *Chicago Sun Times*. Retrieved from https://chicago.suntimes.com/2019/3/25/18355132/the-grid-little-village-s-second-magnificent-mile-captures-heart-of-mexico

Zamudio, M.I. (2020, May 6). Testing Lags in Latino Communities Hit Hardest by COVID-10 in Chicago. *NPR*. Retrieved from www.npr.org/local/309/2020/05/06/851291931/testing-lags-in-

11

SOCIAL DISTANCING AS LENS

Race and Some Instructive Facets of Mass Pathogenic Self-Isolation

Miguel de Oliver

Introduction

"We have a right to protect ourselves. Everybody does," declared Bill (not his real name), referring to illegal Mexican immigrants with coronavirus who were rumored to be overrunning Texas. He lifted his coffee and smirked, "But *whatever*. Short-term it doesn't make any difference to me anyways. *I'm outta here!* I'm off to a little vacation to the Scottish Highlands. I've had tickets for months."

"*Ahhhhhhhhh …*" I uttered with false hesitation.

"The EU just blocked incoming travel from the US. Didn't you know? Nobody tops Uncle Sam in terms of corona cases worldwide. You might call it *national* distancing. The Europeans can't have maskless fools from the US running wild, shedding virus *à la Trump*."

"*Whatttttttt?*" Bill skeptically stated. Silence fell as he quickly pulled out his phone to access the internet and verify what I said. *Jackasses!* he angrily sniped in disbelief. "It's gotta be a '*get-Americans*' thing. Stinks of bile."

Nowhere in his face was there any consciousness of hypocrisy.

Reflexive manias about disease and the diseased, about the presumptively virtuous and the invariably degenerate, are readily exposed by the pandemic of 2020.

Epidemiological Social Distancing and Race

The social distancing that has been broadly implemented on an international scale in response to the coronavirus pandemic is a policy response to the outbreak of a contagious disease; it is clearly envisioned to be practiced by every citizen irrespective of race or ethnicity. But there is a difference between the universality of its application and the universality of its experience; for while the objectives of pandemic-focused social separation are epidemiological, it takes place within a

DOI: 10.4324/9781003268710-11

society already riven with endemic forms of social separation that must necessarily distort its implementation.

Racism is fundamentally a form of social distancing, where a whole class of stigmatized "others" are variably marginalized in a broad array of formal and informal spheres of interaction. This is not to say that pandemic-inspired "social distancing" is racist. Hardly. Deploying space as a preventative measure is a logical response to a physically transmissible threat to public health. But it is instructive to note that the therapeutic objective of pandemic-focused social distancing—the promotion of the general well-being—is also the historical rationale of racist social distancing practiced by White America. The threat to the public well-being with respect to the coronavirus is an infected body, and the threat to the public well-being in a racist culture is the non-White body. This conjunction can therefore be instructive for mainstream society, as the experience of being casually alienated as a threatening body—a reality that is fundamental to the experience of visible minorities—suddenly becomes palpable to members of the mainstream during epidemiological social distancing.

The commonalities between epidemiological social distancing and historical racism explains why ethnic minority groups have long been reflexively perceived by mainstream populations as sponsors of disease (e.g., Kiple & Kiple, 1980; Shah, 2001). The response to the 1853 yellow fever epidemic in the United States punitively targeted specific European immigrants. East Asians bore heavy stigmatization during the 2002–2004 SARS outbreak, and Africans during the 2014 Ebola outbreak. The mainstream association between disease and the presence of a racial "other" is perfectly contemporary when noting the assertions by the Trump administration that Mexicans were agents of "tremendous infectious disease …pouring across the border" (Guardian, 2015). Trump's lawyer claimed that "diseases spreading across the country … are causing polio-like paralysis of our children" (in Kloor, 2020). Indeed, 58% of Asian adults say that the coronavirus outbreak, termed the "Kung flu" by Trump, has occasioned more racist outbursts against them. Compared to only 13% for Whites, large proportions of Asian (39%) and Black (38%) adults say the notion of communicable disease associated with their race/ethnicity has discomfited someone around them since the coronavirus outbreak (Pew Research Center, 2020).

Aside from reports of reflexive association between coronavirus and racial minorities, in terms of transmission, there are clearly racial/ethnic dimensions in play. Speaking collectively, racial minorities "are" subject to greater exposure because of their comparative inability to socially distance. But this comparative inability is largely due to the historical and contemporary effects of systemic and spatialized underprivilege; in other words, class differences, not immutable biological or cultural ones. Not only are higher income (disproportionately White) workers able to more readily convert from face-to-face to online work, but they are far less likely to lose their jobs, suffer income loss, and endure dense residential settings (Chiou & Tucker, 2020; Papageorge et al., 2020). Moreover, even the greater access to online resources that the children of the White mainstream enjoy allow them to isolate and better maintain educational continuity during the pandemic (Bacher-Hicks et al., 2020; Horowitz, 2020). Thus, the ever-attendant specter of race emerges in clear relief when showing the intersection between social distancing and the systemic features of racialized social distancing. But there are additional aspects of epidemiological social distancing that—while ubiquitous—are overwhelmingly veiled from mainstream view. The visibility of these forms of social distancing are, like "Bill" referenced at the start of this chapter, greatly dependent on the matter-of-fact racial positioning of an individual within a racialized society.

This chapter will examine two racialized aspects of epidemiological social distancing that readily escape the mainstream consciousness. The first section addresses the recommendation to "shelter-in-place." But the very notion of "place" has been undergoing a dramatic transformation in the last half century in terms of its social functioning, racially differentiating a place's capacity to service the sheltering citizen's multifaceted needs during a sudden intensive period of isolation. And the second section addresses the disruption of identity caused by the respiratory facemask. While the facemask certainly impedes the diffusion of contagion, it is also an article that fundamentally embodies social distancing by both partially obscuring identity (including racial) and—to a revolutionary degree—visually standardizing individuality. For "all," the implications of the facemask are medically salutary; but for "some," the implications are intensively subversive.

Racialized "Place" as Problematic Refuge During Pandemic

"Could you get the owner of the home, please!?" a stranger shouted up to me from the sidewalk as I was on the balcony with brush in hand, working on a painting.

Once in a dire state of decay, the house was an old Victorian that I had been slowly restoring by hand for years; it had a pronounced White neoclassical temple portico, featuring elaborate Corinthian capitals and robust columns seated on broad pedestals. Presently in the United States, the facade is routinely associated with Greco-Roman democracy and public institutions; however, when in private hands, the architectural facade had been the very symbol of classical social distancing—a function any antebellum southern plantation master positioned where I now stood celebrated reflexively.

But—here and now—the little man stood pat on the street below with an expectant smile on his face as he waited to be informed about the presumed real owner of the house.

As will be shown, even during the therapeutic practices of a pandemic there is a social distancing in the very components of the built environment that requires some to look up and others down.

Social distancing is fundamentally a spatial practice—and not space in general, but rather the particularly "localized" expression of space often referred to as "place." "Place" is a specific point in space that is distinguished by particular functional or cultural significance to an individual or set of individuals. Thus, when authorities in early-mid 2019 variably called for individuals to "shelter-in-place" in response to rapid coronavirus spread, the intention was clearly to impede person-to-person transmission of the virus by reducing the spatial connectivity between individuals. But in the mid-20th century, "place" in the United States became a highly racialized concept, in both physical scale and imprinted meaning. While it has been shown that "White" residential areas are—as a vast statistical average—best situated to materially endure the deleterious effects of widespread social distancing, there are additional aspects of racialized place that are aggravated by the broad practice of "shelter-in-place." Two articulations of social distancing have already been articulated: manifest racism and epidemiological social distancing. But there are additional manifestations of social distancing that permeate the modern landscape within which these two forms of social distancing are embedded.

The Preexisting Landscape of Social Distancing

In the mid-late 20th century, during the post-WWII "Golden Era of Capitalism" (1950–1970) in the United States, a landscape of material opulence for a formerly proletarian urban class became the aspirational norm—an aspirational norm that was heavily racialized. Mass flight from the inner city to the suburbs was envisioned as the prerequisite to formally creating a landscape of racial "Whiteness" in contrast to the decaying inner city that was increasingly "non-White" (Brodkin Sacks, 1994; Brown et al., 2003, pp. 77–80; Massey & Denton, 1993). But whether racialized or not, the built landscapes of modernity were elementally saturated with another systemic feature of industrial mass production. Referred to as "alienation" in the mid-19th century, Karl Marx (1932) described a general sense of social separation resulting from the modern (meaning industrial) individual being reduced to an anonymous part of a machine-driven production process and subjected to the spiritual implications of its vast volume of privatized output. Among a society increasingly defined by the consuming practices of its iconic middle-class suburbs, Putnam (1995) notes the advancement of alienation in the United States since the 1950s, characterized as a growing disengagement from civic participation. From church-going to kinship bonds, union membership meetings to parent-teacher association participation, from Boy Scouts and the Red Cross to bowling leagues and an array of fraternal organizations, the fragmentation of civic cohesion is dramatic (see also Nisbet, 1962). de Oliver (2021) refers to this advanced form of disconnectedness as "emporia," being "a sense of disconnectedness, anonymity, and powerlessness arising from the absence of a stable group identity in a consumer culture mediated by electronic mass media platforms." Indeed, the deleterious effects of alienation, and the attendant inability to affirm identity, is at the core of the ascendance of right-wing populism (see Carney, 2019). The centrality of race and "otherness" is front and center in this political movement as a tonic to counter the socially dispersive effects of post-industrial alienation, a movement absolutely committed to the "social distancing" of "others" as local and national policy (i.e., walls, immigration, neighborhoods that require "protecting", and so on).

When told to "shelter in place" during the pandemic, the dichotomy of the non-White inner-city/White periphery provides a critical window to see an intrinsic problem when creating separate landscapes for a virtuous "us" and a problematic "them"—for the co-dependence of these symbolic landscapes is distorted by the broad experience of systemic alienation during a pandemic.

Racialized Places as Coronavirus Refuge

Along with racial minorities, social distancing and variable applications of shelter-in-place have restricted the movements of the White mainstream; the bulk of this White mainstream has been restricted to what many considered materially privileged but alienating and non-peripatetic, low-density landscapes that are over-whelmingly comprised of highly standardized private property. The mass market commercial centers embedded within this landscape that has taken on such a critical social role as gathering place were themselves closed due to the pandemic. The pandemic has only intensified the pervasive alienation of this landscape that—to many—remains concealed beneath the vast patina of mainstream America's conspicuous consumption.

The modern inner city and suburbia are two environments that were simultaneously created as inverse symbols of each other. It is not surprising that the two environments would represent the symbolic poles of identity-response to systemic alienation, especially during the intensified disconnectedness mandated by the pandemic's social distancing. Therefore, one portion of mainstream society perceived the outbreak of disease in large urban centers disproportionately inhabited by racial minorities as a historical expression of disease common to those associated with degeneracy and squalor. Referring to one such intensively Black urban center as a "disgusting rat and rodent infested mess," Trump regularly labeled these urban centers as "anarchist jurisdictions" in "democrat-run cities" and retweeted the call to "Let them rot" (Blum, 2020; Falconer, 2020; Kimball, 2019; Trump, 2020).

In contrast to mainstream conservatives, another portion of the alienated mainstream reacted differently to the inner-city habitus. There has been a growing acknowledgment since the 1970s that iconic White suburbia lacked critical cultural elements of social health. The most notable expression of this dissatisfaction has been the ongoing process of gentrification—that being the return of the middle class to the inner city. A growing body of research has recognized that the inner city seems to have some "irresistible social and existential appeal ... on a deeper level than that of the market ... [that] reflects real middle class needs and desires" (Zukin, 1982, pp. 174–175, 185). For a subset of the suburban mainstream, the increasingly pervasive homogenization of suburbia incited an aesthetic reaction that valued nonconformity, social experimentation, and a sense of spontaneity that demonstrates a "fierce heterogeneity ... devout irrationalism ... [where the self] sees the city as a shadow-show of its own impulses and movements ..., liberating [individuals] ... from the deterministic schemes [in the suburbs] which ought to have led them into a wholly different style of life" (Raban, 1974, pp. 163–165,

168; also see Bridge, 2003; Caulfield, 1989; Lloyd & Clark, 2001). These cultural agendas have been driven by a "new urban ideology" of renewal premised on the "pursuit of difference, diversity, and distinction" (Smith, 1987, p. 168)—for example, the preservation of historic architecture, artistic expressionism, emancipated homosexual association, Bohemian lifestyle, social preservationism, and as a "particularly emancipatory movement for professional middle-class women … tied to suburban incubators" (Butler, 2007, p. 765; Brooks, 2000; Brown-Saracino, 2004; Florida, 2002; Hosmer, 1965; Ley, 2003; Warde, 1991).

Is what is being suggested here that the materially underprivileged and marginalized environments largely inhabited by racial minorities are in fact in possession of therapeutic attributes to modern alienation and to pandemic isolation specifically? Absolutely not. The chronic problems associated with underprivilege that mandate greater police presence and social welfare supports clearly indicate otherwise. But it is "not" the manifest reality of the minority and his/her environs that is critical to the popular perceptions of them in mainstream America but rather the social construction of them by counter-defining them against a virtuous suburban "us" that lacks spiritual nutrition. To alienated suburbs, the lesser perceived conformity of the inner-city environment (greater density, variable land use, demographic pluralism, public art expressionism, public transportation, etc.) is simplistically perceived (once materially upgraded) as a tonic to contemporary ennui, placelessness, and purposelessness.

Amid the vigorous polarization of Republicans and Democrats that even divided policy response to the coronavirus, the perception of an emotionally vital—albeit underprivileged inner city—was plain to see during the Black Lives Matter (BLM) street protests. For days on end, protests emerged in urban centers nationwide in response to the well-documented and casual public murder of George Floyd by Minneapolis police. What was interesting was the composition of the protesters. In contrast to mainstream Republicans who characterized the demonstrations in terms of a wanton disrespect for law and order by liberally disposed citizens, an astonishing proportion (not infrequently a majority) of the protesters were White, and clearly not from the immediate environment. But the social objectives of the average White protester differed notably from those of BLM. While BLM and its overwhelmingly Black constituency were driven by, and focused on, specific policy response to police brutality, the main of the White contingent seemed driven by an authentic but much larger agenda related to human rights, social justice, and the need for individual purpose. With respect to the latter, Black identity, by being constructed as external to the mainstream culture and its material privileges, retains what the racialized but alienated mainstream identity based in suburbia does not: a sense of purpose, mission, and a metanarrative of collective identity associated with being punitively "otherized." Participation in the anti-racist BLM campaign is an emotive endeavor that lends individual purpose even to those in the larger mainstream society who feel beleaguered by the alienation of consumer culture capitalism. But for the average White protester, especially during the intense isolationism of "shelter-in-place," the association is ultimately more personally therapeutic than policy reform-driven. "[M]uch of the White participation is more symbolic than strategic," said Jesse Washington (2020), senior staff writer for *The Undefeated*. As stated by a political science professor in attendance at one protest. "It's incumbent on White people like myself … who have relatively privileged White-collar experiences, to embrace this multigenerational, multiracial movement[.]" Lamenting the long fragmentation of social bonds that convey purpose and identity, he added.

> It is so difficult in our imperfect system to build, mobilize and sustain coalitions. So any time you have a chance to foster this kind of movement, these kind of coalitions, to try to build some positive change, you need to get involved.
>
> *ibid.*

A Boston Globe columnist asserted that

> White participation in the protests seemed driven, in part, by the need to get out of the house. When Floyd died, the nation was nearing its third month in quarantine to stave off the spread of COVID-19. Schools and many businesses were closed, the weather was good, and people had a lot of time on their hands. The protests served both as a place to go and a way to be self-congratulatory about doing the bare minimum for racial justice.
>
> *Graham, 2020*

This was not a solitary or overly skeptical determination. Douglas McAdam, a sociologist who studies social movements at Stanford added that one "reason young people protested is that they had been cooped up in their homes due to the global pandemic" (Logan, 2020). And Erin Logan (ibid.), a staff writer at the *Los Angeles Times*, wrote an article titled "White people have gentrified Black Lives Matter. It's a problem."

Adrenalized by the isolationism of the pandemic, both White and Black protesters shared a stimulating desire for liberation—one from punitive multigenerational effects of racist social distancing and the other from the endemic social distancing of advanced consumer culture. While not visible to the naked eye on the street, the subtle misalignment of the two modes of alienation within the medium of epidemiological social distancing would soon be evident. Among the protests in the immediate wake of the killing of George Floyd, national support for anti-racism spiked, as 45% of White people surveyed said racism was a big problem. But by early August, support had fallen to 33% as it approached its original baseline (see Tesler, 2020). This is not to assert that such White personal participation in vigorous protests amid the pandemic was inauthentic; rather that relief from the intense isolation of "shelter-in-place" restrictions made it possible to see a vast substrate of racialized aesthetics embedded in the "place" of social distancing. Critical to both poles of the White mainstream response to the non-White inner city during the pandemic was the coalescing effect of a palpable and local expression of "us" amid the socially dispersive alienation of the era. Aggravated by the emotionally con-stipating practice of "shelter-in-place," it is difficult not to look at the collective eruption of contrasting sentiments in the White mainstream reaction to the inner-city "place" as two halves of a self-cleaved collective psyche, each flailing from its partitioned insufficiency.

Social Distancing and the Respiratory Mask as Provisional "Game-Changer"

Ahh … if you could take these two bags, I can handle the smaller one.

In the routine experience of the day, I consider myself well-disposed to any-body who might be in need of some spontaneous assistance in public; Open an obstructive door? Return a forgotten possession? Or reach high for an inaccessible can on the top shelf of a grocery store? For these things, I'm your man. Thus, when in the lobby of a hotel hosting a large academic conference, a complete stranger required my assistance, I ordinarily would be happy to oblige. But there was an air of routine presumption in her placid face. And it was furthered by her spontaneous assessment of what would be a convenient division of luggage to be carried by her and myself. My inaction seemed to unnerve her, momentarily conveying the notion that my tall and darkish presence might very well "not" be made safe by my presumed presence as another member of the low-waged servitude that was every-where apparent. The situation was not resolved until I slightly turned to reveal the nametag showing my presence there—like herself—as a conference attendee.

Such occurrences have infinite permutations.

At a conference in Chicago, a security guard approached to demand to know if I had a room. Long in experience, these type of events are only of concern to me now when the expectant person is armed, as this guard was. Sometimes I speak, other times I do not, but I always look irreverently at the gun, and make sure the bearer is aware of me doing so.

The reader might very well ask "What do these anecdotal experiences have to do with the coronavirus pandemic, and the respiratory mask specifically?" The answer is that—to many, and to the main of society during the pandemic—the respiratory mask would seem to be just a tedious but obligatory clothing accessory scarcely larger than a folded table napkin. But—to some—it can be so much more.

Unlike the preceding portion of this chapter, there is a paucity of scholar-ship examining race in conjunction with the novelty of mass mask wearing. Consequently, I hope the reader is tolerant of pertinent scholarship in this section being combined with the anecdotal experience of the author.

Social distancing is a policy whose objectives are achieved by the deployment of space between individuals so as to preclude the spreading of a contagion. Replace space with a piece of fabric, and the respiratory mask does the same—it is the most "personal" imprimatur of social distancing's alienation of the individual. But it is a sublime irony that the facemask and hygienic spacing share so much more. While both the facemask and hygienic spacing alienate bodies from other bodies, both also alienate individual identity from others. Consistent with the historical feminine veil, the facemask's effective deletion of the face—and the personality for which it is the paramount representation—is the result. During the comparatively short span of pandemic isolation, the mask is a momentary game-changer with respect to the casual reproduction of public race hierarchy.

To the racially marginalized of society, the respiratory mask is much more than a deterrent to aerosol contagion; it is a backstage pass to an egalitarian state of individuality that they regularly see but have scarcely ever experienced. For the effect of simply covering the chin and mouth to the low bridge of the nose unexpectedly obscures much more of one's public racial markers than is generally realized. The "gaiter" is the equivalent of what was once called a bandana, a neck scarf, or neckerchief; it extends from the back of the head completely obscuring the neck and the entire lower half of the face, further anonymizing the individual. I immediately seized upon the utility of the gaiter; for when a pair of sunglasses are combined with full-sleeved shirt and pants, a casual hat, and the hands tucked comfortably in the pocket, it is remarkable how ethnically standardized the male human form becomes.

The first time I put on a gaiter mask, I was spontaneously reminded of another long-forgotten and entirely sudden sensation of liberation. When I was a youngster, the manifest reality had always been that I was clearly seen as a secondary class of child, compassionately tolerated at best, a being to be restricted to the periphery of any gathering, a garnishing contrast to what an idealized child's appearance "could" be. To a notable portion of the racial mainstream, the darker-complected child is less a charming bundle of innocence and more a being whose premature size renders them a temporarily unimposing representative of a problematic race. However harsh such an observation might seem to the White mainstream, corroboration of this sentiment is increasingly apparent in the innumerable online videos of police treatment of underage minorities, a treatment reflective of mainstream apprehension, and often initiated by their calls. In light of this, the reader might realize the equalitarian state of grace that such a child might momentarily experience during Halloween; for this holiday was truly a transcendent experience. Halloween allowed any child to comprehensively camouflage him/herself within the vestments of a fictional character. Once fully costumed, I was suddenly like every other kid—an animated child comprised simply of two non-racialized arms, legs, a torso, and a head. It was spontaneously liberating, a democracy of juvenile individuality. The sweetness of a bag full of treats was easily overshadowed by this exotic state of reputable anonymity. And thus the reader might understand how—during a mask-wearing pandemic—the attainment of this default state of public individuality by a dark male would be seen as a refreshing elevation to equalitarian respectability. A profusion of citizens in masked parity meant—for the darker-complected male—that casually wandering about one's mainstream neighborhood would not elicit general alerts of a potential criminal on Nextdoor; entering a banking establishment would not promptly stiffen the spine of the security guard; going to a precinct to vote in a grade-school building would not evoke consternation of a threat to "our youth"; and—as articulated at the beginning of this section—standing in hotel lobbies at academic conferences might curtail servile demands or armed inquiries.

In his 1897 autoethnographic work, *The Souls of Black Folk*, W. E. B. Du Bois (1994) coined the term "double consciousness." Du Bois was referring to the schizophrenic condition to which the visible racial "other" was subject; it is the involuntary perspective of being the devalued "other" while simultaneously seeing oneself through the racialized perspective of others; the latter being inevitable as the visible minority had always been reared and immersed within the majority culture that, in its general practices, patterns, and preferences, casually affirms the subordinate status of darker skin color. While contradictory impulses are native to the human psychological condition, Du Bois was conveying that for racial minorities the contradictory conceptions of self are rarely submerged deep in the obscurity of the psyche that—for the mainstream—was anchored in reputable identity. The routine perception of self for the racial minority was subject to the continuous and inexorable psychological discord of the double consciousness.

The wearing of the respiratory facemask crystallizes for many racial minorities the schizophrenic condition of Du Bois' double consciousness. However curtailed during the self-isolationism of the coronavirus pandemic, individuals still venture into public to purchase the essential supplies of daily existence. But in a circumstance where routine participation in society is in part visually democratized and anonymized by respiratory masks, the existential threat is "no longer" the traditionally racial "other"; rather, the existential threat becomes the individual "not" wearing a mask. It has been interesting to be within a group of masked individuals standing in a widely spaced line to purchase items when a maskless individual appears, especially if that individual approaches too close. Flouting the public good simply by his/her presence, the maskless "other" strikingly evokes the same muted and spontaneous consternation as the historical "Black man" within definitive White spaces—an existential threat defined by his organic presence, an agent of disruption that compromises any benign predictability of the moment. At a minimum, the maskless individual during the pandemic is a self-indulgent spreader of insecurity. For well-masked minorities, the double consciousness gains a further degree of clarity during a pandemic; now, as a provisional member of the hygienic majority, the well-masked racial minority can actually see and participate, through muted consternation and stolen glances, in the spontaneous affirmation of a miscreant "other" that is not him/herself. Historical race relations might well be different if the Enlightenment document so iconic to the American experience had started "We the *Masked* People."

The mask's ability to make clear Du Bois' double consciousness is perhaps most impactful for the White mainstream. The partial nullification of being a readily perceived member of the standard-bearing race/ethnicity into just another masked stranger cannot be considered an advancement in a society stratified by race/ethnicity. The demotion of the mainstream individual from a person to a masked threat was expressed by conservative former reality TV star Judge Jeanine Pirro. Like many of her ideological disposition, rather than interpreting the mask as a prophylactic health measure, she reflexively construed the mask in social terms, decrying its anonymizing effect. "The point of the mask is to basically kind of dehumanize," she said. "[I]ts to, you know, frighten people. You don't know who's behind the mask" (in Dixon, 2020).

The regressive public attributes that the mainstream mask wearer has been demoted to takes on even more transformational angst when his/her ideology had always assigned propriety to race and class. For when the casual race-conscious mainstream individual is not wearing a mask in commercial settings, s/he suddenly becomes the embodiment of spontaneous consternation. As Du Bois' double consciousness describes, the maskless White conservative simultaneously experiences a comprehensive rejectionism as a problematic "other" from the very mainstream sensibility within which they themselves have long been personally considered "normal" and familiar. It has been interesting to see in person and on innumerable videos online mask-free members of the White mainstream become suddenly aware of the racial "double consciousness."

During the pandemic, the maskless member of the White mainstream perfectly illustrates in small what Emily Bazelon (2018), staff writer at the *New York Times*, asserts is a growing reality: White people "are losing the luxury of non-self-awareness, an emotionally complicated shift that we are not always taking well." And the discomforting circumstance is adrenalized by the advancing tide of systemic alienation and identity crisis that has already been endemic for decades. It is no surprise that the portion of the White mainstream that is the most alienated—and therefore most reliant on peremptory privilege tied to an immutable physical trait like skin color—would have the greatest collective resistance to the symbolic and performative identity deletion that the respiratory mask implies. Thus, several studies find that White Republican-leaning counties, which are comparatively less diverse and registering less per capita income, are the most resistant to social distancing recommendations and quarantine protocols in general (Allcott et al., 2020; Anderson, 2020; Barrios & Hochberg, 2020; Engle et al., 2020; Painter & Qiu, 2020; Wright et al., 2020). But more specifically, it is the core of right-wing populism so vigorously in ascendance at present that registers the highest degree of alienation. This alienation encompasses not only people's relationship to each other but also to a historical identity, and to a sense of purpose and direction in life for themselves and their entire reference group. Thus, Republicans as a whole identified as feeling the most alienated (Harris Poll, 2016; PR Newswire, 2016), and Trump supporters in excess of that. Those who say that they often feel like a "stranger in their own land" were 3.5 times more likely to favor Trump (Public Religion Research Institute, 2017). And the multiple forms of disconnectedness are dramatic. White working-class Trump supporters of all ages were much less likely than their college-educated peers to participate in a broad array of social connectivity activities such as sports teams, book clubs, or neighborhood associations; 55% of the White working class versus 31% of college-educated Whites said they seldom or never participated in those kinds of activities (Green, 2017). Stemming from the waning of these social linkages, the core of right-wing populist support reports an acute sense of vulnerability with respect to social identity (Barber & Pope, 2019, p. 53; also see Ellis & Stimson, 2012; Greene, 1999; Grossmann & Hopkins, 2016); and therefore, this demographic segment registers the most resistance to wearing the identity-deleting respiratory facemask. Dramatically lower than either Democrats or Independents, Republicans (48%) were the least likely to wear a protective mask every time when leaving home or being in contact with other people (71% and 86%, respectively; NBC News/SurveyMonkey, 2020). They were also the most likely (27%) to strongly or somewhat oppose wearing a mask in general when compared with Democrats (3%; Associated Press-NORC Center for Public Affairs Research, 2020; also see Gallup Panel, 2020).

The most rudimentary function of the respiratory mask is as a prophylactic barrier to what is perceived as a hazard. And thus, the mask cannot be therefore thematically discerned from the agenda of those demographic segments of the population who reflexively resort to therapeutic barriers as a preservation of their identity, such as a border wall, the legalistic equivalent that is the Muslim immigration ban, or the protective barrier that Trump asserted "saved" the White suburbs from the penetration of "others." Anti-Obama birtherism, the "Chinese virus," chants to racial minorities to "go back home," and the specter of advancing Mexican rapists are all predicated on the utility of a therapeutic barrier to preserve the righteous. Thus, when the White maskless individual is personally identified as an individual who needs to be behind a very public therapeutic barrier, the schizophrenia of the double consciousness is aggravated by the corresponding passion these individuals manifest themselves when they chanted the same exclusion to perceived "others." At this early point in the pandemic, there doesn't seem to be any readily available research to quantify the potency of the maskless White person's "reaction" to being "otherized." But the outrage is clearly heated—an outrage from the sudden exposure to Du Bois' double consciousness for a population without the historical and quotidian familiarity with 'othering' that racial minorities have.

Finding oneself tossed unceremoniously on the disreputable side of the national mask manifests in many forms.

"You don't look 'American,'" she said.

It was an odd statement to make on the first meet of a blind date. It was not stated with malice or conscious disregard, just a self-indulgent curiosity that was comfortably seated on the presumption that she was entitled to make such a statement about my racial identity on our first encounter. In light of her knowledge that I was professionally conversant in issues of space and identity, it appeared to have been said so as to demonstrate her own cultural literacy as a divorced homemaker of quality. "Maybe from southern India or whereabouts. *Maybe*," she added with discernment.

A deep breath and a moment to therapeutically exhale is—at this point in life—an entitlement I've granted myself.

"Ma'am," I responded.

"In fact—in contrast to me—it is *you* who doesn't look vaguely like the historical inhabitants of this continent. You appear more like I've seen in Europe. Indeed, not even "western" Europe. I'd say central eastern Europe .... *ahhhhh* .... Slovakia comes to mind ... part of the latter wave of European immigrants arriving uninvited from 1883 to 2014."

There was no such subset of White Eastern European physiognomy that I was familiar with. But when encountering such presumptive statements from the racial mainstream, I feel entitled in my response to such fanciful liberties since scornful language or corrective brutality are ill-advised and unproductive reactions.

The woman seemed to be caught short by the statement. Her discomfort was palpable; for it was "her" who was unexpectedly now positioned on the other side of the national mask. And worse still, quietly suspended on her face was the realization that she could not even claim the cosmetic pretext of historical immigration accuracy or superior professional pedigree on the subject to justify her casual act of "othering."

While the respiratory mask has clear and rational epidemiological purposes in the short term, it cannot help but harmonize with historical forms of social distancing that long precede it.

References

Allcott, H., Boxell, L., Conway, J., Gentzkow, M., Thaler, M., & Yang, D. (2020). Polarization and Public Health: Partisan Differences in Social Distancing During COVID-19. *National Center for Biotechnology Information*. Retrieved from www.ncbi.nlm.nih.gov/pmc/articles/PMC7409721/

Anderson, M. (2020). Early Evidence on Social Distancing in Response to COVID-19 in the United States. *SSRN*. Retrieved from https://papers.ssrn.com/sol3/papers.cfm?abstract_id=3569368

Associated Press-NORC Center for Public Affairs Research. (2020, July 23). 3 in 4 Americans Back Requiring Wearing Masks. Retrieved from https://apnews.com/article/ap-top-news-understanding-the-outbreak-health-politics-lifestyle-9126a38ef22c244f9ca18f9584061f8d

Bacher-Hicks, A., Goodman, J., & Mulhern, C. (2020). Inequality in Household Adaptation to Schooling Shocks: COVID-Induced Online Learning Engagement in Real Time. *National Bureau of Economic Research*, Working Paper No. 27555. Retrieved from www.nber.org/papers/w27555

Barber, M., & Pope, J. C. (2019). Does Party Trump Ideology? Disentangling Party and Ideology in America. *American Political Science Review, 113*(1), 38–54.

Barrios, J. M., & Hochberg, Y. V. (2020). Risk Perception through the Lens of Politics in the Time of the COVID-19 Pandemic. *University of Chicago, Becker Friedman Institute for Economics Working Paper*. Retrieved from https://bfi.uchicago.edu/working-paper/risk-perception-through-the-lens-of-politics-in-the-time-of-the-covid-19-pandemic/

Bazelon, E. (2018, June 13). White People Are Noticing Something New: Their Own Whiteness. *The New York Times*. Retrieved from www.nytimes.com/2018/06/13/magazine/white-people-are-noticing-something-new-their-own-whiteness.html

Blum, J. (2020, August 17). Trump Amplifies Ugly Attack on "Democrat." *HuffPost*, Retrieved from www.huffpost.com/entry/trump-democrat-cities_n_5f39e66bc5b65bbd8c8ef9c5

Bridge, G. (2003). Time Space Trajectories in Provincial Gentrification. *Urban Studies, 40*(12), 2545–2556.

Brodkin Sacks, K. (1994). How Did Jews Become White Folks? In S. Gregory & R. Sanjek (Eds.), *Race* (pp. 78–102). New Brunswick: Rutgers University Press.

Brooks, D. (2000). *Bobos in Paradise: The New Upper Class and How They Got There.* New York: Simon & Schuster.

Brown, M. K. et al. (2003). *Whitewashing Race: The Myth of a Color-Blind Society.* Berkeley: University of California Press.

Brown-Saracino, J. (2004). Social Preservationists and the Quest for Authentic Community. *City & Community, 3*(2), 135–156.

Butler, T. (2007). Re-Urbanizing London Docklands: Gentrification, Suburbanization or New Urbanism? *International Journal of Urban and Regional Research, 31*(4), 759–781.

Carney, T. P. (2019). *Alienated America: Why Some Places Thrive While Others Collapse.* New York: Harper.

Caulfield, J. (1989). Gentrification and Desire. *Canadian Review of Sociology and Anthropology, 26*, 617–632.

Chiou, L., & Tucker, C. (2020). Social Distancing, Internet Access and Inequality. *National Bureau of Economic Research*, Working Paper No. 26982. Retrieved from www.nber.org/papers/w26982

de Oliver, M. (2021, May 21). Emporia and the Exclusion Identity: Conservative Populist Alienation in the US and Its Anti-Immigrationism. *International Journal of Politics, Culture, and Society.* Retrieved from http://doi.org/10.1007/s10767-021-09397-5

Dixon, B. (2020). Brianna Keilar's Masterful Take Down of Trump and Fox News. *The Benjamin Dixon Show*, Time stamp: 2:02. Retrieved from www.youtube.com/watch?v=NVhmEsEkQqs&app=desktop

Du Bois, W. E. B. (1994). *The Souls of Black Folk.* New York: Gramercy Books.

Ellis, C., & Stimson, J. A. (2012). *Ideology in America.* New York: Cambridge University Press.

Engle, S., Stromme, J., & Zhou, A. (2020). Staying at Home: Mobility Effects of COVID-19. *VoxEu.* Retrieved from https://voxeu.org/article/staying-home-mobility-effects-covid-19

Falconer, R. (2020, September 3). Trump Issues Memo to Cut Funding from 'Anarchist' Democratic Cities. *Axios.* Retrieved from www.axios.com/trump-memo-cut-funding-anarchist-democratic-cities-ac658965-a427-4149-87f4-58c1f9a8506a.html

Florida, R. L. (2002). *The Rise of the Creative Class: And How It's Transforming Work, Leisure, Community and Everyday Life.* New York: Basic Books.

Gallup Panel. (2020, July 13). Americans' Face Mask Usage Varies Greatly by Demographics. Retrieved from https://news.gallup.com/poll/315590/americans-face-mask-usage-varies-greatly-demographics.aspx

Graham, R. (2020, September 1). Support for Black Lives Matter Is Dropping—among White Americans: Three Months after George Floyd's Killing, Fewer White People Believe That Racism Is a Big Problem. *The Boston Globe.* Retrieved from www.bostonglobe.com/2020/09/01/opinion/support-black-lives-matter-is-dropping-among-white-americans/

Green, E. (2017, March 5). The Death of Community and the Rise of Trump. *The Atlantic.* Retrieved from www.theatlantic.com/politics/archive/2017/03/religiously-unaffiliated-white-americans/518340/

Greene, S. (1999). Understanding Party Identification: A Social Identity Approach. *Political Psychology, 20*(2), 393–403.

Grossmann, M., & Hopkins, D. A. (2016). *Asymmetric Politics: Ideological Republicans and Group Interest Democrats.* New York: Oxford University Press.

Guardian. (2015, July 6). Donald Trump: Mexican Migrants Bring "Tremendous Infectious Disease" to US. *The Guardian*. Retrieved from www.theguardian.com/us-news/2015/jul/06/donald-trump-mexican-immigrants-tremendous-infectious-disease

Harris Poll. (2016). Americans' Sense of Alienation Remains at Record High. Poll Taken May 31-June 2 Among 2,019 Adults aged 18+. *The Harris Poll*. Retrieved from https://theharrispoll.com/in-the-midst-of-the-contentious-presidential-primary-elections-the-harris-poll-measured-how-alienated-americans-feel-as-part-of-a-long-term-trend-the-last-time-alienation-was-measured-was-in-novemb/

Horowitz, J. (2020, April 15). Lower-Income Parents Most Concerned About Their Children Falling Behind Amid COVID-19 School Closures. *Pew Research Center*. A total of 4,917 panelists conducted April 7 to April 12, 2020. Retrieved from www.pewresearch.org/fact-tank/2020/04/15/lower-income-parents-most-concerned-about-their-children-falling-behind-amid-covid-19-school-closures/

Hosmer, C. B. (1965). *Presence of the Past*. New York: G.P. Putnam's Sons.

Kimball, S. (2019, July 27). Trump calls Baltimore a 'disgusting, rat and rodent infested mess' in attack on Rep. Elijah Cummings. *CNBC*. Retrieved from www.cnbc.com/2019/07/27/trump-calls-baltimore-a-disgusting-rat-and-rodent-infested-mess-in-attack-on-rep-elijah-cummings.html

Kiple, K., & Kiple, V. (1980). The African Connection: Slavery, Disease and Racism. *Phylon*, *41*(3), 211–222.

Kloor, K. (2020, January 17). The #MAGA Lawyer behind Michael Flynn's Scorched-Earth Legal Strategy. *Politico*. Retrieved from www.politico.com/news/magazine/2020/01/17/maga-lawyer-behind-michael-flynn-legal-strategy-098712

Ley, D. (2003). Artists, Aestheticisation and the Field of Gentrification. *Urban Studies, 40*, 2527–2544.

Lloyd, R., & Clark, T. N. (2001). The City as an Entertainment Machine. *Research in Urban Sociology: Critical Perspectives on Urban Redevelopment, 6*, 359–380.

Logan, E. B. (2020, September 4). White People Have Gentrified Black Lives Matter. It's a Problem. *Los Angeles Times*. Retrieved from www.latimes.com/opinion/story/2020-09-04/black-lives-matter-white-people-portland-protests-nfl

Marx, K. (1932). Economic & Philosophic Manuscripts of 1844. Translated: By Martin Milligan From the German Text, Revised by Dirk J. Struik, Contained in Marx/Engels, Gesamtausgabe. Retrieved from www.marxists.org/archive/marx/works/download/pdf/Economic-Philosophic-Manuscripts-1844.pdf

Massey, D., & Denton, M. (1993). *American Apartheid: Segregation and the Making of the Underclass*. Cambridge, MA: Harvard University Press.

NBC News/SurveyMonkey. (2020). Coronavirus Concerns Remain Steady. Retrieved from www.surveymonkey.com/curiosity/nbc-poll-covid-july26/

Nisbet, R. A. (1962). *The Quest for Community: A Study in the Ethics of Order and Freedom*. New York: Oxford University Press.

Painter, M., & Qiu, T. (2020, May 11). Political Beliefs Affect Compliance with COVID-19 Social Distancing Orders, *VoxEU*. Retrieved from https://voxeu.org/article/political-beliefs-and-compliance-social-distancing-orders

Papageorge, N. et al. (2020). Socio-Demographic Factors Associated with Self-Protecting Behavior During the COVID-19 Pandemic. *National Bureau of Economic Research*, Working Paper 27378. Retrieved from www.nber.org/papers/w27378

Pew Research Center. (2020). Many Black and Asian Americans Say They Have Experienced Discrimination Amid the COVID-19 Outbreak. July 1 survey of 9,654 U.S. adults conducted from June 4-10. Retrieved from www.pewsocialtrends.org/2020/07/01/many-black-and-asian-americans-say-they-have-experienced-discrimination-amid-the-covid-19-outbreak/

PR Newswire. (2016). Americans' Sense of Alienation Remains at Record High. Retrieved from www.prnewswire.com/news-releases/americans-sense-of-alienation-remains-at-record-high-300305687.html

Public Religion Research Institute. (2017, May 5). Beyond Economics: Fears of Cultural Displacement Pushed the White Working Class to Trump. *PRRI/The Atlantic Report.* Washington, DC. Retrieved from www.prri.org/research/white-working-class-attitudes-economy-trade-immigration-election-donald-trump/

Putnam, R. D. (1995). Bowling Alone: America's Declining Social Capital. *Journal of Democracy, January,* 65–78.

Raban, J. (1974). *Soft City.* London: Hamish Hamilton.

Shah, N. (2001). *Contagious Divides: Epidemics and Race in San Francisco's Chinatown.* Berkeley: University of California Press.

Smith, N. (1987). Of Yuppies and Housing: Gentrification, Social Structuring and the Urban Dream. *Environment and Planning D: Society and Space, 5,* 151–172.

Tesler, M. (2020, August 9). Support for Black Lives Matter Surged during Protests, but Is Waning among White Americans. *FiveThirtyEight.* Retrieved from https://fivethirtyeight.com/features/support-for-black-lives-matter-surged-during-protests-but-is-waning-among-white-americans/

Trump, D. (2020, September 3). Memorandum on Reviewing Funding to State and Local Government Recipients That Are Permitting Anarchy, Violence, and Destruction in American Cities. Retrieved from www.whitehouse.gov/presidential-actions/memorandum-reviewing-funding-state-local-government-recipients-permitting-anarchy-violence-destruction-american-cities/

Warde, A. (1991). Gentrification as Consumption Issues of Class and Gender. *Environment and Planning D: Society and Space, 6,* 75–95.

Washington, J. (2020, June 18). Why Did Black Lives Matter Protests Attract Unprecedented White Support? *The Undefeated.* Retrieved from https://theundefeated.com/features/why-did-black-lives-matter-protests-attract-unprecedented-white-support/

Wright, A. L., Sonin, K., Driscoll, J., & Wilson, J. (2020). *Poverty and Economic Dislocation Reduce Compliance with COVID-19 Shelter-in-Place Protocols.* University of Chicago. Retrieved from https://bfi.uchicago.edu/working-paper/poverty-and-economic-dislocation-reduce-compliance-with-covid-19-shelter-in-place-protocols/

Zukin, S. (1982). *Loft Living: Culture and Capital in Urban Change.* Baltimore: Johns Hopkins University Press.

12

"TO MAKE LIVE AND LET DIE"

Vaccine Nationalism, Vulnerable Solidarity, and Global Inequalities in the Age of COVID-19

Jordan Liz

Introduction

In September 2020, Oxfam International estimated that wealthy nations representing 13% of the world's population had already purchased 51% of the expected doses of the five leading COVID-19 vaccine candidates. Oxfam further estimated that approximately 61% of the world's population will not have access to a vaccine until at least 2022 (Tabacek, 2020). The Center for Global Development similarly predicts that it will take until September 2023 for enough vaccine doses to be produced to inoculate all of humanity; while the Serum Institute in India, the largest vaccine producer in the world, predicts that it will take until the end of 2024 (Bacchus, 2020). This drastic juxtaposition between the vaccine haves and haves-not is the byproduct of "vaccine nationalism." Vaccine nationalism refers to a series of practices whereby a country attempts to secure vaccines for its citizens before they are made available to other countries. Vaccine nationalism has been widely criticized by officials from the United Nations (UN) and World Health Organization (WHO). As WHO chief Tedros Adhanom Ghebreyesus remarked in December 2020, vaccines "must be shared equally as global public goods, not as private commodities that widen inequalities and become yet another reason some people are left behind" (Lederer, 2020). This point is worth emphasizing. The challenges created by COVID-19 are multifaceted and impact diverse populations, whether in the United States or abroad, in ways that are inextricably linked to historical and structural inequalities that cut across race, sex/gender, class, among many other factors. Within this context, vaccine nationalism functions as yet another marginalizing and oppressive force on those already marginalized and oppressed.

This chapter examines how vaccine nationalism operates according to a biopolitical logic aimed at safeguarding the lives of some, while treating the lives

DOI: 10.4324/9781003268710-12

of others as expendable. Vaccine nationalism represents a dangerous globalization of biopolitics precisely at a time when the international community should be banding together to combat the COVID-19 pandemic. The rest of the chapter is divided into four sections: the first section provides a brief overview of the literature on vaccine nationalism. In particular, it notes that, whether for moral, political, public health, and even economic reasons, there is a growing consensus that such practices are ultimately detrimental to global stability and the interests of so-called "developed" nations. Despite this, the trend toward vaccine nationalism continues. To explain this tension, the second section provides an overview of biopolitics, focusing on its relationship to nationalism. The third section examines how vaccine nationalism, as a biopolitical project, functions to endanger the lives of those living in predominately non-White and impoverished nations, as well as serving as the basis for new forms of stigmatization and discrimination. Finally, by way of conclusion, the final section turns its attention to the WHO's global vaccine distribution effort, the COVID-19 Vaccine Global Access Facility (abbreviated COVAX), and the possibility of achieving vaccine multilateralism. Here I draw upon Myisha Cherry's work on "vulnerable solidarity" to examine how a biopolitical framework may contribute toward that end (Cherry, 2017).

The Problems of Vaccine Nationalism

Across the growing literature on vaccine nationalism, broad consensus is quickly emerging around one specific point—unfettered vaccine nationalism should be avoided. Ezekiel Emanuel and his colleagues argue that vaccine nationalism is morally reprehensible since it neglects core values of "benefiting people and limiting harm, prioritizing the disadvantaged, and equal moral concern" for individuals (Emanuel et al., 2020, pp. 1309–1310). Instead, they propose a Fair Priority Model that ties vaccine distribution to preventing death, especially premature death, and reducing serious economic and social deprivations. While this model has garnered significant praise, there are some who argue that *limited* vaccine nationalism may be morally justifiable. For instance, Reidar Lie and Franklin Miller argue that the Fair Priority Model and the WHO's model are untenable since "national governments have both a right and a duty to secure access to a COVID-19 vaccine for their citizens first" (Lie & Miller, 2020). Similarly, Kyle Ferguson and Arthur Caplan argue that limited national partiality in allocating vaccines is a core component of justice (Ferguson & Caplan, 2020). Even Emanuel and his colleagues recognize that some degree of national partiality may be morally defensible by appealing to the moral worth of "associative ties" (Emanuel et al., 2020, p. 1309). Nevertheless, none of these scholars advocate for *unrestricted* vaccine nationalism given its disregard for cosmopolitan duties of benevolence, fairness, and equity.

From a political perspective, vaccine nationalism has been condemned as detrimental to global politics and international relations. Colin Carlson and Alexandra Phelan argue that, by undermining equitable distribution, vaccine nationalism could see a total state-shift in global connectedness, as some countries become essentially impossible to travel to or from. This situation will be compounded if countries require vaccination certificates for entry without parallel equitable global vaccine-access. Fragmentation begets fragmentation, without multilateral cooperation, COVID-19 could redraw the world map.

Carlson and Phelan, 2020, p. 545

The implementation of travel restrictions and vaccination certificates (or immunity passports) is likely to exacerbate existing racial, ethnic, gender, and socioeconomic inequalities throughout the world (Liz, 2021; Schmidt, 2020). Moreover, this fragmentation could undermine international efforts to curb the spread of COVID-19—an effort that will become increasingly important as new variants of the virus emerge. As David Fidler argues, vaccine nationalism creates "a gap between science and politics that makes the pandemic worse and undermines what science and health diplomacy could achieve" (Fidler, 2020, p. 749). The longer the pandemic extends, and the more these restrictions are normalized, the more difficult global coordination may become. This will impact the global response to both COVID-19 as well as future outbreaks. Notably, travel restrictions are one of the few incentives under WHO's International Health Regulations to promote rapid notification of emerging global public health emergencies. The widespread implementation of travel restrictions due to COVID-19 undermines this incentive, and thus may lead to delays that put every country at greater risk during future pandemics (Carlson & Phelan, 2020).

Vaccine nationalism has also been criticized as undermining economic recovery efforts. As José Guimón and Rajneesh Narula write, addressing the COVID-19 pandemic exposes "the underlying contradiction between the sovereignty and interest of nation states and the borderless world shaped by growing interdependence of the scientific community and economic actors" (Guimón & Narula, 2020, p. 41). The interconnectedness of national economies makes rejecting vaccine nationalism in each party's economic self-interest. According to a study conducted by the non-profit RAND Corporation, vaccine nationalism could cost the global economy upward of $1.2 trillion a year in terms of gross domestic product (GDP). By this report's estimation, if wealthy countries paid for the vaccines needed by the poorest, the benefit-to-cost ratio would be 4.8:1, or for every dollar spent on a vaccine, the GDP of developed countries would increase by $4.80 (Hafner et al., 2020). Similarly, the World Economic Forum estimates that the cost of vaccine nationalism to high-income countries will be $119 billion per year, whereas the cost of supplying low-income countries with the vaccine would be an estimated $25 billion (Kretchmer, 2020). Even from the perspective of vaccine manufacturing and development, vaccine nationalism poses a serious problem. As Thomas Bollyky and Chad P. Brown explain, vaccines are the byproduct of a complex and intricate network that relies on international cooperation. As such, vaccine nationalism "will have profound and far-reaching consequences. Without global coordination, countries may bid against one another, driving up the price of vaccines and related materials" (Bollyky & Brown, 2020, p. 97).

Beyond these considerations, there is a more pressing and even more obvious objection against vaccine nationalism: unless the entire world has access to the vaccine, the *pandemic* cannot end. Already new variants are emerging that are more infectious and may even be resistant to currently available vaccines (Cohen, 2021). The longer the developing world—a population that accounts for the majority of humanity—is left without access to the vaccine, the more likely new variants will emerge that could potentially prolong the pandemic and lead to the deaths of thousands, if not millions. From a public health perspective, these are clear reasons for rejecting vaccine nationalism. And yet, the trend continues. The question then is: why? If vaccine nationalism is detrimental for moral, political, economic, and public health reasons, then why are so many countries so vehemently pursuing it? While some of this may be due to short-sightedness, unrestrained self-interestedness, or even an inability—or unwillingness—to recognize the extent to which each country depends on others, such nationalism may also stem from a more problematic base: the failure to recognize the lives of foreign Others as equally as important as the lives of one's own citizens.[1] Especially in light of the reality of global racism, colonialism, and other forms of prejudice—many of which have been historically and contemporarily rationalized within the very language of nationalism—this consideration cannot be readily discarded (Balibar, 2011). To explore this further, I now turn to an overview of biopolitics and its relationship to nationalism.

Biopolitics, State Racism, and Nationalism

For Michel Foucault, biopolitics refers to the techniques used by modern states to manage, control, and regulate the life and health of populations. For instance, during the COVID-19 pandemic, travel restrictions barring entry to non-citizens, social distancing guidelines, mask-wearing mandates, and shelter-in-place orders are all examples of biopolitical technologies (Sylvia IV, 2020; Wagner et al., 2021). Now, a key function of biopolitical governance is the designation of which lives should be protected, and which should be left strategically exposed to harm, subjugation, and death (Foucault, 2003).[2] For instance, the failure of the state to enact legislation that takes meaningful steps to address centuries of structural racism, sexism, and other forms of prejudice all serve to maintain marginalized groups within a perpetual state of vulnerability, hardship, and suffering (Cherry, 2017).

To hasten these deaths, Foucault argues that the state must become racist. As he writes, state racism

> is primarily a way of introducing a break into the domain of life that is under power's control: the break between what must live and what must die. The appearance within the biological continuum of the human race of races, the distinction among races, the hierarchy of races, the fact that certain races are

described as good and that others, in contrast, are described as inferior: all this is a way of fragmenting the field of the biological that power controls.

Foucault, 2003, p. 255

It is a way of delineating how the state will use its power "to make live" those whose lives are considered valuable, and "to let die" those who it does not (Foucault, 2003, p. 239). These divisions are fabricated and maintained via discourse, or ways of speaking and thinking that shape what people consider to be "normal" and even what they hold to be true (Foucault, 2003, 2010). For instance, the discourse of "the illegal immigrant" invading the country perpetuates and nurtures the belief that undocumented immigrants are dangerous and must be eliminated. It achieves this even though immigrants, regardless of their legal status, have a lower crime rate and criminal incarceration rate than U.S. citizens (Landgrave & Nowrasteh, 2019). Since those statistics are incompatible with "the illegal immigrant" discourse, however, they are casted aside as "fake news." At the same time, this discourse serves as justification for the vast array of immigration enforcement, surveillance, and disciplinary mechanisms that collectively function to endanger the lives of undocumented immigrants.

As this example demonstrates, state racism is not limited to U.S.- ethnic and racial categorizations. Within a biopolitical framework, "the illegal immigrant" *is* a racialized subject: they represent a population that has been discursively transformed into a biological and existential threat to the nation and its citizens (Valdez, 2016; Yeng, 2013). As William Schinkel explains, citizenship is not a mere legal designation, but rather refers to a series of mechanisms that classify and organize people. For instance, "civic citizenship" distinguishes between those who have political rights and civil liberties from those who are denied such freedom; "social citizenship" distinguishes between those who are integrated within and acculturated to the economic, social, and cultural norms of society from those who are not; "moral citizenship" distinguishes between those who are "good" citizens from those who are "bad," etc (Schinkel, 2010). In each case, citizenship "attaches to bodies certain territorialized privileges and life-chances, ranging from the freedoms of civic citizenship to the biopolitical possibilities of the welfare state that are part of 'social citizenship'" (Schinkel 2010, p. 165). As such, citizenship, as a series of biopolitical technologies, demarcates which populations should live and which should be left to die. This applies to populations *both* within and across nations. It allows for both undocumented immigrants *and* minorities groups, such as African Americans, to be targets of biopolitics, whether by denying citizenship or subjugating groups to a second-class citizenship. During the COVID-19 pandemic, the biopolitics of citizenship can thus help explain both the racial disparities of the vaccine distribution effort, as well as efforts to deny vaccine access to undocumented frontline workers (Armus, 2021; Doherty & Kenen, 2021).

In general, the division between "the citizen," on the one hand, and "the foreigner" or "the outsider," on the other, serves to maintain a dynamic, whereby the nation is inherently "juxtaposed to a domain 'outside society,' in which 'non-integrated' individuals resides—marked as such by a spatial metaphor (inside/outside) which rhetorically emphasizes the divide between 'society' and its others" (Schinkel, 2010, p. 166). For Nick Vaughan-Williams, such juxtapositions represent instances of an "inclusive exclusion," whereby those who are excluded from the political community remain nevertheless related to it as potential threats that the state and citizens must perpetually guard against (Vaughan-Williams, 2009, p. 734). In maintaining these inclusive exclusions, biopolitics not only divides but also builds solidarity and unity. It provides the foundation for a national identity grounded in the belief that society must be defended against "the foreigner" or "the outsider." Moreover, because this "outsider" is not only separate from the political community, but "inferior," "bad," and "dangerous," it cements the status of the national population as "superior," even "exceptional." Perhaps ironically, this superiority discursively positions the nation as a constant target, whether from terrorist organizations or foreign nations. As such, it serves to justify more spending on law enforcement, military defense, and counterterrorism, as well as increased efforts to protect U.S. citizenship (e.g., calls to repeal birthright citizenship) (Valdez, 2016; Yeng, 2013).

COVID-19 and the Biopolitics of Vaccine Nationalism

Throughout the pandemic, citizenship status provides the underlying basis for willingly allowing the death of hundreds of thousands to occur without impunity. In the name of defending the nation, each country is "justified" in acquiring as much of the vaccine as is necessary to vaccinate their entire population as soon as possible. Vaccine nationalism, alongside other protectionist policies deployed during the pandemic, promotes an arms race wherein each nation is pitted against each other in a struggle to end the outbreak within their own borders.[3] The rest of this section examines the biopolitical consequences of vaccine nationalism on those living in developing countries, as well as how vaccine nationalism may generate new forms of discrimination against biopolitical "outsiders."

COVID-19, the Developing World, and "Letting Die"

COVID-19 has been devastating to developing countries. In 2020, COVID-19 was the leading cause of death in Peru, Brazil, Chile, and Panama; and the second leading cause in Mexico, Bolivia, Colombia, and Costa Rica (Beaubien, 2020). According to the Organization for Economic Co-operation and Development (OECD), COVID-19 deaths in Asian-Pacific countries have steadily increased since late March. By October 2020, the region accounted for approximately 12% of total COVID-19 deaths worldwide (OCED/WHO, 2020). To date, after the United States, India, Brazil, and Mexico have suffered the most deaths from the pandemic, with Latin America and Asia being the worst-hit regions (Horton, 2020). In January 2021, the Africa Centers for Disease Control and Prevention reported that the average COVID-19 case fatality rate rose to 2.5% across the continent, with

21 countries reporting case fatality rates greater than 3%. The worldwide average, at that point, was 2.2% (Campbell, 2021). Moreover, while developed countries such as the United States and United Kingdom have consistently reported the highest overall mortality rates, developing countries have reported the larger share of COVID-19 deaths among young and middle-aged adults (Chauvin et al., 2020). Studies have found that poor medical infrastructure, residential overcrowding, and higher rates of informal employment in these countries have contributed to higher infection rates among the non-elderly population. Moreover, higher prevalence of preexisting conditions has contributed to lower recovery rates among those infected (Chauvin et al., 2020). Given the underdeveloped public health infrastructure, and the lack of widespread testing in many developing countries, these figures may underestimate the true disease burden.

Without access to a vaccine, these rates are likely to worsen as new variants of the virus emerge, fragile healthcare systems are increasingly overburdened, and scarce medical resources are drained. As Owen Dyer notes, while wealthy countries will likely donate unneeded doses of the vaccine, they will first wait and see how well those vaccines perform (especially against emerging variants) and for how long they confer immunity (Dyer, 2020). This outcome, however, is far from necessary. As Mohga Kamal Yanni from the People Vaccine Alliance notes, "Rich countries have enough doses to vaccinate everyone nearly three times over, whilst poor countries don't have enough to even reach health workers and people at risk" (Oxfam International, 2020). By holding onto surplus vaccines, Western states exercise control within their own sovereign borders and over developing countries as well. Domestically, it ensures that there is enough to "make live" their national population; while internationally, it enables, what Lauren Berlant refers to as, a "slow death." For Berlant, slow death "refers to the physical wearing out of a population and the deterioration of people in that population that is very nearly a defining condition of their experience and historical existence" (Berlant, 2007, p. 754). Slow death is more than a mere acknowledgment that all humans are gradually moving toward death, but rather the recognition that the lives of some are systematically and structurally maintained in permanent states of debilitation. For Berlant, slow death blurs the lines between life and death. It is "a condition of being worn out by the activity of reproducing life" (Berlant, 2007, p. 759). The longer the pandemic persists within developing countries, the more difficult and exhausting the mere act of surviving becomes. Moreover, as the pandemic becomes increasingly a crisis exclusive to developing countries, the more likely it is to become normalized internationally as another difficult and unfortunate aspect of "normal" of life in those regions—a situation in which developed nations may *altruistically* intervene, but ultimately are regarded as lacking any obligation to do so. As such, developed nations can maintain a state of crisis and death abroad, while reaping the psychic rewards of appearing humanitarian.

Vaccine nationalism threatens to transform the COVID-19 pandemic into a series of localized epidemics. Even with the vaccine, COVID-19, like influenza, may become endemic around the world and even require yearly vaccination (Lavine et al., 2021; Phillips, 2021). In the long run, the only difference may be how easily countries are able to cope and for which strains of the virus are vaccines regularly produced. There is already evidence suggesting that the Oxford/AstraZeneca vaccine may be less effective for treating the B.1.351 variant of COVID-19 that emerged in South Africa (Cohen, 2021). If regional variants emerge that do not impact wealthy countries, then production of suitable vaccines will likely be delayed. This is already the global norm for pharmaceutical innovations. As Rino Rappuoli, chief scientist at GlaxoSmithKline's vaccine division, explains, the substantial amount of funding provided by wealthy nations was a major factor in producing the COVID-19 vaccine with such unprecedented speed. As he succinctly put it, "Unless you put in the money, there's no way to accelerate" (Ball, 2020). For Tankut Atuk, the perpetual undertreating of the sick and dying by pharmaceutical companies is another key aspect to the "slow death" that occurs in those regions (Atuk, 2020). Whether Ebola, malaria, or measles, epidemics and pandemics have wreaked havoc in developing countries for decades. In the face of this suffering, the inability to finance lifesaving treatments serves as a perverse justification for the inaction of pharmaceutical companies. This situation is further—and intentionally—exacerbated by developed nations. For instance, wealthy nations, including the United Kingdom and European Union (EU), vehemently opposed bids by India and South Africa to suspend patents and intellectual property related to the production of COVID-19 vaccines and treatment. These waivers would have made it easier for developing countries to produce the vaccine themselves. Developed nations, however, opposed the measure alleging that it would stifle innovation in the pharmaceutical industry (Pandey, 2021). While the United States initially opposed such measures, in light of the worsening COVID-19 crisis in India, the Biden administration eventually began supporting calls to lift waivers. This decision was met by intense criticism by pharmaceutical companies and world leaders from developed nations. In particular, many noted that the United States could immediately help foreign nations by lifting its export bans on raw materials necessary for global vaccine production (Casert & Hatton, 2021). The denial of access to intellectual property or necessary raw materials constitutes a biopolitical maneuver to ensure that global medical resources are not used to "make live" the "bad" race.

Slow death in developing countries is facilitated by a lack of economic incentive from multibillion pharmaceutical companies, as well as callous and manipulative political and economic interventions by developed countries. Vaccine nationalism threatens to further exacerbate this by prolonging the dire economic, social, and political impacts of COVID-19. According to the United Nations Development Program (UNDP), income losses in developing countries are estimated to exceed $220 billion in 2020 (UNDP, 2020). Similarly, Daniel Gurara, Stefania Fabrizio, and Johannes Wiegand find that without international support from wealthy countries, lasting damages seems unavoidable. Among these, they cite the possibility of long-term economic "scarring," or the permanent loss of productive capacity, as particularly troubling. Scarring risks worsening health and educational outcomes, creating more poverty, and exacerbating gender inequalities across developing countries

(Gurara et al., 2020). Already dire economic conditions have led to a rise in child labor, child trafficking, and child marriage, threatening to undo years of progress and endangering millions of children in the poorest countries (Ellis-Petersen & Chaurasia, 2020; Gettleman & Raj, 2020). In practicing vaccine nationalism, developed countries extend this suffering, whether deliberately or indifferently. They "scar" all aspects of life in developing countries: biological, economic, social, and political. In the process, it deepens the extent to which developing countries will depend upon foreign aid and political intervention from wealthy nations and corporations. Without access to a vaccine, developing nations will become further entrenched within global biopolitical systems of control and exploitation.

"Reasonable" Discrimination, Vaccine Nationalism, and COVID-19

Vaccine nationalism represents a powerful biopolitical maneuver that takes advantage of a novel pathogen to exert control over foreign bodies without any *direct* intervention. At the same time, it provides a built-in justification: the duty to protect one's citizens by prioritizing their needs over those of other countries. Many political theorists and philosophers have argued that liberalism justifies discriminating against non-citizens, or those excluded from the hypothetical social contract that grounds the political community (Song, 2018; Walzer, 1984).[4]

This right to exclude has historically and contemporarily been used to justify discriminating against people of color. For instance, while the xenophobic Trumpian "America First" discourse calls for an end to all "illegal" immigration, it is actually targeted at immigrants from the so-called "shithole" countries (Dawsey, 2018). For this reason, proponents never reference the hundreds of thousands undocumented immigrants from Canada and European countries living in the United States (Migration Policy Institute, 2018). These discourses further the biopolitical projects of these nations. As Sarah Pedigo Kulzer and Ryan Phillips argue, by enacting travel bans and calling for the cessation of asylum processing of people from "dangerous" countries, these populations are suspended "into a state of exception in which their lives are being disallowed to the point of death" (Kulzer & Phillips, 2020). Vaccine nationalism—as a mechanism for extending the pandemic in specific countries and regions—may similarly be used to conceal state racism under the veneer of reasonable precaution. This "reasonable" discrimination not only serves to justify immigration bans but also empowers its citizens to discriminate free of any moral constraints. Within this discourse, being wary of people from developing countries is not morally reprehensible, it is "reasonable" since "those people" from "those countries" are more likely to be carriers given the prevalence of the virus in their home countries. These discourses transform and pathologize foreign bodies— and those that "look foreign"—as mobile COVID-19 vectors, thereby normalizing their exclusion from society. Moreover, because of the emergence of distinct regional variants, even if all U.S. citizens are vaccinated, refugees and other migrants could continue to be discursively configured as potential biohazards.

Already several human rights advocacy groups have warned that developed nations are using the pandemic to justify discrimination against refugees, asylum-seekers, and other migrants. For instance, Charanya Krishnaswami, Advocacy Director for the Americas at Amnesty International USA, criticized the Trump administration arguing that their "ban on asylum-seekers from Mexico has nothing to do with making Americans safer from the coronavirus pandemic. President Trump is engaging in fear-mongering to justify racist and discriminatory policies whose only purpose is to demonize people seeking safety" (Amnesty International, 2020). Insofar as vaccine nationalism places the power to end overseas outbreaks in the hands of developed countries, they can deliberately maintain this discourse for years to come. This will have effects internationally as well as domestically. Within the United States, the pandemic has already led to greater xenophobia and racism against undocumented immigrants and people of color, especially Asians and Asian Americans (Human Rights Watch, 2020). The EU Agency for Fundamental Rights (FRA) has likewise found that the pandemic is being consistently exploited as a pretext for discrimination, hate speech, and hate crimes against various groups, including Asians, Roma, Muslims, and asylum-seekers (European Union Agency for Fundamental Rights, 2020). As such, vaccine nationalism, like other forms of nationalism, operates to build solidarity among those the state aims to "make live."

COVAX, Vaccine Multilateralism, and Vulnerable Solidarity

In April 2020, the WHO, in conjunction with various partner organizations, launched COVAX. Among the central functions of COVAX is to provide enough vaccines to inoculate an estimated 20% of the population of the 92 poorest countries in the world. To achieve this, it aims to have two billion doses available by the end of 2021 (Berkley, 2020). On February 24, 2021, the first shipment of free vaccines under this program landed in Ghana (Steinhauser, 2021). Under the Trump administration, the United States withdrew from the WHO and declined to join COVAX; however, the Biden administration reversed these decisions and pledged four billion dollars in funding. The United States will donate two billion dollars in 2021, and the additional two billion will be released over two years *if* the other participating donors fulfill their pledges (Rauhala et al., 2021). While the United States' decision to join the global partnership is a major step forward for the initiative, COVAX still faces an estimated $27 billion funding gap for COVID-19 tests, drugs, and vaccines for 2021 (Farge, 2021). Moreover, while COVAX endorses and promotes the values of vaccine multilateralism and global solidarity, many of its partnering developed nations are simultaneously engaging in vaccine nationalism. The United States, United Kingdom, and Australia have preordered enough vaccines to inoculate their entire populations twice over; and Canada has preordered enough to vaccinate 500% of its population (Twohey et al., 2020).

Initially, this scenario appears contradictory: why would countries simultaneously engage in vaccine nationalism—a biopolitical project intended to "make live" their populations while "letting die" foreign nations—and vaccine multilateralism—an altruistic humanitarian endeavor to ensure that all nations are able to recover from the pandemic? While developed countries are donating billions of dollars to purchase vaccines for other nations, they are spending far more purchasing vaccines for themselves, acquiring more vaccines than is necessary given their population size, preventing developing countries from producing the vaccine themselves, and failing to donate enough to maintain the funding levels required to achieve COVAX's mission.

The net result of COVAX will be making developing nations *more* dependent on developed nations, thereby exacerbating the power inequality between them. Even if COVAX is successful, its goal is only to provide vaccines for 20% of the population of 92 developing countries. Given the limited assistance offered by COVAX, in conjunction with the worsening economic situation in those regions, developing countries will ultimately have to rely on donations from developed nations to vaccinate their entire populations. Thus, vaccine nationalism morphs into a vaccine diplomacy that further widens the power asymmetry between the wealthiest and the poorest nations. The inability of COVAX to constitute a true form of vaccine multilateralism is unsurprising. As Schinkel argues, biopolitical divisions operative within Western notions of citizenship undermine "currently fashionable pleas for 'world citizenship' or 'cosmopolitan citizenship'" (Schinkel, 2010, p. 170). Despite this, a biopolitical perspective may offer us a path toward genuine vaccine multilateralism by demonstrating the need to forge a "vulnerable solidarity." For Myisha Cherry, this "is solidarity that is formed based on the vulnerability that we all face as citizens to be targeted and/or affected by state racism and state violence" (Cherry, 2017, p. 360). This is not simply an acknowledgment that every human is biologically and existentially vulnerable to harm and injury. Rather, it involves recognizing that within a biopolitical state, any group can be potentially racialized, and thereby subjected to state violence. As such, everyone has an interest in resisting attacks and harms performed by the state.

For Cherry, this is true even if one does not currently belong to a group discursively designated as "inferior" or "undesirable." As she writes,

> Vulnerable solidarity opens up the bonds of trusts among "vulnerable" groups, which may be difficult to do with groups defined by their super race and subrace identities. Instead of joining a cause because it has a direct impact on our social positioning now, people will join causes because they will know that all injustices have an impact on us all; if not directly, indirectly, if not now, in the future.
>
> *Cherry, 2017, pp. 360–361*

While Cherry's account focuses predominately on state racism and biopolitics within a single country, as the foregoing analysis shows, biopolitical governance is not limited by sovereign borders. Anyone, anywhere, whether now or later, can become racialized. This entails that not only are developing nations susceptible to the effects of state racism, but so too are developed nations. For instance, in January

2021, the European Union placed temporary controls enabling member nations to halt exports of vaccines if vaccine makers fail to honor their contracts. These controls were implemented following shipment delays by AstraZeneca. In March 2021, Italy evoked these controls to block a shipment of 250,000 doses of the Oxford/AstraZeneca vaccine headed to Australia. While the Australian government condemned the action, the French government supported Italy's move and even indicated that it may do the same (Amaro, 2021). Here, Italy's decision is intended to "make live" its own population, while "letting die" the Australian population—this is biopolitics among developed nations. The more the COVID-19 vaccine, and other resources used to combat the pandemic, are transformed into a biopolitical arms race and further entrenched into systems of controls, the more vulnerable *each* country will become. While developing countries will suffer the most, developed nations cannot count themselves absolutely safe. Only by rejecting biopolitical logics and embracing that everyone's life must matter, regardless of race, sex, sexuality, and even nationality, can true vaccine multilateralism arise. Otherwise, global efforts such as COVAX will continue to offer partial humanitarian gestures, while widening inequalities that make the developing world more liable to exploitation and domination.

Notes

1 As Evelyn Glenn argues, the category of "the citizen" is not neutral with regard to race, sex/gender, sexuality, class, among other factors (Glenn, 2000). While this chapter focuses predominately on the citizen/non-citizen divide, this should not be taken to mean that *all* citizens are treated equally by the state.

2 Two points here are worth emphasizing. First, biopolitical accounts do not require denying the reality of state-sanctioned killings. Within the United States, the death penalty and the killing of unarmed Black people by law enforcement represent two important examples of this. Rather, the point is to describe how, in addition to these forms of killings, the state kills by creating and maintaining systems that operate passively and habitually expose marginalized groups to death and illness. Second, despite the emphasis on exposure, biopolitics is not devoid of direct violence. For instance, in 2020, a whistle-blower alleged that women held at U.S. Immigration and Customs Enforcement detention centers were being forced to undergo hysterectomies (Paul, 2020). Such acts are part of a longer history, and present, of forced sterilizations within the United States that have been disproportionately targeted against people of color, especially women. They represent an important example of biopolitics—of how the state manages the life and survival of those deemed "inferior" or "bad," not by directly killing them, but via the control of their bodies and reproductive capacities (Murphy, 2012).

3 While vaccine nationalism has garnered much of the critical attention, it is not the only instance of global biopolitics during the pandemic. For example, in April 2020, then-President Trump invoked the Defense Production Act to redirect surgical masks manufactured by 3M abroad to the United States (Swanson et al., 2020).

4 Importantly, even within this literature, there are exceptions. For instance, Michael Walzer believes that nations must adhere to the Principle of Mutual Aid. Under this principle, nations are morally obligated to help non-citizens in dire need, such as asylum-seekers and refugees, so long as doing so is minimally risky and low cost (Walzer, 1984).

References

Amaro, S. (2021). Europe Facing 'Uphill Battle' with COVID Vaccines as Italy Blocks AstraZeneca Shipment. *CNBC*. Retrieved from www.cnbc.com/2021/03/05/eu-covid-vaccine-under-spotlight-as-italy-blocks-shipment-to-australia.html

Amnesty International. (2020). USA: Trump Administration Using Coronavirus Pandemic to Justify Discriminatory an on Asylum-Seekers at Southern Border. *Amnesty International*. Retrieved from www.amnesty.org/en/latest/news/2020/03/usa-trump-coronavirus-pandemic-discriminatory-ban-asylum-seekers/

Armus, T. (2021). Nebraska Governor Says Citizens, Legal Residents will get Vaccine Priority over Undocumented Immigrants. *The Washington Post*. Retrieved from www.washingtonpost.com/nation/2021/01/06/nebraska-covid-vaccine-immigrants-meatpacking/

Atuk, T. (2020). Pathopolitics: Pathologies and Biopolitics of PrEP. *Frontiers in Sociology*, *5*(1), 1–13.

Bacchus, J. (2020). The Antidote to Vaccine Nationalism. *Centre for International Governance Innovation*. Retrieved from www.cigionline.org/articles/antidote-vaccine-nationalism

Balibar, E. (2011). Racism and Nationalism. In E. Balibar & I. Wallerstein (Eds.), *Race, Nation, Class: Ambiguous Identities (Radical Thinkers)* (pp. 37–67). New York: Verso.

Ball, P. (2020). The Lightning-Fast Quest for COVID Vaccines—and What It Means for Other Diseases. *Nature*. doi:10.1038/d41586-020-03626-1. Retrieved from www.nature.com/articles/d41586-020-03626-1

Beaubien, J. (2020). COVID-19 Is Now Leading Killer in 5 Latin American Nations. *NPR*. Retrieved from www.npr.org/sections/goatsandsoda/2020/12/18/947792819/chart-covid-19-is-now-leading-killer-in-5-latin-american-nations

Berkley, S. (2020). COVAX Explained. *Gavi, the Vaccine Alliance*. Retrieved from www.gavi.org/vaccineswork/covax-explained

Berlant, L. (2007). Slow Death (Sovereignty, Obesity, Lateral Agency). *Critical Inquiry, 33*(4), 754–780. doi:10.1086/521568

Bollyky, T. J., & Brown, C. P. (2020). The Tragedy of Vaccine Nationalism: Only Cooperation Can End the Pandemic. *Foreign Affairs, 99*(5), 96–108.

Campbell, J. (2021). COVID-19 Death Rate Rising in Africa. *Council on Foreign Relations*. Retrieved from www.cfr.org/blog/covid-19-death-rate-rising-africa

Carlson, C., & Phelan, A. (2020). A Choice between Two Futures for Pandemic Recovery. *The Lancet: Planetary Health, 4*(12), 545–546. Retrieved from www.thelancet.com/journals/lanplh/article/PIIS2542-5196(20)30245-X/fulltext

Casert, R., & Hatton, B. (2021). EU says US Stand on Patent Virus Waiver Is No 'Magic Bullet.' *AP News*. Retrieved from https://apnews.com/article/europe-technology-patents-coronavirus-pandemic-health-570081abd85da67f009f24ecda7cd998

Chauvin, J. P., Annabelle, F., & Herrera, L. N. (2020). The Younger Age Profile of COVID-19 Deaths in Developing Countries. *Inter-American Development Bank*. Retrieved from https://publications.iadb.org/publications/english/document/The-Younger-Age-Profile-of-COVID-19-Deaths-in-Developing-Countries.pdf

Cherry, M. (2017). State Racism, State Violence, and Vulnerable Solidarity. In N. Zack (Ed.), *The Oxford Handbook on Philosophy and Race* (pp. 353–363). Oxford: Oxford University Press.

Cohen, J. (2021). South Africa Suspends Use of AstraZeneca's COVID-19 Vaccine after It Fails to Clearly Stop Virus Variant. *Science*. Retrieved from www.sciencemag.org/news/2021/02/south-africa-suspends-use-astrazenecas-covid-19-vaccine-after-it-fails-clearly-stop

Dawsey, J. (2018). Trump Derides Protections for Immigrants from 'Shithole' Countries. *The Washington Post*. Retrieved from www.washingtonpost.com/politics/trump-attacks-protections-for-immigrants-from-shithole-countries-in-oval-office-meeting/2018/01/11/bfc0725c-f711-11e7-91af-31ac729add94_story.html

Doherty, T., & Kenen, J. (2021). Just 5 Percent of Vaccinations Have Gone to Black Americans, Despite Equity Efforts. Retrieved from www.politico.com/news/2021/02/01/covid-vaccine-racial-disparities-464387

Dyer, O. (2020). COVID-19: Many Poor Countries Will See Almost no Vaccine Next Year, Aid Groups Warn. *BMJ*. Retrieved from www.bmj.com/content/371/bmj.m4809

Ellis-Petersen, H., & Chaurasia, M. (2020). COVID-19 Prompts "Enormous Rise" in Demand for Cheap Child Labor in India. *The Guardian*. Retrieved from www.theguardian.com/world/2020/oct/13/covid-19-prompts-enormous-rise-in-demand-for-cheap-child-labour-in-india

Emanuel, E. J., Persad, G., Kern, A., Buchanan, A., Fabre, C., Halliday, D., Health, J., & et al. (2020). An Ethical Framework for Global Vaccine Allocation. *Science, 369*(6509), 1309–1312.

European Union Agency for Fundamental Rights. (2020). *Coronavirus Pandemic in the EU: Fundamental Rights Implications*. Retrieved from https://fra.europa.eu/sites/default/files/fra_uploads/fra-2020-coronavirus-pandemic-eu-bulletin-july_en.pdf

Farge, E. (2021). U.S. Alone Won't Fill COVAX Funding Gap, Lead Official Says. *Reuters*. Retrieved from www.reuters.com/article/us-health-coronavirus-who-covax-idUSKBN29R1Q3

Ferguson, K., & Caplan, A. (2020). Love Thy Neighbor? Allocating Vaccines in a World of Competing Obligations. *Journal of Medical Ethics, 47*(12), 1–4.

Fidler, D. P. (2020). Vaccine Nationalism's Politics. *Science (American Association for the Advancement of Science), 369*(6505), 749.

Foucault, M. (2003). *"Society Must Be Defended": Lectures at the Collège de France, 1975-1976* (D. Macey, Trans.). New York: Picador.

Foucault, M. (2010). *The Archaeology of Knowledge: And the Discourse on Language* (A. M. S. Smith, Trans.). New York: Vintage Books.

Gettleman, J., & Raj, S. (2020). As COVID-19 Closes Schools, the World's Children Go To Work. *The New York Times*. Retrieved from www.nytimes.com/2020/09/27/world/asia/covid-19-india-children-school-education-labor.html

Glenn, E. (2000). Citizenship and Inequality: Historical and Global Perspectives. *Social Problems, 47*(1), 1–20.

Guimón, J., & Narula, R. (2020). Ending the COVID-19 Pandemic Requires More International Collaboration. *Research Technology Management, 63*(5), 38–41.

Gurara, D., Fabrizio, S., & Wiegand, J. (2020). COVID-19: Without Help, Low-Income Developing Countries Risk a Lost Decade, *IMF Blog*. Retrieved from blogs.imf.org/2020/08/27/covid-19-without-help-low-income-developing-countries-risk-a-lost-decade/

Hafner, M., Yerushalmi, E., Fays, C., Dufresne, E., & Stolk, C. (2020). COVID-19 and the Cost of Vaccine Nationalism. *RAND Corporation*. Retrieved from www.rand.org/pubs/research_reports/RRA769-1.html

Horton, J. (2020). Coronavirus: What Are the Numbers Out of Latin America? *BBC News*. Retrieved from www.bbc.com/news/world-latin-america-52711458.

Human Rights Watch. (2020). COVID-19 Fueling Anti-Asian Racism and Xenophobia Worldwide. Retrieved from www.hrw.org/news/2020/05/12/covid-19-fueling-anti-asian-racism-and-xenophobia-worldwide

Kretchmer, H. (2020). Vaccine Nationalism—and How It Could Affect Us All. *World Economic Forum*. Retrieved from www.weforum.org/agenda/2021/01/what-is-vaccine-nationalism-coronavirus-its-affects-covid-19-pandemic/.

Kulzer, S. P., & Phillips, R. (2020). Those Who Must Die: Syrian Refugees in the Age of National Security. *Human Rights Review, 21*(1), 139–157.

Landgrave, M., & Nowrasteh, A. (2019). *Criminal Immigrants in 2017: Their Numbers, Demographics, and Countries of Origin.* Retrieved from www.cato.org/publications/immigration-research-policy-brief/criminal-immigrants-2017-their-numbers-demographics

Lavine, J. S., Bjornstad, O. N., & Antia, R. (2021). Immunological Characteristics Govern the Transition of COVID-19 to Endemicity. *Science, 371*(6530), 741–745.

Lederer, E. (2020). UN Chief Warns 'Vaccine Nationalism' Is Moving at Full Speed. *AP News.* Retrieved from https://apnews.com/article/health-coronavirus-pandemic-antonio-guterres-africa-united-nations-f02e0245d56259040643abe37e564fd0.

Lie, R. K., & Miller, F. G. (2020). Allocating a COVID-19 Vaccine: Balancing National and International Responsibilities. *The Milbank Quarterly.* Retrieved from www.milbank.org/quarterly/articles/allocating-a-covid-19-vaccine-balancing-national-and-international-responsibilities/.

Liz, J. (2021). COVID-19, Immunoprivilege and Structural Inequalities. *History and Philosophy of the Life Sciences, 43*(1), 1–6.

Migration Policy Institute. (2018). *Profile of the Unauthorized Population: United States.* Retrieved from www.migrationpolicy.org/data/unauthorized-immigrant-population/state/US

Murphy, M. (2012). *Seizing the Means of Reproduction: Entanglements of Feminism, Health, and Technoscience.* Durham: Duke University Press.

Organization for Economic Co-operation and Development (OECD)/World Health Organization (WHO). (2020). Health at a Glance: Asia/Pacific 2020: Measuring Progress Towards Universal Health Coverage. Retrieved from www.oecd-ilibrary.org/docserver/26b007cd-en.pdf?expires=1614823645&id=id&accname=guest&checksum=674D63FF7C8C073B0CA28CAA9C4B8B98

Oxfam International. (2020). Campaigners Warn that 9 Out of 10 People in Poor Countries Are Set to Miss Out on COVID-19 Vaccine Next Year. *Oxfam International.* Retrieved from www.oxfam.org/en/press-releases/campaigners-warn-9-out-10-people-poor-countries-are-set-miss-out-covid-19-vaccine

Pandey, A. (2021). Rich Countries Block India, South Africa's Bid to Ban COVID Vaccine Patents. *DW.* Retrieved from www.dw.com/en/rich-countries-block-india-south-africas-bid-to-ban-covid-vaccine-patents/a-56460175

Paul, K. (2020). Ice Detainees Faced Medical Neglect and Hysterectomies, Whistleblower Alleges. Retrieved from www.theguardian.com/us-news/2020/sep/14/ice-detainees-hysterectomies-medical-neglect-irwin-georgia

Phillips, N. (2021). The Coronavirus Is Here to Stay—Here's What That Means. *Nature.* Retrieved from www.nature.com/articles/d41586-021-00396-2

Rauhala, E., Cunningham, E., & Taylor, A. (2021). White House Announces $4 Billion in Funding for COVAX, The Global Vaccine Effort That Trump Spurned. *The Washington Post.* Retrieved from www.washingtonpost.com/world/2021/02/18/5-percent-vaccine-donations-france/

Schinkel, W. (2010). From Zoëpolitics to Biopolitics: Citizenship and the Construction of "Society." *European Journal of Social Theory, 13*(2), 155–172.

Schmidt, I. M. (2020). Immunity-Based Licenses and the Politics of the Body. *Medical Humanities Blog.* Retrieved from https://blogs.bmj.com/medical-humanities/?p=2472.

Song, S. (2018). Political Theories of Migration. *Annual Review of Political Science, 21*(1), 385–402.

Steinhauser, G. (2021). Ghana Is First Nation to Get Free COVID-19 Vaccines Under COVAX Plan. *The Wall Street Journal.* Retrieved from www.wsj.com/articles/first-free-covid-vaccines-from-who-backed-covax-arrive-in-ghana-11614155319

Swanson, A., Kanno-Youngs, Z., & Haberman, M. (2020). Trump Seeks to Block 3M Mask Exports and Grab Masks from Its Overseas Customers. *The New York Times.* Retrieved from www.nytimes.com/2020/04/03/us/politics/coronavirus-trump-3m-masks.html

Sylvia VI, J. J., VI. (2020). The Biopolitics of Social Distancing. *Social Media + Society, 6*(3), 1–4.

Tabacek, K. (2020). Small Group of Rich Nations Have Bought Up More Than Half the Future Supply of Leading COVID-19 Vaccine Contenders. *Oxfam International.* Retrieved from www.oxfam.org/en/press-releases/small-group-rich-nations-have-bought-more-half-future-supply-leading-covid-19

Twohey, M., Collins, K. & Thomas, K. (2020). With First Dibs on Vaccines, Rich Countries Have 'Cleared the Shelves.' *The New York Times.* Retrieved from https://www.nytimes.com/2020/12/15/us/coronavirus-vaccine-doses-reserved.html

United Nations Development Program. (2020). COVID-19: Looming Crisis in Developing Countries Threatens to Devastate Economies and Ramp up Inequality. *UNDP.* Retrieved from www.undp.org/content/undp/en/home/news-centre/news/2020/COVID19_Crisis_in_developing_countries_threatens_devastate_economies.html

Valdez, I. (2016). Punishment, Race, and the Organization of U.S. Immigration Exclusion. *Political Research Quarterly, 69*(4), 640–654.

Vaughan-Williams, N. (2009). The Generalized Bio-Political Border? Re-Conceptualizing the Limits of Sovereign Power. *Review of International Studies, 35*(4), 729–749.

Wagner, A., Matulewska, A., & Marusek, S. (2021). Pandemica Panoptica: Biopolitical Management of Viral Spread in the Age of COVID-19. *International Journal for the Semiotics of Law—Revue International De Sémiotique Juridique, 0*(0), 1–37.

Walzer, M. (1984). *Spheres of Justice: A Defense of Pluralism and Equality.* New York: Basic Books.

Yeng, S. (2013). *The Biopolitics of Race: State Racism and US Immigration.* Lanham: Lexington Books.

13

LOOKING AHEAD

Sharon A. Navarro and Samantha L. Hernandez

Introduction

Structural approaches to inequality are linked to normative ideals of democracy. Once we recognize that inequalities across positions in an economic structure do not simply reflect the distribution of individual attributes, but are to a significant extent the result of the exercise of power, then, in addition to the issue of equal opportunity, the distribution of power becomes a salient normative concern. The question of fairness of inequalities is thus not simply a question of the opportunities people have in gaining rewards in the economic system, but of the fairness of who gets to exercise critical forms of power that shape those inequalities. As more research has emerged about COVID-19 and its effects on minorities, the role that structural racism has played in furthering inequalities during the pandemic has become increasingly apparent.

Racial and ethnic minorities are at a particular disadvantage as many already assume the status of a marginalized group. In the earliest days of the COVID-19 pandemic, scholars like Amy Schoenecker and Elizabeth Alejo, in Chapter 10, examined a community in Chicago that was overwhelmingly populated with low-wage and informal Latinx workers. They reported higher instances of COVID-19 infections among Latinx workers who were considered essential or engaged in informal work. These were workers who were unable to stay at home even if they were exposed to the virus because their survival depended on their labor. These findings are consistent with Selden and Berdahl's (2020) study on disparities in health, employment, and household composition. They concluded that in many areas of the United States, non-Hispanic Blacks and Hispanic are more than twice as likely as non-Hispanic Whites to die from COVID-19 because of exposure. In fact, the Centers for Disease Control and Prevention (CDC) found that as of October 2021, COVID-19 hospitalization rates for Hispanics and Blacks population were

DOI: 10.4324/9781003268710-13

25% and 16%, respectively. The magnitude of these disparities has focused renewed attention on the consequences of long-standing structural inequality along racial/ ethnic lines (CDC, 2021). Scholars like Williams (2001) argues that racial segregation is a fundamental cause of racial disparities in health. The physical separation of the races by forcing residents to stay in certain areas is an institutional mechanism of racism that was designed to protect Whites from social interaction with Blacks and other racial minorities. The effects of this finding are consistent with de Oliver's in Chapter 11, where he concludes that Latinx masking and spacing/isolation is not perceived as a privilege, but met with suspicion and mental distress not shared by non-Hispanic, Black, or Asian Americans. In fact, King-Meadows et al., Chapter 6, centers ethnoracial identity and economic status as added layers in understanding how mental distress and anxiety color the COVID-19 experience.

Bagheri and Yates, in Chapter 9, argue that even though many states implemented stay-at-home orders in an attempt to contain COVID-19, the lens through which we examine ethnic and racial disparities misses gender all together. In other words, because we, as political scientists, tend to focus on the racial and ethnic disparities as exacerbated by COVID-19, we overlook the struggles of COVID-19 on women as mothers. Jun and Zhang, in Chapter 8, argue that COVID-19 and its related effects are completely devoid of the Asian experience. Jun and Zhang write about Asian Americans organizing themselves against hate crimes, by coalescing with other advocacy groups, publicizing biases, and violence. They propose structural solutions—policy, research, practice, and activism—to combat Asian discrimination and hate.

The pandemic disrupted education nationwide, calling on public outcry on the existing racial and economic disparities and creating the potential for a lost generation. Even before the outbreak, students in vulnerable communities, particularly predominately Black, Latinx, and Indigenous and other majority-minority areas were already facing inequality in everything from resources to student-teacher ratios and to extracurricular activities. Chapters 2 and 3, by Parker Moore et al. and McGlynn and Stout, respectively, problematized the deep educational deficit in remote learning and the gaps in resources, funding, and technology that will have an adverse effect on intellectual development for generations to come.

In news media, reporting is understood to play a central role during national security and health emergencies (Klemm et al., 2016; Pieri, 2019). News coverage communicates risks to readers and listeners and shapes public perceptions through the amount, content, and tone of reporting. In Chapter 4, Gordon-Brilla et al. notes that the COVID-19 pandemic changed the way (social) media was used, it also changed the way people viewed George Floyd's death, and the way in which the Black Lives Matter movement created a collective conscience about racism as a pandemic. These authors point to the use of social media as a precondition for policy change. Similarly, in Chapters 5 and 7, Gardner et al. and Martinez suggest that both COVID-19 and the response to the death of George Floyd have reminded everyone about the entangled character of the biopolitical world and where we live and die. But it has also reminded us about the continuing salience of national spaces, including the contradictory roles occupied by national governments and their involvements in political mobilization and de-mobilization of a healthcare crisis. These authors write about the power of communication as a de-marginalizing agent for all communities.

In Chapter 12, Liz writes about the long history of powerful countries, such as the United States, securing vaccines at the expense of less wealthy countries; it is short-sighted, ineffective, and deadly. Ultimately, wealthy countries have a critical interest and arguably also a moral responsibility in assisting global vaccination. These inequalities reveal a fundamentally flawed view of global health, and our global economy more broadly, in which vaccines are treated as a market commodity rather than as a public good.

Despite governmental claims "that we are all in this together," COVID-19 turned out to be anything but an evenhanded pandemic. Rather, its impact has been profoundly unequally distributed: in the United States, it has disproportionately affected minorities, women, poor people, and people working in low paid but "essential" occupations. The collective chapters in this edited volume have provided a glimpse as to how the pandemic has so far impacted communities of color.

An outbreak can emerge all of a sudden or sometimes there may be signs beforehand. Active surveillance and infection control measures are extremely important but may not be enough all of the time. Below are recommendations that are not perfect nor an inclusive list of solutions as to how to thwart continued marginalization during humanitarian crises, like a pandemic. They were drawn from the findings of the chapters in this volume, yet represent just some of the ways in which we might move toward a more just society. It is important that humanitarian crises like COVID-19 never exacerbate the inequalities faced by various minority communities, including women.

- Accessible healthcare. It is important to understand how an individual's racial and ethnic economic position or status in society intersect with mental health, vaccine access, and how this can affect their future. Different communities experience events differently and those experiences need to be recognized, validated, and addressed. Every individual, regardless of the color of their skin, should receive the same quality of healthcare.
- Social media use to spread correct information. Using social media to promote public awareness about health disparities by race, ethnicity, and gender is essential to shoring up support for developing just social policy like ending the digital divide. Health providers could use social media as a tool to obtain emotional, informational, and peer support.
- Cultural education. Recognizing the importance of education and training of cultural humility to reduce provider bias, prejudice, and stereotypes. The narratives also incorporate a necessity to go beyond awareness to combat institutional racism and promote integration and racial equality.
- Education. There is a need for a stronger and improved education system across demographic (such as race and gender) groups. Stakeholders need to come

together to resolve issues where the government fails to address the digital divide. It is imperative that we utilize digital technology to expand opportunities for student learning.

- Economic opportunity. This requires a systemic reinvestment in underprivileged people and neighborhoods, job creation, workforce development, income equality, and economic literacy. This could mean relocating food security systems within other community-based institutions to address food needs when schools or community centers close. It could also mean ensuring essential workers are guaranteed appropriate compensation.
- Gendered lens. Scientist, researchers, journalist, and policymakers need to ensure that every humanitarian crisis is viewed from a gendered lens. It is important to understand that humanitarian crises impact men and women in very different ways. Consequently, we need to examine how race, ethnicity, and gender are shaped by humanitarian issues like COVID-19.
- National moral responsibility. The United States should develop a common plan to produce and distribute vaccines internationally with concrete commitments to pool technology, invoke patent waivers, and invest in rapid production (Mayta et al., 2021). In addition, all national and international institutions should be connected with each other, work together, share experiences, and publish guidelines for general population, healthcare facilities, local authorities, public service facilities, and so on.
- Requiring demographic data. The creation of policies that standardize and disaggregate state-level data by race/ethnicity are vital to understanding how governmental entities and the medical community can ensure an equitable-based response and recovery efforts. Scientific researchers and healthcare professionals need to advocate for the demographic data so that they can better serve those in need.
- Elected officials. Constituents need to hold elected officials and policymakers accountable by demanding equality across all sectors of the economy and across all communities of color and minority women through elections, candidate selection, or protests. Community activists and practitioners should serve as community watchdogs and work to actively address inequities.
- Address historical trauma. Discussions involving healing historical structural racism are not the most comfortable and should not be taken lightly. Conversations could foster deeper efforts toward inclusive critical consciousness that have the potential to raise awareness and spur on community action, particularly for residents who are most affected by historical and contemporary trauma stemming from structural racism.
- Communication accessibility. Government entities at every level should have a policy implemented to include messaging in appropriate languages (i.e., Spanish translation, etc.) and modes of accessibility (i.e., including signers for the hearing impaired), so that medically necessary information has the potential to reach every community equally. Community practitioners need to demand these changes of their elected officials and government entities.

By ensuring equity is integrated across all public spaces and sectors, all communities will be stronger, healthier, and more resilient. The power for change is in our communities. Community practitioners should utilize all of their community organizing skills, including digital organizing networks, social media, and access to big data sources, to serve as community watchdogs and advocates for efforts that promote increased participation of all within our political systems and demand a just society. Finally, the collective chapters in this edited volume clearly illustrate the devastating and unequal impact of COVID-19 on people of color and minority women. The potential to prevent any future, unnecessary marginalization, especially among communities of color, should strongly motivate policymakers, researchers, and the community members everywhere to face structural racism head on.

References

Center for Disease Control and Prevention. (2021). COVID-19 Hospitalization by Race and Ethnicity in United States. CDC Case Surveillance Restricted Access Detailed Data. Retrieved from https://healthequitytracker.org/exploredata?gclid=CjwKCAiAm7OMBhAQEiwArvGi3GZZf-e4EbwDBHHFhmb0hc18rsKHyo8yqUypC2SL-nbTe2Pm0fzJ3hoC2TAQAvD_BwE&dt1=hospitalizations

Klemm C., Das E., & Hartmann, T. (2016). Swine Flu and Hype: A Systemic Review of Media Dramatization of the H1N1 Influenza Pandemic. *Journal of Risk Research, 19*(1), 1–20.

Mayta, R., Shailaja, K. K., & Nyongo, A. (2021, June 17). Vaccine Nationalism Is Killing Us. We Need an Internationalist Approach. *The Guardian.* Retrieved from www.theguardian.com/commentisfree/2021/jun/17/covid-vaccine-nationalism-internationalist-approach

Pieri, E. (2019). Media Framing and the Threat of Global Pandemics: The Ebola Crisis in UK Media and Policy Response. *Social Research Online, 24,* 73–92.

Selden, Thomas M. & Terceira A. Berdahl. (2020). Covid-19 And Racial/Ethnic Disparities in Health Risks, Employment, and Household Composition. *Health Affairs 3(*9): https://doi.org/10.1377/hlthaff.2020.00897

Williams, D. R. (2001). Racial Residential Segregation: A Fundamental Cause of Racial Disparities in Health. *Public Health Reports, 116*(5), 404–416.

INDEX

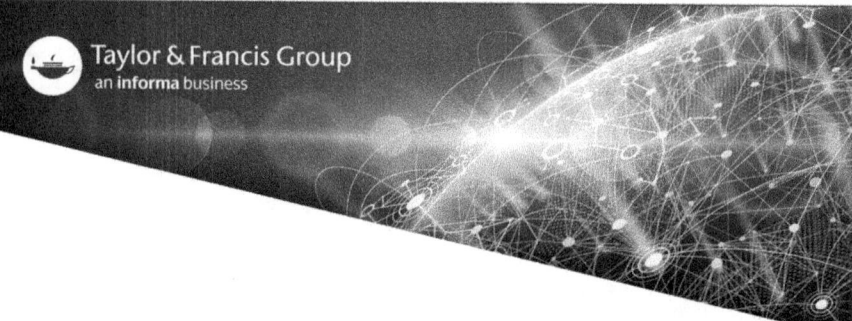
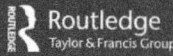
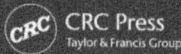